Disclaimer

The information on this book is not intended to diagnose or treat any disease or condition. The author is not a health practitioner and is not offering advice. No content in this book has been evaluated or approved by the FDA. Following any information is at your own risk.

Do your own thorough research before following any herbal advice. Be aware of interactions (drug or herbal), allergy, sensitivity or underlying conditions before proceeding with following any health information.

By continuing to read this book you agree to be responsible for yourself, do your own research, make your own choices and not to hold the author responsible for your own actions.

Some of the plants, mentioned in the book, might be under protection in your area. Inform yourself and follow regional and national regulations, before you collect them.

Table of Contents

Introduction

Something that has long interested me is how many people "can't see the forest for the trees", or in the case of herbalists, can't see the trees for the herbs. The old saying, of course, refers to people who get so caught up in detail or definitions, that they cannot see the larger picture. Such is certainly the case for many herbalists, who overlook the medicinal value of trees. Why is this? Well, it likely stems from the multiple meanings of the word "herb". An herb may refer to any tender, green plant of the herbaceous layer – the low growing wildflowers and weeds, the annuals and bi-annuals, which include not only many of our medicinal plants, but also or garden vegetables and wild foods. An herb may also refer to any plant used to season or flavor food. To the herbalist the word, herb, generally means any plant useful medicinally. Simply put, if a plant can help make one healthy or even … shall we be so bold as to say, "treat or cure" any sickness, disease or complaint, it is an herb.

Of course, we cannot legally say any plant can be used to treat or cure (etc) any illness. That is the law… no matter how stupid and misguided it certainly is, it is still the law. If we disobey, people with guns and regulators with fines will show us exactly what it means to live "in the land of the free and the home of the brave." Supposedly, many laws and regulations were passed from 1920 or so, on to protect the American people from tainted food and fraudulent drugs. In 2021, a free American cannot buy raw/unpasteurized milk in most states, vaccines are being mandated against religious and health concerns and we have seen health food stores raided by SWAT teams, guns drawn and bullets firing, to ensure that no one says that ginseng may put a bit of pep in your step…. No, my ancestors did not cross the ocean on ancient, wooden ships and fight multiple wars for this… but, there you have it. As the late President Reagan said, "The scariest words in the English Language are, we are from the government, and we are here to help."

That said, here, I must offer my disclaimer:

The information in this book is not intended to diagnose or treat any disease or condition. I am not a health practitioner and am not offering advice. No content on this site has been evaluated or

Read that and embrace it or go no further. If you use any herb, whether recommended by me or anyone else, you are treating yourself... and as the old saying goes about the man who represents himself legally, you maybe "have a fool" for a doctor. Frankly, as I often say, I won't even guarantee that anything I write in this book or elsewhere, is true. Do your own research.

But, back to trees. It is a bit odd that we mainly think of weeds and wildflowers when we consider the subject of herbs. Many trees are not only as potently medicinal as a plant from the herbaceous layer, but much more so! Consider the "YARFAS". The late herbalist, Michael Moore identified so many astringent herbs in the Rose family, that he called them Yet Another Rose Family Astringent. So, to him, Potentilla was just another YARFA. That name is in fairly common use among many herbalists, as Moore was the leading teacher of Herbal Medicine in his day. Frankly, I don't like it. Who knows, maybe I can convince my students, and those who read my articles, to respect the integrity of the individual plant... Regardless, I took Moore's classes and learned a great deal from him – my opinion is not a criticism of his opinion. We have different perspectives. But, what if I told you that when you need a YARFA, the herbaceous layer is usually not the best place to look?!

Truly, very few green plants have as much tannic astringency as the bark of several trees. In the modern world, would you be better served driving out to a meadow and looking for Potentilla or going to your back yard, city park or sidewalk and scraping off some oak bark? Well, if you have severe diarrhea, you are weak and can't get far from the bathroom... I think the oak, dogwood or pine, etc, etc, may be more convenient. Call me crazy, but in such a situation, I don't want to take a hike! The same is certainly true for bleeding, sore throat, congestion, spasmodic coughs and so many other things for which trees are useful

Of course, there are many trees. In my native state of North Carolina, we have more than 400 common trees, both indigenous and introduced… and, that does not include shrubs/bushes! The very identity of my state is so closely tied to Pine Trees, that not only is our state tree the Longleaf Pine, but North Carolinians are called "Tarheels", in recognition that the tar made from pine sap was once the major industry, sealing ships for their Atlantic voyages. If anyone were to doubt the impact of trees to the North Carolinian, have him visit us in spring, when tree pollens form yellow clouds thicker than any smoke, fog or urban smog! Whether the pines of the eastern part of the state, or the hardwoods that birthed the furniture and timber industry in the central and western regions of North Carolina, we are certainly a tree state!

In this book, I will offer the medicinal values of most of the trees that grow in the eastern, Continental US – east of the Mississippi river. However, most of these trees grow throughout Canada and most of Europe, into Asia and beyond. Simply stated, most trees that grow in North of the Equator and below the Artic, grow most everywhere in that region. Many common trees grow in the Southern hemisphere, too. But, I have no business writing about the trees of Australia or the Amazon… I don't know these trees. They may have some that grow here, but I have very few unique to such regions, and no indigenous. Here, we have mountains similar to upstate New York and coastal regions that are at the very least, similar to norther Florida. We have hardwood forests, swamps and sandhills. Botanists of a few generations ago found North Carolina a paradise of diversity, but I will not limit my exposition to my home state. My goals will be to present most trees growing east of the Mississippi, in the temperate regions…. Fortunately, though, I do not have to journey far from home. I will however, always giver sentimental preference to the Southern Magnolia and the iconic Live Oak.

If your idea of medicinal herbs is little green plants, you will certainly find some surprises here! Trees can be strong medicine. I hope to change the way you view the world around you. I grew up in the mountain forests and the coastal swamps. I have always been fascinated by trees. I have practiced herbal medicine for more than 25 years, but I have spent my life among the trees… my formal education includes not only credentials as a Master Herbalist, but certifications in Forestry, as well. As such, I can offer a very practical presentation on the medicinal uses of trees.

That said, the medicinal use of trees has a very long use and I think it far more important to present them in the context of history. For me, it is far more convincing if someone can show me that an herb has been used traditionally for a specific purpose. Simply put, I trust the collective wisdom of a hundred or a thousand generations of human history than I do the opinion of an individual or a "new discovery". The Bible states, "There is nothing new under the sun." The discoveries of herbalists, from time immemorial have been handed down from herbalist to herbalist and tested by each generation. New uses for herbs, as they are discovered, are added to the vast knowledge of the various traditions and tested by those who follow.

Where possible, I have chosen to keep my mouth shut and quote the great herbalists, from varying traditions – Greek and Roman, Monastic Medicine, German Folk Medicine, British, Native American, Eclectic, the herbal revivalists of the 1960s-80s, Organic Gardeners, Field Guides and Botanists, Scientists and Doctors. I don't like to make much noise in the woods anyway....

By the way, the Cover Photo is of the historic Angel Oak on John's Island, SC. This iconic tree is estimated to up to 500 years old. The photo is used with permission, and was shared with me by Joel Sayre, thanks to the recommendation of his sister, Jenny Talbot.

So, let's take a hike and look at the trees!

Abies, Fir

Twenty four varieties of Abies are used medicinally: Abies alba - Silver Fir, Abies amabilis - Red Fir, Abies balsamea – Balsam Fir, Abies cephalonica – Grecian Fir, Abies concolor - Colorado Fir, Abies delavayi, Abies firma - Momi Fir, Abies fraseri - She Balsam, Abies grandis - Grand Fir, Abies homolepis - Nikko Fir, Abies lasiocarpa - Subalpine Fir, Abies magnifica - Californian Red Fir, Abies nordmanniana - Caucasian Fir, Abies pindrow - West Himalayan Fir, Abies procera - Noble Fir, Abies recurvata, Abies religiosa - Sacred Fir, Abies sachalinensis, Abies sibirica - Siberian Fir, Abies spectabilis - Himalayan Fir, Abies squamata - Flaky Fir, Abies veitchii - Veitch Fir, Abies veitchii sikokiana

Only the Fraser Fir grows in my region.

The needles, resin, roots, bark and branches are used.

This is a mountain tree. It grows in nine counties in North Carolina, but just two counties each in Virginia and Tennessee… only one county in Georgia. However, cultivated firs are truly abundant. This is one of the main trees grown on farms as a Christmas tree.

The primary medicinal use of the firs is as an astringent. As such, it is extremely useful because it both tightens tissue and increases blood flow. We will discuss the astringency of several trees, but this is one that is particularly effective against anything from sore throats to dysentery, especially when there is danger of the tissue becoming "boggy". In cases of severe, chronic or intense inflammation, the inflamed tissue can suffer serious damage. Boggy tissue occurs when the tissue loses its tone. It often develops a purplish hue and loses its ability to tighten back up. It is flaccid and filled with fluid. When this happens for instance. in the throat, the results can be deadly. The astringency of this tree not only tightens the tissue and reduces swelling, but its ability to increase blood circulation to the affected area both helps transport the fluid away from the site of inflammation and speeds healing.

Dioscorides included Abies under Pine:

Moist resin also comes out of the pine tree and the pitch tree brought from Gallia and Hetruria. Previously it was sometimes brought from Colophon from which it had its surname of colophonia, as well as from Galatia (which is near the Alps) which

the inhabitants of that place in their proper tongue call the larch tree. This is particularly good (taken in a linctusn [syrup] or alone) for lasting coughs. They are also different in colour for one is white, another of oil colour, and another looks like honey, such as that of the larch tree. Moist resin also comes out of the cypress tree, good for the same purposes. Of that which is dry there is some called strobilina [from pine cones], elaterium, peucine and pituine. Choose that which smells sweetest and is clear — neither too dry nor too moist, but like wax and brittle. Of these that of the pitch tree and fir tree excel, for they have a sweet smell and resemble frankincense in their odour. The best are brought out of Pityusa (an island which lies near Spain), but that from the pitch tree, strobilus [pine cones] and the cypress are of a meaner sort and are not the same in strength as the others, yet they are made use of for the same purposes. Lentiscina matches terminthos in strength.

Saint Hildegard von Bingen, likely the most wise and profound herbalist of all time, wrote of Fir around 1100 AD:

When the tree is green and has not yet lost its sap, as in March or even May, take the bark and leaves of this tree, and even some of its wood, and cut it into tiny bits. Add half as much sage and then boil this until it thickens. Then add cow's butter, prepared in May, and strain it through a cloth, making an ointment. If someone ails in his head so that he is virgitiget, raving or mad, and if his heart is failing in strength, first anoint his heart well with this ointment. Then, having shaved his head, anoint his head with the same ointment. Repeat this on the second and third day, and his head will recover its health, and he will return to his senses. If someone ails in his spleen, first anoint his heart with this ointment, because of the weakness of his heart. Soon afterward, anoint his stomach, if that is where the pain is, or his spleen, if he is ailing there. The ointment will pass through the skin with its strength, so that he will be cured quickly.

For one who is congested in his chest, who coughs, and who even ails in his lungs so that they are swollen and beginning to be putrescent, burn the wood of the fir tree, when it is fresh and the sap is still in it, until it is ash. Let nothing else be added to this ash. Into these ashes put twice as much burnet saxifrage and the same amount of fennel, and half as much licorice as saxifrage. Cook this together in good wine with some honey. Strain it through a cloth to *make a spiced wine. Drunk often, it will purge the chest, restore the lungs to health, and therefore cure the person.*

"Virgitiget" is an old German term that can mean anything from paralysis to rheumatism or arthritis. Saint Hildegard also recommends Fir for venereal Crabs, and for swollen lips and mouth.

The British herbalist and plant collector, John Gerard wrote of Fir in 1597:

A. The liquid resin of the Fir tree called turpentine, looseth the belly, driveth forth hot choleric humours, cleanseth and mundifieth the kidneys, provoketh urine, and driveth forth the stone and gravel.

B. The same taken with sugar and the powder of Nutmegs, cureth the strangury, stayeth the Gonorrhoea or the involuntary issue of man's nature, called the running of the reins, and the white flux in women.

C. It is very profitable for all green and fresh wounds, especially the wounds of the head: for it healeth and cleanseth mightily, especially if it be washed in Plantain water, and afterward Rose water, the yolk of an egg put thereto, with the powders of olibanum and mastic finely searced, adding thereto a little saffron.

The puckish and rebellious Nicholas Culpepper, who infuriated the British medical and academic establishments by translating their medical books and formulas from Latin, into the English language of the common Englishman, was more effusive in his unique style. He further upset the educated classes by including astrology, folklore and the "Doctrine of Signatures into his works; the Doctrine of Signatures being the belief that God designed herbs so that the appearance of the plant would indicate its medicinal use. Writing in 1652:

Government and virtues. Jupiter owns this tree. The leaves and tops of both sorts are used in diet-drinks for the scurvy, for which they are highly commended by the inhabitants of the northern countries. It is said a good quantity of them are put into Brunswick mum. From this tree, of which there grow great numbers in several parts of Germany, is gotten the Strasburg turpentine, which is clearer, of a pale colour, and of a thinner consistence than Venice turpentine, of a bitterish taste, and of a pleasant smell, a little like lemon-peel. It is of a mollifying, healing, and cleansing nature; and, besides its uses outwardly in wounds and ulcers, is a good diuretic, and of great use in a gonorrhoeœa and the fluor albus; given in glysters, mixed with the yolk of an egg it is very serviceable against the stone and gravel. It is likewise a good pectoral, and often given in affections of the breast and lungs.

Tar is likewise the product of these trees, which are cut into pieces, and piled up in a heap, and being set on fire at the top, the resinous liquor is driven out by the heat of the fire, and, running down, is received into trenches made for it, and so put into the casks; and by boiling is hardened into pitch.

Tar is by some accounted a good pectoral medicine, and used for obstructions of the lungs, and shortness of breath.

From the young branches of this tree is produced the famous spruce beer; and the juice which runs from the trunk upon its being tapped, is what is sold in the shops here under the name of the Balm of Gilead. The young tops of this tree make an excellent antiscorbutic either infused or boiled in beer or wine; experience has sufficiently confirmed their efficacy in that distemper in our American plantations, where the inhabitants used to be severely afflicted with it, who since they have taken to brewing a kind of liquor of molasses, in which they boil the young fir-tops in the room of hops, they are very little troubled with the scurvy; and many of our sailors whose diet on board of ships makes them subject to it, have had reason to commend that liquor. This tree yields two resinous substances; a thin liquid sort, which comes forth from the young firs, and is known in the shops by the name of Strasburg turpentine; and a dry substance resembling frankincense, to which it is not unlike in quality.

An Irish Herbal (written in 1735) states:

The leaves and top of this tree can be used against scurvy. The turpentine, or liquid resin extracted from this tree is somewhat purgative, and also provoking urine and is beneficial to the bladder, kidneys and arthritic conditions. It is good for wounds, being healing and cleansing.

Fr. Künzle wrote of Fir in 1911, showing its use in the tradition of German Folk Medicine:

Finely chop green fir tree twigs or, if you can't get them, European spruce (picea abies) will also do and you chop it thinly. Fill 8-10 baskets and put them in the patient's bedroom or, if there is not enough space, hang them up like lamps; every evening before going to bed, stir and shake every basket so that the scent comes out.

If the twigs no longer smell after three to four weeks, replace them filled with the fresh ones. I have seen tuberculosis patients who could only move with the help of sticks cured in this way. In mountainous areas a much stronger and more effective variety of pines thrives, namely the dwarf mountain pine; it is hardly as tall as a man, but it spreads countless branches that crawl over the rocks up to the top of the tree line.

Speaking of a man who was successfully treating tuberculosis, he wrote:

Uelis Sepp goes outside three times a day, into the healthy, dust-free air, if it is possible, he should stand under a fir tree, slowly and deeply breathes in with an open mouth and spreads out arms like on a cross so that the chest is expanded; as soon as his lungs are completely full, he folds both his hands as tightly as he can on his chest and breathes out; he repeats that ten to twelve times, always before taking a meal. This exercise ensures that the illness no longer destroys his lungs and so that those still healthy parts of the lungs remain intact.

Every hour Uelis Sepp takes a sip of the medicine made according to the recipe for lung patients. He can eat whatever he wants.

The kidneys and bladder of the lung patients usually work badly; as a result, entangled urine substances get into the lungs and new mucus is produced every day; no cure is possible before the kidneys and the bladder start working properly. The tea for lung patients drunk 2-3 weeks could help to make the kidneys and bladder function; Furthermore, warm herbs such as marjoram, thyme, mint and nettles are placed as a poultice as close as possible to the kidneys and to the bladder, and this bandage is worn for three to four weeks and during the cold season continuously. 10 - 20 warm hip baths in boiled pine or fir twigs strengthen the cure. This would make the kidneys and the bladder start working properly; more urine comes out; no more new mucus would develop in the lungs; the old mucus is excreted; without mucus, the Tuberculosis bacteria cannot multiply so quickly, the lungs become stronger and overcome the crisis.

In case of a very advanced tuberculosis, however, there is no guarantee that this remedy will help.

The Thomsonian System of Medicine, published in 1905, states:

BALSAM FIR. Abies Balsamea.

This balsam is obtained from a tree known in all parts of the country; it is taken from small blisters which form in the bark. It is of a very healing nature and is good to remove internal soreness. In cases where the mucous membrane is irritated it should not be given, but is very good in relaxed and torpid cases, as in cystic and renal congestions, gleet, etc. In bronchial and pulmonary congestions it is a stimulating expectorant. It is an excellent remedy for aged persons suffering from congestion of the kidneys as it then acts as a kidney tonic. In old coughs it is also excellent. Dose: It should be given only when mixed with glycerine and honey. One ounce Balsam Fir, Glycerine and Honey, each four ounces; flavor to suit, mix thoroughly, and give one teaspoonful four times a day

King's American Dispensatory, 1898 tells us:

Abies Canadensis.—Hemlock Spruce.

Action, Medical Uses, and Dosage.—A strong decoction of the bark of this tree is beneficial in leucorrhoea, prolapsus uteri, prolapsus ani, diarrhoea, etc., administered internally, and used in enema; it is likewise of service as a local application in gangrene, and in aphthous, and other oral ulcerations.

The essential oil of this tree, the oil of hemlock, has occasionally been used by pregnant females to cause miscarriage, but serious effects are apt to follow therefrom. As a liniment this oil has been used in croup, rheumatism, and other affections requiring a stimulating local application. The essence (oil) of hemlock is diuretic and highly stimulant. Dr. W. K. Everson states it to be a superior remedy in gastric irritation to allay vomiting in cholera morbus, etc.

The dose is 5 or 10 drops in water, every 10 or 20 minutes, until relief is afforded.

The alcoholic preparations of this drug usually pass under the name of Pinus canadensis. Such preparations are of much value where a mild stimulant and astringent is required, and especially in catarrhal disorders of the mucous tissues, with marked pallidity and relaxation. It is likewise of value in passive hemorrhages and is useful topically in scalds and burns. Tincture, 5 to 30 drops; specific Pinus canadensis, 2 to 10 drops, preferably in equal parts of water and glycerin; the oil, 2 to 5 drops.

Specific Indications and Uses.—General asthenic state, with feeble digestion, vascular weakness, and pale mucous membranes; broncho-pulmonary irritation, with profuse secretions; coughs and colds; renal torpor; pyrosis and gastric irritation, with vomiting and diarrhoea; some cutaneous affections. Never to be used in inflammatory or sthenic conditions.

Mrs. Grieves wrote of Abies in her A Modern Herbal, written in 1931:

Abies Nigra.—Black Spruce.

Action and Medical Uses.—An aqueous decoction of the young branches, strained and concentrated, forms the well-known Essence of Spruce, which enters into the formation of Spruce Beer, an agreeable and salutary summer beverage, possessing diuretic and anti-scorbutic properties, and valuable on board ships. Spruce Beer may be made as follows: Take of ginger, sassafras bark, and guaiacum shavings, each, 2 ounces; hops, 4 ounces; essence of spruce, 10 ounces; water, 4 gallons; mix them and boil for 10 or 15 minutes, then strain. Add 10 gallons of warm water, 3 quarts of molasses, and 12 fluid ounces of yeast, and allow it to ferment. While fermentation is going on, put the fluid in strong bottles and cork them well.

ESSENCE OF SPRUCE is a viscid, molasses-like liquid, having a somewhat sour and bitterish, astringent taste.

Plants for a Future states:

Medicinal use of Balsam Fir: The resin obtained from the balsam fir (see "Uses notes" below) has been used throughout the world and is a very effective antiseptic and healing agent. It is used as a healing and analgesic protective covering for burns, bruises, wounds and sores. It is also used to treat sore nipples and is said to be one of the best curatives for a sore throat. The buds, resin, and/or sap are used in folk remedies for treating cancers, corns, and warts. The resin is also antiscorbutic, diaphoretic, diuretic, stimulant and tonic. It is used internally in propriety mixtures to treat coughs and diarrhoea, though taken in excess it is purgative. A warm liquid of the gummy sap was drunk as a treatment for gonorrhoea. A tea made from the leaves is antiscorbutic. It is used in the treatment of coughs, colds and fevers. The leaves and young shoots are best harvested in the spring and dried for later use. This plant was widely used medicinally by various North American Indian tribes. The resin was used as an antiseptic healing agent applied externally to wounds, sores, bites etc., it was used as an inhalant to treat headaches and was also taken internally to treat colds, sore throats and various other complaints.

Traditional and Healing Herbal Beers tells us:

Like cedar, fir has traditionally been used by many indigenous cultures as a spirit medicine. It is commonly used in sweat lodges and for its antiscorbutic actions. It is also a traditional indigenous medicine for high fever, weight loss, anemia, lack of energy and appetite. .. It has traditionally been used for urinary tract infections, coughs and colds, external wounds, asthma, and as an analgesic for wounds, burns, sores and ulcers. Like pine, it is strong and may irritate mucous membranes.

Peterson Field Guides Eastern and Central Medicinal Plants tells us of balsam fir:

Canada balsam an oleoresin is collected by cutting bark blisters or pockets in would July through August used as an antiseptic an in creams and ointments for piles and root canal sealers diuretic it may irritate mucous membranes American Indians applied the residence as an analgesic for burns sores bruises and wounds leaf tea used for coughs cold and asthma the olio resin is a pale yellow to greenish yellow transparent an pleasantly scented it is primarily commercial application and has been a ceiling agent for mounting microscope slides warning the resident may cause dermatitis in some individuals

Fraser fir she balsam: Cherokees used the resin for chess helmets coughs sore throats urinary tract infections and wounds

Eastern hemlock: American Indians used tea made from leafy twigs for kidney elements in steam bass from rheumatism colds and coughs and into induced sweating inner bark tea used for colds fevers diarrhea coughs stomach troubles and scurvy externally used as a wash for rheumatism and stop bleeding bark is very astringent formally used as a pollsters for bleeding wounds and in tanning Leathers.

Botany In a Day states:

Fir contains turpentine, made of essential oils and resin. The oleo resin is stimulant, diuretic and sometimes diaphoretic and externally rubefacient. The needles can be used as an aromatic bath for rheumatism and nervous diseases. Steeped fir needles make one of my favorite wilderness teas.

Acer, The Maples

At least thirty Maples are used medicinally: Acer acuminatum, Acer argutum, Acer caesium, Acer campestre - Field Maple, Acer carpinifolium - Hornbeam Maple, Acer circinatum - Vine Maple, Acer crataegifolium - Hawthorn-Leaved Maple, Acer distylum, Acer ginnala - Amur Maple, Acer glabrum - Rock Maple, Acer interius - Box Elder, Acer macrophyllum - Oregon Maple, Acer mono Synonym: Acer pictum, Acer negundo - Box Elder, Acer oblongum, Acer palmatum - Japanese Maple, Acer pensylvanicum – Moosewood, Acer platanoides - Norway Maple, Acer pseudoplatanus – Sycamore, Acer rubrum - Red Maple, Acer saccharinum - Silver Maple, Acer saccharum - Sugar Maple, Acer saccharum grandidentatum - Big-Tooth Maple, Acer saccharum nigrum - Black Maple, Acer spicatum - Mountain Maple, Acer sterculiaceum, Acer tataricum - Tatarian Maple, Acer ukurunduense caudatum

Eleven varieties of Maple grow in my region: Acer floridanum (Southern Sugar Maple), Acer leucoderme (Chalk Maple), Acer negundo var. negundo (Eastern Boxelder, Ash-leaved Maple), Acer negundo var. texanum (Texas Boxelder, Ash-leaved Maple), Acer nigrum (Black Maple), Acer pensylvanicum (Striped Maple), Acer rubrum var. rubrum (Red Maple), Acer rubrum var. trilobum (Carolina Red Maple), Acer saccharinum (Silver Maple), Acer saccharum (Sugar Maple), Acer spicatum (Mountain Maple)

Naturalized are: Acer ginnala (Amur Maple), Acer palmatum (Japanese Maple) and Acer platanoides (Norway Maple)

An infusion of the bark of the Maples, especially the Red Maple, Acer Rubrum, is used for its astringent properties. It has traditionally been used for treating sore eyes. It has also been used to help ease cramps and as a remedy in cases of dysentery or severe diarrhea. It may also be useful externally, to tread bruises, swellings and skin inflammations.

A charcoal made from the Vine Maple was used in the treatment of polio. A tea made from the wood and bark of Rock Maple is said to be effective against nausea.

The Moosewood, Acer Pensylvanicum, has the longest and most documented history of use. It has been found effective for a number of ailments. Generally, a tea is made of the inner bark. This tea is useful for coughs, cold, bronchitis and kidney infections. As a wash, it has been used for swellings.

The Sugar Maple is said to be good used as a tonic tea, diuretic and expectorant. It is said to cleanse the liver and kidneys. It is also recommended as a blood cleanser and expectorant for clearing congestion of the lungs.

The Mountain Maple has a long history of use as a poultice for wounds. It is also said to help stop internal hemorrhages, taken as a tea.

Overall, the chief value of the Maple (beyond firewood and furniture) is its sugar. These trees (along with several others) may be tapped in early spring to collect the sap as it rises. This sap may be fermented and turned into a delicious and healthful maple wine or beer. To this, birch twigs, spruce tips, sassafras roots etc may be added for vitamins and as a "spring tonic". Most often though, the sap is cooked down, unfermented, into syrup or sugar. Along with honey, Maple Syrup is likely the most pure and healthful of sweeteners. The sap is rich in minerals. It may help regulate blood sugar, is immune-supportive, anti-inflammatory and is good for gastric ulcers.

Maple nuts are also of interest. Although small, they are very nutritious and quite tasty. No breeding has been done for nut production. But, if you are diligent, you may find a big, old Maple tree that produces many pounds of lentil sized maple nuts each fall. They can be eaten like sunflower seeds. The spring leaves of several varieties, especially Japanese Maple, are a tasty spring snack when small and tender. They are often used as an edible garnish in higher end Asian restaurants.

Gerard stated in his Herbal tells us :

What use the Maple hath in medicine we find nothing written of the Grecians, but Pliny in his 14th book, 8th chapter affirmeth, that the root pounded and applied, is a singular remedy for the pain of the liver. Serenus Sammonicus writeth, that it is drunk with wine against the pains of the side:

Si latus immeritum morbo tentatur acuto,

Accensum tinges lapidem stridentibus undis.

Hinc bibis: aut Aceris radicem tundis, & una

Cum vino capis: hoc præsens medicamen habetur.

Thy harmless side if sharp disease invade,

In hissing water quench a heated stone:

This drink. Or Maple root in powder made,

Take off in wine, a present med'cine known.

Culpepper wrote:

It is under the dominion of Jupiter. The decoction either of the leaves or bark, must needs strengthen the liver much, and so you shall find it to do, if you use it. It is excellently good to open obstructions both of the liver and spleen, and eases pains of the sides thence proceeding.

An Irish Herbal states:

The roots pounded in wine and drunk are beneficial for the pains in the side.

Plants for A Future tells us:

Medicinal use of Sugar Maple: A tea made from the inner bark is a blood tonic, diuretic and expectorant. It has been used in the treatment of coughs, diarrhoea etc. A compound infusion of the bark has been used as drops in treating blindness. The sap has been used for treating sore eyes. The inner bark has been used as an expectorant and cough remedy. Maple syrup is used in cough syrups and is also said to be a liver tonic and kidney cleanser.

The Rodale Herb Book states, " .. there is considerable evidence of the Indians using and extract of the bark of several sorts of the maples for sore eyes."

Sacred and Herbal Healing Beers tells us:

Indigenous cultures have traditionally used maple (sap and bark) for skin conditions such as hives and stubborn wounds, as a wash, a decoction for kidney trouble, as a cough remedy, as a diuretic, for cramping, as a blood purifier, as a tonic and as an astringent for bleeding. Oddly, in spite of the pervasiveness and importance of this tree, there is less information on its medicinal use than any other American herb I know of.

Peterson Field Guides Eastern and Central Medicinal Plants states:

Boxelder: American Indians use the inner bark tea as in an emedic inducing vomiting. Sap boiled down as sugar source.

Striped Maple: American Indians used inner bark tea for colds, coughs, bronchitis, kidney infections, gonorrhea, spitting of blood; wash used for swollen limbs. Inner bark tea was used as a wash for paralysis. Historically, bark tea was used as a folk remedy for skin eruptions, taken internally and applied as an external wash. Leaf

*and twig tea used both to allay or induce nausea, and induce
vomiting, depending on dosage.*

*Sugar Maple: American Indians used inner bark tea for coughs,
diarrhea; diuretic, expectorant, blood purifier. Maple syrup said to
be a liver tonic and kidney cleanser and used in cough syrup.
During the Maple sap gathering process in spring, New Englanders
drank the sap collected in buckets has a spring tonic.*

Maple may not be our most medicinal tree, but it is nutritious and
useful. A few trees could make enough Maple wine/beer, whether
distilled or not, for all the tinctures and herbalist would need.
Therefore, it should not be overlooked, as herbal beers and wines,
as well as tinctures, are often or most effective means of preserving
and delivering medicinal herbs.

Aesculus, Buckeye

Ten varieties of Buckeye are used medicinally: Aesculus californica
- Californian Buckeye, Aesculus flava - Sweet Buckeye, Aesculus
glabra - Ohio Buckeye, Aesculus hippocastanum - Horse Chestnut,
Aesculus chinensis - Chinese Horse Chestnut, Aesculus indica -
Indian Horse Chestnut, Aesculus parviflora, Aesculus pavia - Red
Buckeye, Aesculus turbinata - Japanese Horse Chestnut, Aesculus
x carnea - Red Horse Chestnut

Of the above, only three are native to my region, Aesculus flava
(Yellow Buckeye), Aesculus pavia (Red Buckeye) and Aesculus
sylvatica (Painted Buckeye), with one naturalized, Aesculus
hippocastanum (Horsechestnut). They are remarkably tough trees.
Even as seedlings, they are weedy and very hard to kill. You can
cut them down to the ground, and they simply grow right back!
Their fruit looks like chestnuts, but is inedible for humans. They are
good for firewood, and may be coppiced. Generally, though,
Buckeyes are considered a nuisance… they tend to pop up in one's
hedges and landscape and are very difficult to remove. For that
reason, I was very glad to learn of the herbal use of the Buckeye
tree!

Useful parts are the peeled seed or live, inner bark. The bark can be taken from pruned branches. It is used for poor circulation and claudication (swelling of the ankles). Improves the charge of venous capillaries and veins. Blood rising from the legs is thick and when you stand a lot, fluid pools in the feet and ankles. Buckeye is good for venous congestion in the legs - purple, spidery veins. It can be used topically and internally. Buckeye can be used as a tea with witch hazel or hyssop and is best Combined with Butcher's Broom.

Caution should be used with any internal use of Buckeye, but very small amounts of the tincture may be useful for spasmodic coughs and bronchial tightness.

Externally, Buckeye is most often used for varicose veins, hemorrhoids and rheumatism.

The Buckeye, or "horse chestnut" has long been used as an astringent and anti-inflammatory herb. It is analgesic and diuretic, hemostatic and vasoconstrictive, tonifying the veins.   The root may be useful for chest pains.

Mrs. Grieves lists its medicinal uses as:

The bark has tonic, narcotic and febrifuge properties and is used in intermittent fevers, given in an infusion of 1 OZ. to the pint, in tablespoonful doses, three or four times daily. As an external application to ulcers, this infusion has also been used with success.

The fruits have been employed in the treatment of rheumatism and neuralgia, and also in rectal complaints and for haemorrhoids.

Brother Aloysius wrote of Horse Chestnut:

The horse chestnuts and the flowers are used medicinally. The fresh plucked flowers, steeped in 75 percent alcohol, are an excellent remedy for rheumatic pain; the affected area should be rubbed twice daily with this tincture. Chestnut powder, carried in a linen bag over the heart, is to be recommended for cramps; very finely powdered chestnut is an excellent snuff; the powder is also most efficacious taken internally for colic and cramps. The dose it 2 to 3 pinches per day. Chestnut powder mixed with vinegar and barley meal, cures hardened breasts and dissolved the clotted milk.

The powder alone is an excellent remedy for headaches and eye complaints, it should be sniffed up the nose.

Resources of the Southern Fields and Forests states:

AESCULACEAE. (The Horse Chestnut Tribe).

The seeds contain a great quantity of nutritive starch; also a sufficient amount of potash to be useful as cosmetics, or as a substitute for soap.

HORSE CHESTNUT ; BUCKEYE, (Aesculus pavia, L.)

Diffused. I have observed it in Greenville, Fairfield and Charleston Districts; vicinity of Charleston, Bach.; North Carolina. Fl. May.Shec. Flora Carol. 105; Griffith's Med. Bot. 214. The fruit is about the size of a small lemon, and of a beautifully polished mahogany color externally; it contains a great deal of starch. Dr. Woodhouse prepared a half a pint from the nuts, which retained its color for two years. It is superior to the famous Portland starch, and does not impart a yellow color to cloth. It is said that the washing from this is narcotic and poisonous. Dr. McDowol tried the powder of the rind, and states that ten grains were equivalent to three of opium; a strong decoction is recommended as a lotion to gangrenous ulcers. A strong decoction of the root is said to relieve toothache when held in the mouth. The fresh kernels, macerated in water, mixed with wheat flour into a stiff paste and thrown in pools of standing water, intoxicate fish, so that they float on the surface, and may be taken; reviving, however, when placed in fresh water. I am informed that large quantities were formerly caught in this way in the swamps along the Santee River. See, also, Ell. Bot. Med. Notes. The roots are preferred even to soap for washing and whitening woollens, blankets, and dyed cottons—the colors of which are improved by the process. Satins washed in this manner and carefully ironed, look almost as well as new. The Buckeye has been used in St. John's, Berkeley, S. C, (186.3,) to fix the color of cotton fabrics, muslins, etc., when alum ox gall, sugar of lead, etc., had proved inefficient. Bedsteads made of the horse chestnut are said not to be infested by bugs. I am told that in the West they use the buckeye to prevent piles, worn about the loins as an amulet!

King's American Dispensatory, 1898 tells us:

Aesculus.—Ohio Buckeye.

Action, Medical Uses, and Dosage.—This agent influences the nervous and circulatory systems, having a selective affinity for the portal circulation. In over-doses it affects the cerebro-spinal system somewhat after the manner of nux vomica. Dizziness, fixation of the eyes, impairment of vision, vomiting, wry-neck, opisthotonos, stupor, and tympanites are among its effects. In lethal doses these symptoms are increased, coma supervenes, and death finally takes place. The dried powder of the nut inhaled causes violent sneezing. The action of buckeye is similar to, but more powerful than that of the horse-chestnut (A. Hippocastanum), though some think it less powerful than the latter in its effects upon the portal circulation. It probably acts more powerfully on the spinal than upon the sympathetic nerves. When an excited circulation, with frequent pulse, depends upon disorders of the respiratory and sympathetic nerves, it acts as a decided sedative. The difficult breathing of non-paroxysmal asthma, where the dyspnoea is persistent, but does not amount to a paroxysm, is markedly benefited by aesculus glabra, while in coughs, associated with post-manubrial constriction—a sensation of grasping and tightening—its action is positive. The latter sensation without the cough quickly yields to it. Phthisis, bronchitis, etc., with dyspnoea and oppression, are palliated by it. Intestinal uneasiness and irritation, with a sense of contraction and colic-like pains in the region of the umbilicus, are indications for its use. It is asserted valuable in intestinal dyspepsia with these symptoms, and in hepatic congestion and chronic constipation. Its control over the portal circulation and its attendant disorders is pronounced, and as a remedy for hemorrhoids depending upon portal derangements, it has attained a reputation. A sense of constriction in the rectum is the guide to its use. In female disorders, with tumid and enlarged cervix uteri, with too frequent and profuse menstruation, it may be employed with advantage. Owing to its powerful action upon the nervous system the drug will repay study. It has been employed with asserted success in rheumatism and as a stimulant in paralysis. The dose of specific aesculus glabra is from 1 to 5 drops.

Specific Indications and Uses.—A sensation of grasping or constriction in the post-manubrial space, or at the supra-sternal notch; cough of spasmodic character, with but little expectoration; asthma, with continual dyspnoea, non-paroxysmal; tightness in the chest and about the heart; bronchial irritation with constriction;

sense of constriction, tightness or uneasiness in the rectum, accompanied or not with hemorrhoids; intestinal irritation with constriction and colicky pains near the umbilicus.

Related Species.—Aesculus pavia, Linné. Red buckeye. United States. Southern states, from Georgia and Virginia westward.

Jolanta Wittib writes of Horse Chestnut:

I use the seeds of Horse chestnut. It is my home medicine, my laundry liquid, my dishwasher and material for creative activities with children and grandchildren. As a home medicine, I make a tincture from fresh chestnut seeds. I fill 1/3 of a jar with chopped chestnut seeds, add high percentage alcohol, keep it tightly closed for at least two weeks, and shake it daily. Then I strain the liquid and pour it into a dark bottle for storing. I use it as a prevention for varicose veins. My father and mother suffered a lot from varicose veins. So far I am very lucky and I have no problems at all. Is it thanks to this tincture or to my habit to sit with legs up, whenever I have a chance....

I love nature and I am really conscious of the damage we humans cause by polluting nature and ourselves, thus I systematically try to replace all the synthetic and nature polluting laundry, washing and cleaning liquids and powders in my home. I want to contribute to preserving nature. I want my grandchildren to learn how to cherish nature, to be able to enjoy the green, the fresh, the beautiful. Telling is one, teaching by example is something else. I try to teach by example.

For my laundry I use either dark green ivy (hedera) leaves, or fresh or dried Sweet William herb or horse chestnut seeds. I cannot imagine laundry with any synthetic powder or liquid anymore.

As this is a chapter about chestnut - here is my recipe:

Collect chestnuts, chop them fresh (do not remove the brown shell), dry well and store in tightly

closed jars. For a laundry you pour 300 ml of boiling water onto 3 spoons full of dried chestnuts, let it soak for about 30 minutes, strain the liquid through a sieve and pour it into the washing machine. Do not throw away the thick mass. You can use it once or twice again for washing if you do more laundry in the coming days.

Peterson Field Guides Eastern and Central Medicinal Plants tells us of the Buckeye family:

The Ohio Buckeye, aesculus glabara: Traditionally, powdered nut in minute doses used for spasmodic cough, asthma with tight chest, intestinal irritations. External tea or ointment used for rheumatism and piles. American Indians put ground nuts in streams to stupify fish, which floated to the surface for easy harvest. Warning: nuts toxic, causing severe gastric irritation. Still, Indians made food from them after elaborate processing.

Horsechestnut, aesculus hippocastanum: as in A. glabara; Also, peeled roasted nuts of this tree were brewed for diarrhea, prostate ailments. Thought to increase blood circulation. In Europe, preparations of the seeds are believed to prevent thrombosis, and are used to treat varicose veins and hemorrhoids; thought to help strengthen weak veins and arteries. Also used in gastritis and gastroenteritis. Leaf tea tonic; use for fevers. Flower tincture used on rheumatic joints. Bark tea astringent; used in malaria, dysentery, externally, for lupus and skin ulcers. Warning: outer husks poisonous; All parts can be toxic. Fatalities reported. Seeds (nuts) contain 30 to 60% starch, but can be used as a foodstuff only after the toxins have been removed.

The Physician's Desk Reference for Herbal Medicines notes that, "Health risks or side effects following the proper administration of designated therapeutic dosages are not recorded." However, it cautions that Horse Chestnut/Buckeye may interact negatively with persons taking warfarin, salicylates and other drugs with anti-coagulant properties, and that, "The intake of larger quantities of Horse Chestnut seeds (in one case of a child with 5 seeds) can bring about vomiting, diarrhea, severe thirst, reddening of the face, enlargement of the pupils, vision and consciousness disorders."

Ailanthus altissima, Tree-of-heaven

Tree of Heaven is has been naturalized in my region.

Mrs. Grieves lists Tree of Heaven as:

Antispasmodic, cardiac depressant, astringent. The effect produced by Hetet when experimenting on dogs, was copious stools and the discharge of worms. The resin purges, but rarely acts as an anthelmintic. In China the bark is popular for dysentery and other bowel complaints. A smaller dose of the oleoresin produces similar results and keeps better than the bark.

The vapours of the evaporating extract have a prostrating effect, as have the emanations from the blossoms, while the action upon patients of powder or extract is disagreeable and nauseating, though they have been successfully used in dysentery and diarrhoea, gonorrhoea, leucorrhoea, prolapsus ani, etc., and also as a taenifuge.

The infusion may be given in sweetened orange-flower or other aromatic water, to lessen the bitterness and resultant sickness. Though it produces vomiting and great relaxation, it is stated not to be poisonous.

A tincture of the root-bark has been used successfully in cardiac palpitation, asthma and epilepsy.

The action of the trees in malarial districts is considered to resemble that of the Eucalyptus.

The statement that the resin is purgative has been disputed, some asserting that it is inert.

King's American Dispensatory, 1898 tells us:

Action, Medical Uses, and Dosage.—The bark of ailanthus has been employed by Roberts, Dugat, and others, both in the recent and dried state, as a remedy for dysentery and diarrhoea; also in gonorrhoea, leucorrhoea, prolapsus ani, etc. Fifty grammes of the root-bark are infused for a short time in 75 grammes of hot water, then strained, and when cold, administered in teaspoonful doses, night and morning. To lessen the disagreeable impression following its use, as well as to mask its bitterness, it may be administered in sweetened orange-flower water, or in some other aromatic.

Professor Hetet, of the Toulon Naval School, states in Jour. de Chim. Med., December, 1859, that the leaves and bark, in powder, or in the form of an aqueous or of an alcoholic extract, will remove tapeworm; but he found its action upon patients to be very disagreeable and nauseating, somewhat like that occasioned by tobacco upon young smokers. Dupuis has also found it useful as a taenifuge. In the September number of the Eclectic Medical Journal, for 1875, p. 393, Dr. H. L. True, of Ohio, states, that from his observations, the bark is not poisonous, but produces vomiting, great relaxation, and a deathlike sickness, which symptoms gradually pass away. He has successfully employed a tincture of the root-bark in cardiac palpitation, obstinate singultus, asthma, and epilepsy. Its use in epilepsy has gained in reputation. It should be studied for its action in sick and nervous headache, with nausea, and an indescribable burning sensation in the forehead. Webster states, "the remedy, in 2x dilution, will cure malignant sore throat, ulcerated tonsils, and other tonsillar inflammations, marked by adynamia and persistency." He states that he has been pleased with it in putrid, malignant, typhoid scarlatina, with dusky, carmine eruption, high temperature, pungent surface, pulse small and extremely rapid, with thirst, delirium, and coma. The tongue is dusky, parched, and fissured; sores upon the teeth; and the urine discharges involuntarily. Dose, 1 to 10 drops of the 2x dilution. His uses of the drug were derived from homoeopathy. Dr. True considers the presence of these trees in malarial districts to have a strong action, similar to that of the eucalyptus, in antagonizing those influences that produce intermittents. The dose of the tincture is from 5 to 60 drops, repeated as often as required, or, from 2 to 4 times a day; specific ailanthus, 5 to 20 drops.

Specific Indications and Uses.—Cardiac palpitation; spasmodic or epileptiform muscular contraction.

Plants for A Future sates:

Medicinal use of Tree Of Heaven: The tree of heaven is not often used in Western herbal medicine, though it is more popular in the Orient. Various parts of the plant are used, though the bark is the part most commonly used - however, it contains a glycoside that has not been fully researched and so should be used with caution. The root and stem bark are antispasmodic, astringent, bitter, cardiac depressant, diuretic, emetic, febrifuge, rubefacient and vermifuge. *The vermifuge properties do not act on round worms or earthworms. A nauseatingly bitter herb, it is used internally to treat malaria and fevers, it also slows the heart rate and relaxes spasms. It needs to be used under the supervision of a qualified practitioner since the bark readily causes vomiting. In China, the bark is a popular remedy for dysentery and other complaints of the bowels. In one clinical trial, 81 out of 82 patients were cured of dysentery when they were given this herb. A tincture of the root-bark has been used successfully in the treatment of cardiac palpitations, asthma and epilepsy. Tree-of-heaven is a folk remedy for asthma, cancer, diarrhoea, dysentery, dysmenorrhoea, dysuria, ejaculation (premature), epilepsy, eruption, fever, gonorrhoea, haematochezia, leucorrhoea, malaria, metrorrhagia, sores, spasms, spermatorrhoea, stomachic, tumours of the breast (China), and wet dreams The bark is harvested in the spring and dried for later use. The leaves, bark of the trunk, and roots are put into a wash to treat parasitic ulcers, itch, and eruptions. In Korea, the root bark is used in the treatment of coughs, gastric and intestinal upsets. The stembark is emmenagogue. The leaves are anthelmintic, astringent and deobstruent. The fruit is used in the treatment of bloody stools and dysentery. They have also been used to treat ophthalmic diseases. Extracts from the plant are bactericidal. The tree is used in homeopathic remedies for cancer. A resin extracted from the roots and leaves is a revulsive or vesicant.*

Peterson Field Guides Eastern and Central Medicinal Plants tells us:

Two ounces bark infused in one quart water, given in teaspoonfuls for diarrhea, dysentery, leukorrhea, tapeworm; Used in traditional Chinese medicine. Recently shown could contain at least 3 potent antimalarial compounds. Warning: large doses potentially poisonous. Gardeners who cut the tree may suffer from rashes.

The Physicians' Desk Reference for Herbal Medicine tells us:

An antimalarial action is being tested in an in vitro trial period the active agents also have a stringent, antipyretic, and antispasmodic properties. Unproven uses: in Africa, tree of heaven is used for cramps, asthma, tachycardia, gonorrhea, epilepsy and tapeworm infestation it is increasingly used in the treatment of malaria.

Albizia, Mimosa

Two Mimosas have been naturalized in my region, though neither grow at my elevation. Mimosa is a very important herb, so I make a point of scouting for trees during my travels throughout the summer and gathering flowers from those trees in the spring. Mimosa has the unique ability to reduce mast cells, which are the receptors for histamines in an allergic reaction. In that way, Mimosa is almost a reverse antihistamine that is more effective than mot antihistamines, long term. Mimosa is also a mild narcotic, that can reduce pain and relax the body. Although the leaves and bark may be used, a tincture of the flowers is sweet smelling and tastes reminiscent of watermelon – it is not only among my favorite medicinal herbs but finds its way into the occasional cocktail!

Plants for A Future states:

Medicinal use of Mimosa: The flower heads are carminative, digestive, sedative and tonic. They are used internally in the treatment of insomnia, irritability, breathlessness and poor memory. The flowers are harvested as they open and are dried for later use. The stembark is anodyne, anthelmintic, carminative, discutient, diuretic, oxytocic, sedative, stimulant, tonic, vermifuge and vulnerary. It is used internally in the treatment of insomnia, irritability, boils and carbuncles. Externally, it is applied to injuries and swellings. The bark is harvested in spring or late summer and is dried for later use. A gummy extract obtained from the plant is used as a plaster for abscesses, boils etc and also as a retentive in fractures and sprains.

Alnus, Alder

Sixteen varieties of Alder are used Medicinally: Alnus cordata - Italian Alder, Alnus glutinosa, Alnus hirsute, Alnus incana - Grey Alder, Alnus japonica - Japanese Alder, Alnus maritima - Seaside Alder, Alnus maximowiczii Family, Alnus nepalensis - Nepalese Alder, Alnus nitida, Alnus rhombifolia - White Alder, Alnus rubra - Red Alder, Alnus rugosa - Speckled Alder, Alnus serrulata - Smooth Alder, Alnus sinuata - Sitka Alder, Alnus tenuifolia - Mountain Alder, Alnus viridis crispa - American Green Alder

Of these, only two grow in my region, Alnus serrulata (Hazel Alder, Tag Alder) and Alnus viridis crispa (Mountain Alder, Green Alder)

The most common use of Alder bark is as a source of salicylic acid, the base from which aspirin was created. It is anodyne, febrifuge and analgesic. It is also emetic, astringent, hemostatic, stomatic and tonic. A poultice of the leaves may be used for sores and wounds and is useful against infection.

Saint Hildegard states, " … if someone is a bit ulcerous on his skin, place new, fresh leaves of this tree on the ulcers. During that time it will become smoother."

Gerard wrote of Alder:

A. The leaves of Alder are much used against hot swellings, ulcers, and all inward inflammations, especially of the almonds and kernels of the throat.

B. The bark is much used of poor country dyers, for the dying of coarse cloth, caps, hose, and such like into a black colour, whereunto it serveth very well.

Mrs. Grieves listed of Alder:

Medicinal Action and Uses---Tonic and astringent. A decoction of the bark is useful to bathe swellings and inflammations, especially of the throat, and has been known to cure ague.

Peasants on the Alps are reported to be frequently cured of rheumatism by being covered with bags full of the heated leaves.

Horses, cows, sheep and goats are said to eat it, but swine refuse it. Some state that it is bad for horses, as it turns their tongues black.

An Irish Herbal states:

The bark or rind of it, because of its astringent quality is useful against swellings of the throat. It heals and cauterizes sores and ulcers. … and the leaves of it are made use of against ulcers and all kinds of inflammations.

Brother Aloysius wrote of Alder:

Alder bark is very rich in tannin, which makes it very astringent and febrifuge. The dose is 1/4th cup power in a glass of white wine, taken in the mornings on an empty stomach, while the patient is in bed, as this remedy causes excessive sweating. Decoction of alder is an excellent remedy for inflammation of the throat and tonsils. One should gargle four to six times a day. The fruit (alder buds) should be picked in October and bottled in gin; one tablespoon taken twice a day is a recommended remedy epilepsy. The bluish colored buds, picked in the spring, dried and taken in the form of a tea, are highly recommended for rheumatism. The fresh leaves, pounded and applied to ulcers, take away the burning and cause them to suppurate and heal.

Herbal Remedies of the Lumbee Indians states:

A handful of bark that was peeled from a tree that was knotty and gnarly was boiled down by the Lumbee healers to make a strong tea of deep red color to reduce swellings and sprains, coughs and skin eruptions. Aunt Cat Lowry, a Lumbee midwife and herbal expert, would recommend a tea made from Red Tag Elder to nurse the pains of the mother related to the birthing process. Many healers thought an ingredient in this tea cleared milky urine. For drooping eyes, some healers would rub and blow the decoction of the bark into the eyes or suggest a bark tea for general pain or heart trouble. A hot berry tea was often prescribed to treat fever. Drinking a cold tea from bark shavings was suggested by one healer to help the kidneys act. Lumbee mothers would often give the tea to babies for "thrash" (thrush), a mouth soreness. Sugar was added to the tea by many Lumbee mothers and given to babies for hives or teething. A cold bark tea was prescribed by Lumbee healers to purify the blood and bring down high blood pressure.

Resources of the Southern Fields and Forests states:

The bark is astringent. N. Y. Journal Med. V. 7, 8. It had for a long time been neglected; but in the article referred to the decoction is spoken highly of as an alterative and astringent in scrofula and cutaneous diseases, and it is said to have been very successful in haematuria; in these affections producing beneficial results where all other means had failed. Shec, in his Flora Carol., spoke of the alder tags as being of great service on account of their alterative powers; a decoction of the leaves has also been used to suppress hemorrhage, and they have been found effectual in relieving dyspepsia and bowel complaints. An astringent decoction may be made of the bark, leaves, or tags—acting also as a diuretic. A tincture may also be used. Poultices made of them are used as a local application to tumors, sprains, swellings, etc. The leaves are applied externally to wounds and ulcers. The inner bark of the root is emetic, and it has been given in intermittents.

King's American Dispensatory, 1898 tells us:

Action, Medical Uses, and Dosage.—To the taste tag alder is bitter and astringent. It powerfully increases retrograde metamorphosis and exerts a direct tonic action upon mucous surfaces, aiding digestion and assimilation. It is a true catalytic and a positive anti-putrefactive agent. Locally applied, the decoction stains the skin. The drug stimulates the gastric mucous membrane and causes an increased flow of gastric juice. Applied to the mammae, the leaves are said to decrease the lacteal secretion. It is alterative, emetic, and astringent.

This much neglected, but very important, remedy is a valuable agent in scrofulosis, especially in those cases marked by glandular enlargements and suppuration. Prof. Scudder speaks of it as one of the most valuable of our indigenous remedies, and points to its use in "superficial diseases of the skin and mucous membranes, taking the form of eczema or pustular eruption." Administered internally and applied locally in these conditions, we may expect from alnus the best of results. Impetigo, prurigo, herpes, and scorbutus, are diseases in which alnus will be of great utility. In scurfy tetter of the scalp, in children, it is of much value. The happiest results are obtained from its use in successive crops of boils. It is a good agent in passive hemorrhages, particularly in hematuria, for which a decoction of the cones has also been used, and it is favorably mentioned for purpura hemorrhagica. In marasmus of children, it is a much praised remedy. Combined with rumex crispus, and used locally and internally, it is a good drug in nursing sore mouth of mothers. Alnus is an important drug in indigestion and dyspepsia, when resulting from deficient secretion of gastric juice and debility of the muscular coat of the stomach. It may be associated with specific nux vomica. In diarrhoea, caused by or attended with deficiency of the gastric secretion, it serves an excellent purpose. It has been used with good results as an injection for leucorrhoea, and the leaves may "scatter" indurations of the mammary glands during the nursing period. ¥ Dr. A. D. Ayer reports many cases of periodical hyperaesthetic rhinitis (hay fever) cured by alnus. He recommends a distillate prepared after the manner of distillate of hamamelis. The distillate is first used with an equal bulk of water and snuffed up the nostrils 5 or 6 times daily. It may be increased to full strength in a day or two. If desirous, it may be applied by atomization. At night the nose is smeared with the distillate combined with petrolatum. At the same time give internally: Rx Distillate of alnus, gtt. xv to xxx, in a little water, 1 hour before or after meals. Dr. Ayer also recommends this preparation in the acute stage of gonorrhoea, and as an antidote to rhus poisoning. The remedy is most effectual in infusion (fresh alnus bark, ʒj, aqua Oj); dose, a wine-glassful. Specific alnus, 1 to 20 drops.

Specific Indications and Uses.—The specific use of this remedy is to improve nutrition and increase waste. It is of particular value in scrofula, with feeble vitality, and chronic skin diseases exhibiting scaly or pustular eruptions.

Plants for A Future states:

Medicinal use of Alder: The bark is alterative, astringent, cathartic, febrifuge and tonic. The fresh bark will cause vomiting, so use dried bark for all but emetic purposes. A decoction of the dried bark is used to bathe swellings and inflammations, especially of the mouth and throat. The powdered bark and the leaves have been used as an internal astringent and tonic, whilst the bark has also been used as an internal and external haemostatic against haemorrhage. The dried bark of young twigs are used, or the inner bark of branches 2 - 3 years old. It is harvested in the spring and dried for later use. Boiling the inner bark in vinegar produces a useful wash to treat lice and a range of skin problems such as scabies and scabs. The liquid can also be used as a toothwash. The leaves are astringent, galactogogue and vermifuge. They are used to help reduce breast engorgement in nursing mothers. A decoction of the leaves is used in folk remedies for treating cancer of the breast, duodenum, oesophagus, face, pylorus, pancreas, rectum, throat, tongue, and uterus. The leaves are harvested in the summer and used fresh.

The Rodale Herb Book lists Alder:

The bark and berries are cathartic, similar to cascara in cation. The astringent bark, prepared as a decoction, is used for a gargle for sore throat, to induce circulation, check diarrhea, and for eye drops. Leaves are glutinous and used to cure inflammation. Fresh leaves applied to bare feet, are said to be excellent for burning and itching feet. Also used as a foot bath when brewed as a strong tea.

Sacred and Healing Herbal Beers states:

Alder is rarely used in botanical medicine at this time, though it is a powerful remedy for a number of conditions. It is strongly astringent, the leaves and bark containing 16 percent tannin. ... Traditionally, alder has been used as a vulnerary(wound healer) and stomatic. It tonifies the stomach and small intestine, helping improve food absorption and fat metabolism. It is also a bitte and stimulates gastric secretion. Traditionally, elder has been used with great effectiveness in eye infections, sore throats, mouth infections, stubborn and bleeding wounds, diarrhea and skin irritations. Felter and Lloyd call it a 'positive anti-putrefactive agent,' and a number of traditional medical herbalists note its effectiveness in treating gangrene.

Botany In a Day states:

Alders are very astringent, and the bark is the most potent. The live inner bark from our local alders quickly turns a flaming orange-brown color when exposed to air. The color is from tannic acid. It is a brilliant an permanent dye. Some Native Americans even dyed their hair with it! Other species of Alder may produce darker colors. Medicinally, the alder can be used as a potent astringent for wounds, diarrhea and so forth. Some species produce anti-tumor properties similar to the birches.

The Physicians Desk Reference for Herbal Medicines tells us:

Black Alder: Affects. The decoction is a tonic and has astringent and hemostatic properties, which may be due to the tannins, flavone glycosides, and triterpenes. Unproven uses: Black Alder is used as a decoction for gargles in the treatment of streptococcal sore throat and pharyngitis, and for internal bleeding. The bark is considered to be affective for intermittent fever. No health hazards or side effects or known in conjunction with the proper administration of designated therapeutic dosages.

Amelanchier, Serviceberry

Twenty six varieties of Serviceberry are used medicinally or for fruit: Amelanchier alnifolia – Saskatoon, Amelanchier alnifolia cusickii - Cusick's Serviceberry, Amelanchier alnifolia semiintegrifolia - Pacific Serviceberry, Amelanchier arborea - Downy Serviceberry, Amelanchier asiatica - Korean Juneberry, Amelanchier bartramiana, Amelanchier basalticola, Amelanchier canadensis – Juneberry, Amelanchier confuse, Amelanchier humilis, Amelanchier huroensis, Amelanchier interior, Amelanchier intermedia, Amelanchier laevis - Allegheny Shadberry, Amelanchier lamarckii - Apple Serviceberry, Amelanchier obovalis - Southern Juneberry, Amelanchier ovalis - Snowy Mespilus, Amelanchier ovalis integrifolia, Amelanchier pallida - Pale Serviceberry, Amelanchier parviflora, Amelanchier sanguinea - Roundleaf Serviceberry, Amelanchier spicata, Amelanchier stolonifera - Quebec Berry, Amelanchier utahensis - Utah Serviceberry, Amelanchier weigandii, Amelanchier x grandiflora

Of these, four grow in my region: Amelanchier arborea (Common Serviceberry), Amelanchier canadensis (Canadian Serviceberry), Amelanchier laevis (Allegheny Serviceberry), Amelanchier sanguinea (Roundleaf Serviceberry)

Although there are a couple pf varieties of Serviceberry that grow outside of North America, this is predominately New World medicine. Serviceberry was much used by Native Americans.

According to Plants for a Future:

Saskatoon was quite widely employed as a medicinal herb by the North American Indians, who used it to treat a wide range of minor complaints. It is little used in modern herbalism. An infusion of the inner bark is used as a treatment for snow-blindness. A decoction of the fruit juice is mildly laxative. It has been used in the treatment of upset stomachs, to restore the appetite in children, it is also applied externally as ear and eye drops. A decoction of the roots has been used in the treatment of colds. It has also been used as a treatment for too frequent menstruation. A decoction of the stems, combined with the stems of snowberry (Symphoricarpos spp) is diaphoretic. It has been used to induce sweating in the treatment of fevers, flu etc and also in the treatment of chest pains and lung infections. A decoction of the plant, together with bitter cherry (Prunus emarginata) has been used as a contraceptive. Other recipes involving this plant have also been used as contraceptives including a decoction of the ashes of the plant combined with the ashes of pine branches or buds. A strong decoction of the bark was taken immediately after childbirth to hasten the dropping of the placenta. It was said to help clean out and help heal the woman's insides and also to stop her menstrual periods after the birth, thus acting as a form of birth control.

A tea made from the root bark (mixed with other unspecified herbs) was used as a tonic in the treatment of excessive menstrual bleeding and also to treat diarrhoea. A bath of the bark tea was used on children with worms. An infusion of the root was used to prevent miscarriage after an injury. A compound concoction of the inner bark was used as a disinfectant wash.

A compound infusion of the plant (Downy Serviceberry)has been used as an anthelmintic, in the treatment of diarrhoea and as a spring tonic. An infusion of the bark has been used in the treatment of gonorrhoea.

George Washington is said to have planted Serviceberry at Mount Vernon, but we can only assume his reason for doing so was the fruit. Overall, Serviceberry is a much-underutilized native fruit. Recent research has shown that it may have anti-viral properties that could be useful in combating such viruses as COVID-19

Peterson Field Guides Eastern and Central Medicinal Plants tells us:

Chippewas used root bark tea with other herbs as a tonic for excessive menstrual bleeding, a female tonic and to treat diarrhea. Cherokees used in herb combinations as a digestive tonic. Bath of bark tea used on children with worms.

Aralia Spinosa, Devil's Walking Stick

Now, this one is interesting! I would have considered it more of a shrub than a tree, but several sources list it as a native tree... so, who am I to argue? It is certainly a unique plant and a valuable herb. The Devil's Walking stick grows throughout much of my region, from the mountains down to the piedmont, and even occasionally found in the coastal counties of NC. This Aralia is called Devil's Walking Stick, because it not only grows straight and is the right size and shape for a walking stick, but the trunk is covered in wicked thorns. I have backed into a few, not paying attention in the woods.... NOT FUN! It may also be called Hercules' Club, Prickly Ash or Prickly Elder.

This plant is in the same family as Ginseng. It has long been used medicinally. Early settlers found the berries useful for toothaches, as the plant has analgesic properties. The fresh bark is said to be emetic and purgative. The dried bark is stimulating, alterative, meaning it gradually brings one back to health., and diaphoretic, meaning it helps resolve a fever. The effects of the dried bark put it in the category of the other aralias and ginsengs, it is a mild adaptogen. Adaptogens help the body recover from stress.

Mrs. Grieves referred to Aralia spinosa as "Angelica Tree", stating of its use:

Fresh bark causes/vomiting and purging, but dried is a stimulating alterative. A tincture made from the bark is used for rheumatism, skin diseases and syphilis. The berries in tincture form, lull pain in decayed teeth and in other parts of the body, violent colic and rheumatism, useful in cholera when a cathartic is required in the following compound: 1 drachm compound powdered Jalap, 1 drachm Aralia spinosa, 2 drachms compound rhubarb powder or infused in 1/2, pint boiling water and when cold taken in tablespoonful doses every half-hour. This does not produce choleric discharges. Also a powerful sialogogue and valuable in diseases where mouth and throat get dry, and for sore throat; will relieve difficult breathing and produce moisture if given in very small doses of the powder. The bark, root, and berries can all be utilized.

Traditionally, Aralia Spinosa has been used somewhat interchangeably with Arailia Hispida and shares many of the qualities of Sarsaparilla (smilax) as a mild adaptogen, alterative or general tonic.... In many ways, it is a larger, weaker version of American Spikenard. Aralia racemose, but still quite useful.

Resources of the Southern Fields and Forests states:

TOOTHACHE BUSH; ANGELICA TREE; PKICKLY ASH; PEICKLY ELDER, (Amlia spinosa, L.) Collected in St. John's; rich soils along fences; Charleston, Florida and North Carolina.

Plant often confounded with the Xanthoxylon ; properties somewhat similar. See JC. Fraxineium which is the true Prickly Ash. Ell. Bot. 373 ; Mer. and de L. Diet, de M. Med. i, 379; Coxe, Am. Disp. 100; Shcc. Elora Carol. 191; Frost's Elems. 20; Griffith, Med. Bot. 345. It is a stimulating and very certain diaphoretic, " probably to be preferred to any emetic yet discovered among our native plants." This species is more stimulating than the A. nudicaulis. The infusion of the bark of the root is used in chronic rheumatism and cutaneous eruptions, also employed in lues venerea. Pursh states that a vinous or spirituous infusion of the berries is remarkable for their power in relieving rheumatic pains, and the tincture is also given in Virginia in violent colics. See Dr. Meara's experiments. Merat says, it has been used to allay pain caused by carious teeth. Dose, of the saturated tincture, a tablespoonful three times a day. A decoction is often preferred in rheumatism, made by boiling an ounce of the bark in a quart of water; taken in divided doses several times a day. In South Carolina, this plant is the rattlesnake's master par excellence, according to the negroes; they rely on it almost exclusively as a remedy for the bite of serpents. I am informed that they use the bark of the fresh root in substance, taken internally, also applying it powdered to the wounded part. Dr. Meara advises that the watery infusion, when employed as a diaphoretic, should be made very weak, as it is apt to excite nausea, and cause irritation of the salivary glands.

King's American Dispensatory, 1898 tells us:

Action, Medical Uses, and Dosage.—The fresh bark will produce vomiting and purging; but when dried it is a stimulating alterative, producing a determination toward the surface. The tincture has been used in syphilitic and rheumatic affections, and in some diseases of the skin. The warm infusion, especially when strong, is apt to induce vomiting. The berries in tincture have been found useful in lulling the pain from a decayed tooth; also in various painful affections of other parts. Much use was made of this bark by physicians in Cincinnati during the cholera of 1849-50, in cases where cathartics were required, but where the action of every purgative was difficult to control; the preparation was composed of 1 drachm of compound powder of jalap, 1 drachm of aralia spinosa, and 2 drachms of compound powder of rhubarb. Given in powder, in half-teaspoonful doses; or the powder was infused in half a pint of boiling water, of which infusion, when cold, a tablespoonful was given every half hour. In no case in which it was given did it produce a tendency to looseness or choleraic discharges. It is a powerful sialagogue, and is valuable in diseases where the mouth and throat are dry and parched, as a very small portion of the powder will produce a moisture and relieve difficult breathing; also useful in sore throat. The dose of tincture (bark ℥viij to dilute alcohol Oj) is from 5 to 60 drops, of the infusion (℥ss to aqua Oj) a tablespoonful to a wineglassful.

Asimina triloba, the Pawpaw

This one is easy to identify, because there is only one variety of Pawpaw. Pawpaw is another of our uniquely native plants. I'd love to tell you it has all kinds of impressive, medicinal properties… and it does have some… but its main value is its fruit. The Pawpaw is our native "tropical" fruit, that grows in temperate regions. It was long considered a variety of papaya, but it is a unique and distinct tree. Sometimes called the Custard Apple, this fruit has a tropical flavor, but grows best in the mountains and hills. It is a smallish tree, one that inhabits the under-story. It would be far more common were it not for the practices of real estate and forestry that clear the understory, in favor of tall trees for timber and landscape. Pawpaws like a mixed forest, not a park-like setting or a timber stand.

Two other factors have led to the Pawpaw falling out of favor as a favorite American fruit. The first is simply that knowledge of this fruit has not been passed down through the generations as it was in earlier times. If only we still had intact families, where grandparents and parents took the kids into the woods and meadows to teach them about wild edible and medicinal plants! If families still spent such time together, foraging, hunting, fishing, trapping and gardening, we would likely have far more intact families! The second has to do with market forces. The fruit and vegetables we see in modern grocery stores are not offered for their flavor or nutritional value. No, modern produce is chosen specifically for its ability to withstand shipping long distances while still appearing fresh, and its shelf life. The tomato you buy was likely shipped thousands of miles. The fruit you buy may have come even further. The watermelon is by no means the full flavored, vitamin packed watermelon our grandparents enjoyed… it is chosen for its tough, thick rind and uniform appearance. That it has little flavor is of little concern to modern agri-business. Pawpaws are delicious fruit, but they will not stand shipping. Their shelf life is similar to a ripe banana. They make a fine fruit for local farmer's markets and roadside fruit stands, but rarely, if ever, will you see them in a grocery store.

As for medicinal use, the fruit is laxative when eaten in large amounts. The leaves are diuretic, and make a good poultice for wounds, boils, infections and inflammations. The bark may be used as a digestive bitter. There is also some history of use as a wash in cases of head lice.

41

Of the seeds, Mrs. Grieves writes:

Emetic, for which a saturated tincture of the bruised seeds is employed, dose, 10 to 60 drops. The bark is a bitter tonic and is said to contain a powerful acid, the leaves are used as an application to boils and ulcers.

Pawpaw trees may be purchased from many nurseries that specialize in fruit trees or who cater to Permaculture folks. I hope my readers will consider planting Pawpaws. I'd love to see some of these natives that are becoming all too rare become popular – A Pawpaw, Persimmon and Passionfruit vine in every yard!

Resources of the Southern Fields and Forests states:

Grows in rich soils along streams. I have observed it in Fairfield and Spartanburg districts, South Carolina, and collected it in St. John's; Mr. Elliott says it is found at Beck's ferry, Savannah river, and North Carolina. Fl. May. Diet, de Mat. Med par Mer and de L. tom. i, 311. The rind of the fruit of the A. triloba of Linn, possesses a very active acid; pulp sometimes employed as a topical application in ulcers. Lind. Nat. Syst. Bot. 69. "Juice of unripe fruit is a powerful and efficient vermifuge; the powder of the seeds answers the same purpose; a principal constituent of the juice is fibrin—a product supposed peculiar to animal substances and to fungi." " The tree has, moreover, the property of rendering the toughest animal substances tender by causing a separation of the muscular fibre— its very vapor even does this; newly killed meat suspended over the leaves, and even old hogs and poultry, when fed on the leaves and fruit, become ' tender in a few hours!' " Lind. loc. cit. The sap of the Papaw tree, {Carica papaya), which is extracted from the fruit by incision, is white and excessively viscous. In a specimen from the Isle of France, Yauquelin found a matter having the chemical properties of animal albumen, and lastly, fatty matter. Boussingault. This tree can be found in many parts of the South and I would invite examination into these very curious properties. For an excellent description of the Papaw, see Hooker in the Bot. Magazine, 808. At Pittsburgh, a spirituous liquor has been made from the fruit. Michaux notices that the cellular integument of the bark, and particularly that of the roots, exhales in summer a nauseous odor so strong as to occasion sickness if re- spired in confined air. Am. Sylva.

King's American Dispensatory, 1898 tells us Pawpaw:

Action, Uses, and Dosage.—Emetic, for which purpose a saturated tincture of the bruised seeds is employed, in doses of from 10 to 60 drops. The bark is said to be a bitter tonic and has been used as such in domestic practice. The medical properties of this agent have not been fully investigated.

Peterson Field Guides Eastern and Central Medicinal Plants tells us:

Fruit edible, delicious; also a laxative. Leaves insecticidal, diarrhetic; Applied to abscesses. Seeds emetic, narcotic producing stupor. The powdered seeds, formally applied to the heads of children to control lice, having insecticidal properties. Warning: seeds toxic. Leaves may cause rash.

Baccharis halimifolia, Bush Groundsel

Halimifolia is the only Baccharis found in my region, but four are used in herbal medicine: Baccharis halimifolia - Bush Groundsel, Baccharis patagonica, Baccharis pilularis - Dwarf Chaparral, Baccharis viminea - Mule's Fat

Honestly, I'd like to have a plant called "Mule's Fat" in my landscape just for the name, alone! As for the Bush Groundsel though, it is mainly a hedge plant. This is another I would consider to be more of a shrub.

Medicinally, the Bush Groundsel has been used for coughs and lung ailments. It is demulcent and calming to the lungs.

Betula, Birch

Sixteen varieties of Birch are used medicinally: Betula alleghaniensis – Yellow Birch, Betula alnoides, Betula ermanii - Gold Birch, Betula glandulosa - Scrub Birch, Betula kenaica - Kenai Birch, Betula lenta - Cherry Birch, Betula nana - Dwarf Birch, Betula nigra - River Birch, Betula occidentalis - Water Birch, Betula papyrifera - Paper Birch, Betula pendula - Silver Birch, Betula platyphylla - White Birch, Betula populifolia - Grey Birch, Betula pubescens - White Birch, Betula schmidtii, Betula utilis - Indian Paper

Betula populifolia (Gray Birch) has been naturalized here.

Of these, four varieties grow in my aera: Betula alleghaniensis (Yellow Birch), Betula cordifolia (Mountain Paper Birch), Betula lenta (Sweet Birch, Black Birch, Cherry Birch), Betula nigra (River Birch)

Birch has long use both in herbal medicine and as a beverage. The tips of birch twigs and the bark can be gathered in the spring and used to make Birch Beer, that was very popular in early America. It has a wintergreen-like flavor. Birch can also be tapped like Maple, to gather the sweet sap as it rises. This quality made Birch a veritable beer plant, as it supplied its own water, sugar and flavoring. All that was needed to turn it into beer was yeast, and wild yeasts are not only in the air, but would be on the birch twigs themselves. In a time when clean, drinkable water was scarce, such low alcohol beers and wines were essential to survival.

Bark, leaves, twigs, buds and shoots of Birch are used medicinally. Birch is anti-inflammatory and helps break a fever. It stimulates bile. The bark is astringent. The sap is diuretic. The shoots are laxative. Birch has been used for fevers and colds, as an aid in digestion, for skin conditions such as eczema and psoriasis, rheumatism and arthritis, gout, fluid retention, kidney stones, wounds and sores.

Gerard wrote of Birch:

Concerning the medicinable use of the Birch tree, or his parts, there is nothing extant either in the old or new writers.

This tree, saith Pliny in his 16th book, 18th chapter, *Mirabili candore & tenuitate terribilis magistratum virgis:*["Wonderfully white, and striking fear as the flogging-canes of the magistrates"] for in times past the magistrates' rods were made hereof: and in our time also the schoolmasters and parents do terrify their children with rods made of Birch.

It serveth well to the decking up of houses, and banquetting rooms, for places of pleasure, and beautifying of streets in the cross or gang week, and such like.

Culpepper, in his unique style said:

Government and virtues. It is a tree of Venus, the juice of the leaves, while they are young, or the distilled water of them, or the water that comes from the tree being bored with an auger, and distilled afterwards; any of these being drank for some days together, is available to break the stone in the kidneys and bladder and is good also to wash sore mouths.

Mrs. Grieves tells us:

Various parts of the tree have been applied to medicinal uses. The young shoots and leaves secrete a resinous substance having acid properties, which, combined with alkalies, is said to be a tonic laxative. The leaves have a peculiar, aromatic, agreeable odour and a bitter taste, and have been employed in the form of infusion (Birch Tea) in gout, rheumatism and dropsy, and recommended as a reliable solvent of stone in the kidneys. With the bark they resolve and resist putrefaction. A decoction of them is good for bathing skin eruptions, and is serviceable in dropsy.

The oil is astringent, and is mainly employed for its curative effects in skin affections, especially eczema, but is also used for some Internal maladies.

The inner bark is bitter and astringent, and has been used in intermittent fevers.

The vernal sap is diuretic.

Moxa is made from the yellow, fungous excrescences of the wood, which sometimes swell out from the fissures

An Irish herbal states:

The liquid that is drained off this tree in the springtime is good for dispelling urinary disorders, like stones, pains and bleeding. A decoction of the leaves, when drunk, is considered good for scurvy.

Brother Aloysius wrote of Silver Birch:

The bark is bitter and astringent; the leaves are hot, desiccative, solvent, and stimulative to the appetite. It is recommended for dropsy. The decoction of the leaves, bark and thin twigs is ½ to 1 cup per 2 cups water. People who suffer from nerves or dropsy should take 1 to 2 cups per day.

Fr. Künzle wrote of Birch:

*The man from icy land particularly liked the birch with its fine, delicate foliage, which playfully
moved in the wind. The Dane explained to him that there are forests full of birch where it is very
healthy to sojourn, the leaves are a delicious medicine for urine ailments, the sap of the tree is a
useful drink against edema…. Continued consumption of birch leaves (Betula alba), boiled with wine, drunk in the morning and evening helps against edema.*

… if your rheumatism has not appeared all of a sudden, but has already been there for years, or if you are 60 or more years old yourself, take the full herbal bath on one day, take the juniper on the next day, drink daily tea from birch leaves, Meadowsweet, Spiny restharrow and Lady's bedstraw, take a sip about every hour, then you can be cured in three to six weeks, depending on the depth and length of your illness. I have seen 70-year-old people suffering and distorted from gout got cured after having undergone this treatment in the spa building "Wangs" near Sargans (Switzerland).

Jolanta Wittib wrote in her commentary on Fr. Künzle's book:

I love birch trees. They are so beautiful with their white trunks and the shade they cast is light,

shivering of the leaves in the light breeze on a hot summer day. It is a very robust tree. A
pioneer tree - one of the first ones to start growing after avalanches, mud slides, volcano
eruptions. Birch is so generous and we are given so much from the birch: sap, buds, leaves. Sap is my favorite. Every second spring I am waiting for that moment, when I can drill a small hole into the body of my birch, insert a straw into it and then enjoy the sap - cold, slightly sweet. I take a few Liters from the tree during a period of 5-7 days and then I close the hole, so that the leaves have enough water and minerals.

My day's portion is about 50 Grams on an empty stomach as I want to get the most of it. The
rest I keep in the fridge. It would stay fresh for a day, but then it starts fermenting. I freeze the
rest - it will be for the next year, when I do not exploit my tree.

I use birch water for boosting my immune system, for more energy, which I sometimes lack in
spring. Birch water has many useful minerals. It is also used for the skin and hair. Every man in
German speaking countries would know birch water against hair loss and dandruff.

I collect birch buds round the same time, when I enjoy sap. The right time is when the tops of
the buds turn green. I cut a few twigs, dry them, brush off the buds, powder them in a coffee
grinder and store them in a jar. The powdered buds land on my salad, soup, on bread or are
added to my morning herbal infusion. I use the buds for strengthening my immune system, for
detoxification.

And then come the soft spring leaves. They are part of my salad, or I just eat a few leaves now
and then when I pass a birch tree.

Towards summer, I collect birch leaves - the young and healthy ones. These I dry for my detox
mixtures (they are mild diuretic) and for anti-inflammatory mixtures. And then I leave my birch
in peace, until next spring.

The Thomsonian System of Medicine states of Black Birch:

BLACK BIRCH BARK. Betula Lenta. (Dr. Thomson.)

*A tea made of this bark is useful in curing all complaints of the
bowels and to remove obstructions. It is also of use in dysentery.
This tea, with peach meats or cherry-stone meats, made into a
syrup, is an excellent article to restore patients after having been
reduced by that disease, and to promote the digestion. It is good for
canker and all complaints of the bowels.*
*The leaves can also be used as medicine and are more diuretic
and are very soothing to the entire urinary apparata in cases of
renal and cystic irritation or inflammation. The dose of the tincture is
from 15 to 45 minims. Can be taken in hot or cold water. In hot
water it acts the same as an infusion and is a diaphoretic.*

King's American Dispensatory, 1898 tells us of Birch:

*Action, Medical Uses, and Dosage.—Gently stimulant, diaphoretic,
and astringent. Used in warm infusion wherever a stimulating
diaphoretic is required; also in diarrhoea, dysentery, cholera
infantum, etc. In decoction or syrup it forms an excellent tonic to
restore the tone of the bowels, after an attack of dysentery. Said to
have been used in gravel and female obstructions. Oil of birch will
produce a drunken stupor, vomiting, and death. It has been used in
gonorrhoea, rheumatism, and chronic skin diseases. Dose, 5 to 10
drops.*

Native Plants, Native Healing states:

*The same chemical actions are found in white, black, sweet or river
birch trees. It has layers of bark that resemble the skin, but it is the
inner bark that is medicinal. It is best gathered in the wintertime,
when the sap is flowing and the bark is thicker. There is less
chance at this time of the bark having insect or fungal damage. As
with other barks, it is best gathered when the first days of 40
degrees F or higher weather makes the sap rise. This timing varies
according to droughts and is dependent on water levels and also
the phases of the moon. The bark comes off easier if there is a full
moon, or close to the full moon as the moon is coming up.*

*This signature of this plant is the skin like payers of the bark. This
shows that the tea made from the inner bark is good for skin*

problems. The oils found in birch bark are very similar to those found in human skin. This makes it very soothing to rough, itchy and sensitive skin, when made into a water-based wash. It is used externally to ease skin problems.

The birch water is used as a skin wash for any type of rash, dermatitis, insect bite or sting. It is also used as a wash for sunburn and hemorrhoids. It is good for cradle cap in children or dandruff and scaly scalp of any kind. It is also useful for dogs with mange or dry skin problems, and sebaceous adenitis symptoms of itching, and rough scaly skin, even resulting in hair loss. The water can be used… as an aftershave… It is used on elderly people who develop thing, paper-like skin. It is used once a month on invalids and the elderly as a preventative to keep the skin toned. It can be used for poison ivy and other itchy rashes.

The leaves and bark are made into a tea together. …This tea is used internally, in 1 cup doses as a mild calmative and diuretic. It is used to induce sleep and calm stress, and is very good during menses and for PMS. The tea is also taken to calm the lower back nerves during bouts of sciatica.

A mixture of sassafras, ginseng and birch is used for muscle regrowth, even where the muscle has been severed.

Plants for A Future lists Birch as:

Anti-inflammatory, cholagogue, diaphoretic. The bark is diuretic and laxative. An oil obtained from the inner bark is astringent and is used in the treatment of various skin afflictions, especially eczema and psoriasis. The bark is usually obtained from trees that have been felled for timber and can be distilled at any time of the year. The inner bark is bitter and astringent, it is used in treating intermittent fevers. The vernal sap is diuretic. The buds are balsamic. The young shoots and leaves secrete a resinous substance which has acid properties, when combined with alkalis it is a tonic laxative. The leaves are anticholesterolemic and diuretic. They also contain phytosides, which are effective germicides. An infusion of the leaves is used in the treatment of gout, dropsy and rheumatism, and is recommended as a reliable solvent of kidney stones. The young leaves and leaf buds are harvested in the spring and dried for later use. A decoction of the leaves and bark is used for bathing skin eruptions.

The Rodale Herb book states:

Beer is often made from the sap of sweet birch. A type of oil of wintergreen is distilled from the inner bark and twigs. It is also used for remedies to purify the blood, rheumatism and to expel worms. Applied externally, it is useful for boils and sores.

Rodale's Illustrated Encyclopedia of Herbs states:

Birch contains methyl salicylate, which has counter irritant and analgesic properties. Thus there may be some validity to the folk medicine use of birch to relieve the ache of rheumatism. Try making a tea from the leaves or a decoction of the bark and catkins to apply externally. The skin absorbs methyl salicylate. A poultice can also be used on skin irritations and minor wounds.

Amy Stewart writes of Birch in The Drunken Botanist:

Starting in the early 17th century, several scientists wrote of the use of birch sap in medicinal, or purely recreational, liquors. Flemish physician Johannes Baptista van Helmont wrote that birch sap could be collected in the spring and poured "into the Ale, after the greatest settlement of its boiling or working… He recommended this naturally fermented sap as a treatment for ailments of the kidneys, urinary tract and bowels.

Euell Gibbons gives us a recipe for Birch Beer in his classic work, Stalking The Wild Asparagus:

Measure 4 quarts of finely cut twigs of sweet birch into the bottom of a 5 gallon pot. In a large kettle stir in one gallon of honey into 4 gallons of birch sap and boil this mixture for 1o minutes, then pour over the chopped twigs. When cool, strain to remove the now expended twigs and return the liquid to the crock. Spread 1 cake of soft yeast on a slice of toasted rye bread and float this on top of the beer. Cover with a cloth and let it ferment until the cloudiness just starts to settle. This will usually take about a week, but it depends somewhat on the temperature. Bottle the beer and cap it tightly. Store in a dark place, and serve it cold before meals after the weather gets hot. It has a reputation for stimulating the appetite.

More than a glass or two at a time is likely to stimulate other things, for this beer has a kick like a mule.

Gibbons' Birch beer is a traditional and rustic recipe. You may wish to experiment with more modern brewing techniques such as specific yeasts and fermentation air locks to ensure the beer does not spoil. Traditional "soft drink" techniques can also be used to make a naturally fermented carbonated beverage that has only tiny amounts of alcohol. However, the higher alcohol, traditional Birch beer may be stronger medicinally. Either way, it is a very pleasant way to take your medicinal herbs and a fine reason to toast, "To your health!"

Sacred and Healing Herbal Beers tells us about Birch:

Methyl salicylate, the main active constituent of birch sap and the herb wintergreen, has the delicious and easily recognizable taste we call "wintergreen." Methyl salicylate is similar to aspirin. It is strongly analgesic and anti-inflammatory, being therefore of use in decoction for treating arthritic and rheumatic conditions.

Peterson Field Guides Eastern and Central Medicinal Plants tells us :

Black Birch: our most fragrant Birch was widely used by American Indians, inner bark tea for fevers, stomach aches, lung ailments, twig tea for fever. Essential oil methyl salicylate distilled from bark was used for rheumatism, gout, scrofula, bladder infection, neuralgia; anti-inflammatory, analgesic. To alleviate pain or sore muscles, the oil has been applied as a counter irritant. Essential oil was formerly produced in Appalachia, But now methyl salicylate is produced synthetically using menthol as the precursor. Warning: essential oil toxic. Easily absorbed through the skin period. Fatalities reported

Botany In a Day states:

A tea of the leaves or twigs can be used externally as an astringent wash, or internally for diarrhea or boils. A tea of the twigs is also somewhat anthelmintic. The birches also contained some amount of methyl salicylate oil (like willow and aspirin) making them both diaphoretic an analgesic. The bark and twigs are chopped, then simmered overnight and distilled; it is commonly substituted for Wintergreen oil. A strong tea of the bark or leaves can be used externally as a wash for Poison Ivy or acne, or internally as a mild sedative. A compound called betulinic acid, derived from the bark is being tested on some types of skin cancer.

The Physicians Desk Reference for Herbal Medicine tells us:

Affects of birch leaf: Birch leaves have a mild saluretic effect an are anti pyretic. In animal tests, they have shown to increase the amount of urine.

Unproven Uses: The leaves are used in flushing out therapy for bacterial an inflammatory disease of the urinary tract and for kidney gravel. They are also used in adjunct therapy for rheumatoid arthritis, for increasing amount of urine. In folk medicine the leaves are used as a blood purifier, and for gout and rheumatism. Externally the leaves are used for hair loss and dandruff. No health hazards or side effects are known in conjunction with proper administration of designated therapeutic dosages.

Broussonetia papyrifera, Paper-mulberry has been naturalized in my region. Plants for A Future states:

Medicinal use of Paper Mulberry: Astringent, diuretic, tonic, vulnerary. The leaf juice is diaphoretic and laxative - it is also used in the treatment of dysentery. It is also poulticed onto various skin disorders, bites etc. The stem bark is haemostatic. The fruit is diuretic, ophthalmic, stimulant, stomachic and tonic. The root is cooked with other foods as a galactogogue.

Carpinus, Hornbeam

Four Hornbeams have been used in herbal medicine: Carpinus betulus – Hornbeam, Carpinus caroliniana - American Hornbeam, Carpinus americana, Carpinus cordata Carpinus laxiflora

Only Carpinus caroliniana is native to my area.

Hornbeam is in the Birch family and the uses of these trees are similar. Native Americans were known to have used the bark as an astringent against diarrhea. The leaves may be used to stop bleeding and heal wounds. A Bach Flower Remedy utilizes Hornbeam for tiredness and exhaustion.

Virginia Ironwood, *Ostrya virginiana*, is closely related to the Hornbeams. It also grows in my region. Virginia Ironwood has more traditional use in herbal medicine, also likely finding its source in Native American practice. Its bark is astringent, but also analgesic – used for sore muscles, toothache, bruises and sprains. It is used as a blood tonic and for stopping bleeding and hemorrhage. Ironwood is also used for rheumatism and arthritis, as a soak.

Carya, Hickory

Eighteen varieties of Hickory may have medicinal use: Carya aquatica - Water Hickory, Carya buckleyi, Carya californica, Carya carolinae-septentrionalis - Southern Shagbark, Carya cathayensis - Chinese Hickory, Carya cordiformis – Bitternut, Carya floridana - Scrub Hickory, Carya glabra - Sweet Pignut, Carya glabra megacarpa - Coastal Pignut, Carya illinoinensis, Carya laciniosa - Shellbark Hickory, Carya myristiciformis - Nutmeg Hickory, Carya ovalis - Sweet Pignut, Carya ovata - Shagbark Hickory, Carya pallida - Sand Hickory, Carya texana - Black Hickory, Carya tomentosa – Mockernut, Carya x laneyi

Twelve Hickories are native to my region: Carya aquatica (Water Hickory), Carya carolinae-septentrionalis (Carolina Shagbark Hickory), Carya cordiformis (Bitternut Hickory), Carya glabra var. glabra (Pignut Hickory), Carya glabra var. hirsuta (Hairy Pignut Hickory), Carya glabra var. megacarpa (Coastal Pignut Hickory), Carya laciniosa (Shellbark Hickory), Carya myristiciformis (Nutmeg

Hickory) , Carya ovalis (Red Hickory, Sweet Pignut Hickory), Carya ovata (Shagbark Hickory), Carya pallida (Sand Hickory), Carya tomentosa (Mockernut Hickory)

Carya illinoinensis (Pecan) has been naturalized.

As you can see, Hickories are common and plentiful in North Carolina. Traditionally, their wood has been very valuable both for furniture making and for smoking pork barbecue – two things for which my home state is very well known. The nuts though, are also very tasty, if you have the patience to shell them. The common name, "Mockernut Hickory" is no joke! Hickory is related to Walnut and Pecan, but much closer to walnut in flavor. The Pecan, however, is out most widely grown nut. Pecans are rich, sweet, meaty and easy to shell.

The bark is astringent and good for treating wounds. It is likely, that like Walnut, the leaves may have some vermifuge or anti-parasitic properties. All members of the Juglandaceae family secrete juglone from the roots, a plant hormone that prevents most other plants from growing close enough to the tree to compete for resources such as sunlight, water and space. Traditionally, it is believed the juglones are useful in making the human body inhospitable to worms and other parasites in a similar fashion. Hickory smoke was also used in the curing of meats, to prevent infestation by insects. One thing I know for sure though, hickory smoke makes any meat taste fantastic when cooked low and slow!

Resources of the Southern Fields and Forests states:

The barks are astringent. Mr. Fred. Stearns, of Detroit, has called attention to the bark of the several species of Hickory, in his paper on the medicinal plants of Michigan, published in the Proc. Am. Pharm. Assoc, 1859, p. 249. Mr. Chaffinbury, of the same State, had found great advantage from chewing the inner bark in dyspepsia, and has used a tincture made from the same bark in intermittent fever. Many in the neighborhood used it, the infusion also being found equally effectual. U. S. Disp., 12th Ed.

Castanea, Chestnut

Four varieties of Chestnut that may be found in America are used in herbal medicine: Castanea species - Chestnut Hybrids, Castanea crenata - Japanese Chestnut, Castanea dentata - American Sweet Chestnut, Castanea mollissima - Chinese Chestnut

Native to my region are the Castanea dentata (American Chestnut), Castanea pumila (Chinkapin)

Castanea mollissima (Chinese Chestnut) has been naturalized

The Chinkapin likely has the same medicinal qualities of all other Chestnuts – I consider them interchangeable. It is simply smaller and less well known internationally.

Unfortunately, the American Chestnut, is rarely seen in our time. A blight nearly wiped them all out in the east, a century or so ago. According to legend among the Appalachian Mountain folks, the blight was not a mere coincidence. Chestnuts had been both enjoyed and used as a survival food in the mountains for centuries. As timber interests encroached, and rail cars could carry nut crops to market for profit, landowners became more protective of their Chestnut trees. The old-timers said that the blight was not due to contaminated imports, but from greed – it was a punishment for misusing a wild gift from God meant for all people. Regardless, the blight was devastating. Perhaps, our native Chestnut will adapt eventually. There are some signs that may be beginning to happen. However, we still have chinkapins, naturalized Asian Chestnuts and Asian/American hybrid Chestnuts.

If you grow them intentionally, or look around for wild chinkapins, you can still enjoy Chestnuts. A couple of years ago, I spotted an old homestead on a large acreage in South Carolina. The price was low enough to demand I drive down to take a look. I found a beautiful old, early American farmhouse in the center of 200 acres of cotton fields. Unfortunately, I have a strong toxic reaction to cotton poison, so that ruled the property out for me. But, I still took some time to enjoy exploring the centuries old landscaping – Rose of Sharron bushes, Magnolias, Pecans, Camelias, Daffodils and Irises, Roses, yuccas, Crabapples, Pears... and several Chinkapins. My mother and my dog stayed in the car while I explored. Suddenly, my mother called me over and said, "We have to go!". I was enjoying the flowers and warm spring sunshine... I felt very peaceful and welcome, and was wishing the property would work out in spite of the agricultural chemicals. So, I asked her why. "This place is haunted! I can hear two elderly sisters at the upstairs window, talking... excited to have guests for dinner!"

Well, my mother is a practical, not at all superstitious lady with advanced degrees and retired from a career in clinical Psychology. I was shocked. She was adamant we leave though, and my dog was acting creeped out, too! I'm pretty practical, as well... I often say that I may be the only herbalist who doesn't see fairies or have two-way conversations with plants! But, I did feel very welcome there, as if I was someone's guest in a bygone era, when hospitality was far more valued than it is now. "Well," I answered as we drove away, "I don't doubt you at all. It's a shame though, because those ladies must have been great gardeners to still have such beautiful grounds, especially since no one has lived in that house for over 70 years. I guess they must be still taking care of it. It could be, we'd have gotten along just fine!"

Back to herbs though...

Aside from being a very nutritious and starchy nut, more like a potato than a nut in flavor and texture, and a beautiful wood for paneling, cabinets and furniture, the Chestnut does have medicinal value. The American Chestnut was used to soothe the lungs and as both an expectorant and astringent. This was taken as a tea made from the leaves. The Chinese Chestnut has been used to settle the stomach and to treat diarrhea. Culpepper mentioned the astringency of Chestnut, and its use against bleeding. Mrs. Grieves wrote of its folk use in treating fevers and spasmodic coughs. Long before that, Dioscorides also praised the astringency of Chestnut.

An Irish Herbal states of Chestnuts:

... They are good for chest problems and for arresting the bowels. A paste made from them is good against coughing or spitting of blood.

Fr. Johannes Künzle wrote of Chestnut:

Higher up there was a tall, old chestnut tree with fruits covered in prickly pods. The laplander was beside himself from surprise when the Dane opened the shell and showed him the fruit. "This tree

56

provides food for millions of people because these fruits are extremely nutritious." "But why are these spikes all around?" Without this protection birds and squirrels and insects would eat everything up; the almighty Creator added this protective skin; when the fruit is ripe, it falls to the ground, the protective cover pops up and we can collect it. In the south they have even much taller trees; near the fire-spitting mountain Etna there is a chestnut tree under which 200 riders and their horses have enough space.

Jolanta Wittib Writes:

The southern part of Tirol is proud of sweet chestnut (Castanea sativa). They have beautiful, delicious seeds which one can use in so many ways. Every autumn there is a kind of a gourmet festival called Törggelen: you drink wine and eat roasted sweet chestnuts together with other specialties of the region like ham and cheese and bacon....Many people come just for that. It is very popular. And roasted chestnuts are so delicious.

Resources of the Southern Fields and Forests states:

CHESTNUT, (Castanea vesca, L.) Fairfield District, Florida and northward. In South Carolina only found in upper districts; one of our noblest trees.

The fruit of this tree and the chinquapin (C. ptimila') are well known. Eaten either raw or boiled. The roots contain an astringent principle; that of the chinquapin boiled in milk is much used in the diarrhoea of teething children. I would advise a tea made of this to be used extemporaneously in diarrhoea by soldiers in camp. The late Dr. Nelson Burgess, of Sumter District, S. C, informed me that at the recommendation of Dr. Jones, he has used the decoction of the root and bark of the chinquapin frequently as a substitute for quinine in intermittent and remittent fever, and with decidedly satisfactory results. I mention this hoping that it will be examined by others. I can have no clue to the reasons of its utility, regarding it heretofore simply as an astringent. Hot water is poured over the root and bark, and a large quantity taken during the twenty four hours. Dr. J. S. Unzicker, of Cincinnati, reports the use of a decoction of the leaves of the chestnut in hooping cough. He says that he has given it in about thirty cases, in all of which it gave decided relief in two weeks. He uses a decoction made with three to four drachms of the leaves in a pint of water given ad libitum. Caulophyllin, in doses of one-fourth to four grains, has also been much used recently in this disease and in asthma. Boston Med. and vSurg. J., Jan., 1868. See, also. Bates in Tilden's J. Mat. Med. Sept., 1868, article containing a history of the Blue Cohosh, (Caulophyllum.).

King's American Dispensatory, 1898 tells us of ChestnutL

Action, Medical Uses, and Dosage.—Chestnut leaves appear to have been brought into notice, as a therapeutical agent, by Mr. G. C. Close, in a statement before the American Pharmaceutical Association, in 1862. Subsequently, they were employed by the late Dr. J. S. Unzicker, of Cincinnati, who valued them highly in the treatment of whooping-cough; since which, most favorable reports have been made by other physicians, as to their value. These leaves have, thus far, been employed mainly in the treatment of pertussis, in which malady they have proved remarkably efficient; but their manner of action has not yet been determined. It is very probable that they may be found useful in other irritable or excitable conditions of the respiratory nerves. Dr. Unzicker employed an infusion of the leaves, an ounce to a pint of boiling water, and administered this in tablespoonful, or small wineglassful doses, repeated several times a day. The fluid extract, when properly made, will be found reliable; its dose is from ½ to 1 fluid drachm, repeated 3, 4, or 5 times daily. Chestnut bark appears to possess astringent and tonic properties, and is used in some sections of our country as a popular remedy for fever and ague. Other forms of paroxysmal or convulsive cough resembling pertussis have been cured with it. Prof. Scudder (Spec. Med., p. 103), suggests a trial of the remedy in cases exhibiting unsteadiness of gait and a disposition to turn to one side.

Catalpa

Two varieties of Catalpa have been naturalized in my region, Catalpa bignonioides (Southern Catalpa) and Catalpa speciosa (Northern Catalpa).

King's American Dispensatory, 1898 tells us of Catalpa:

Action, Medical Uses, and Dosage.—It is stated that poisonous emanations issue from this tree, but we have no knowledge of any serious effects resulting from an exposure thereto. The pods and seeds have been employed in decoction in chronic bronchial affections, spasmodic asthma, and dyspnoea, and certain forms of functional heart disease; 6 or 8 ounces to a pint of water, and given in tablespoonful doses, repeated every 1 or 2 hours. The leaves, bruised, and applied as a cataplasm, have been used in irritable scrofulous ulcers; they appear to possess anodyne properties. The bark has been employed internally, in powder, or in decoction, in scrofulous maladies, and as an anthelmintic. The juice of the leaves, as well as of the root, has been beneficially employed as a local application in the several forms of strumous ophthalmia, as well as in certain cutaneous affections. From the statements that have been made as to the toxic properties of this tree, and which have not yet been satisfactorily demonstrated, it would be advisable to use some prudence and care in the internal administration of any of its preparations. Dose of specific catalpa, fraction of a drop to 20 drops.

Plants for A Future states:

Medicinal use of Indian Bean Tree: A tea made from the bark has been used as an antiseptic, antidote to snake bites, laxative, sedative and vermifuge. As well as having a sedative effect, the plant also has a mild narcotic action, though it never causes a dazed condition. It has therefore been used with advantage in preparations with other herbs for the treatment of whooping cough in children, it is also used to treat asthma and spasmodic coughs in children. The bark has been used as a substitute for quinine in treating malaria. The leaves are used as a poultice on wounds and abrasions. A tea made from the seeds is used in the treatment of asthma and bronchitis and is applied externally to wounds. The pods are sedative and are thought to have cardioactive properties. Distilled water made from the pods, mixed with eyebright (Euphrasia officinalis) and rue (Ruta graveolens) is a valuable eye lotion in the treatment of trachoma and conjunctivitis.

Peterson Field Guides Eastern and Central Medicinal Plants tells us:

Common catalpa: bark tea formally used as antiseptic, snakebite antidote, laxative, sedative, worm expellant. Leaves poulticed on wounds, abrasions. Seed tea used for asthma, bronchitis; externally, for wounds. Pods sedative, thought to possess cardioactive properties.

Celtis, Hackberry

Seventeen varieties of Hackberry are used in herbal medicine: Celtis australis - Nettle Tree, Celtis boninensis, Celtis bungeana, Celtis caucasica, Celtis glycycarpa, Celtis jessoensis, Celtis koraiensis, Celtis laevigata – Sugarberry, Celtis laveillei, Celtis lindheimeri - Palo Blanco, Celtis occidentalis – Hackberry, Celtis pallida - Desert Hackberry, Celtis reticulata – Paloblanco, Celtis sinensis, Celtis tenuifolia - Small Hackberry, Celtis tetrandra, Celtis tournefortii

Only three varieties are native to my area: Celtis laevigata var. laevigata (Sugarberry), Celtis occidentalis var. occidentalis (Common Hackberry), Celtis tenuifolia (Dwarf Hackberry)

Naturalized is Celtis sinensis (Chinese Hackberry)

According to Plants for A Future, "An extract obtained from the wood has been used in the treatment of jaundice. A decoction of the bark has been used in the treatment of sore throats. When combined with powdered shells it has been used to treat VD." Unfortunately, they do not inform us which venereal disease may be treated with Hackberry.

It seems that Hackberry was much utilized by Native American tribes as an antioxidant rich food. American folk use seems to stem from that tradition. As of yet though, I have found very little recorded information its historic use. It seems we have some tasty experimentation to undertake in future!

Cercis Canadensis, Redbud

This is another tree with little recorded herbal use, but it is an extremely valuable part of the landscape. It is a beautiful ornamental, an edible, a nitrogen fixing fertilizer and medicinal. Redbud is usually the first flowering tree to appear in the spring, often a month before the similarly sized Dogwood. Its bright, magenta flowers stand out in stark contrast to both the barren landscape and its own dark trunk. Unlike most other trees and bushes, the flowers are not only born on the ends of twigs and stems, but clusters of flowers appear all over the limbs and even the trunk of the tree!

The flowers are a nutritious edible, tasting much like garden peas. In earlier times, this part of spring was known as "the hunger season." It was the time when the winter store of food was dwindling, if not exhausted, but the garden was not yet producing. Who knows how many lives the Redbud may have saved? Who knows how many cases of vitamin deficiency it may have prevented? The deer certainly know this, as they will walk upright, on their hind legs, eating as many of the lower flowers as they can reach!

Redbud is one of the few trees in the legume family, as evidenced by the bean like pods that hang dry on its branches all winter. Legumes have a remarkably important characteristic – they take nitrogen from the air and "fix" it in the soil. The tens of thousands of members of the legume family – beans, peas, peanuts, locust and mimosa trees, wisteria, kudzu, etc., are not only "self fertile" in terms of providing their own nutrition, but provide nitrogen for all manner of plant growth. Having Redbuds in your landscape will help fertilize your property, saving you money and effort and giving you food, herbs and flowers. They are trees that require little to no maintenance. If ever there was a "giving tree", Redbud is one!

Medicinally, the bark is astringent with the inner bark said to be most potent. A tea made from the bark is used for fevers and diarrhea. It has also been used in folk medicine for coughs and congestion.

Beyond that, the bees LOVE it! Legend states that Redbud was the tree on which Judas hanged himself after betraying Christ. I doubt that very much though, as it is not a large tree and the limbs are not very strong. A folk name though is still, "Judas Tree."

Resources of the Southern Fields and Forests states:

REDBUD; JUDAS TEEE, {Cercis canadensis, Ij.) Swamps vicinity of Charleston ; collected in St. John's; N. C. Fl. March. Shec, Flora Carol. 380. " The wood is of great value for mechanical purposes, as it polishes exceedingly well, and is admirably veined with black and green." Mills, in his Statistics of S. C, states that the blossoms are used as a salad. Pithecolobium ungiiis-cati, Benth. Inga U7iquis-cati, Willd. S. Fla. Chap. Said to be a good remedy in urinary complaints and obstruction of the liver and spleen; a decoction of the bark is very astringent. Macfadyen.

Peterson Field Guides Eastern and Central Medicinal Plants tells us:

Inner bark tea highly astringent. An obscure medicinal agent once used for diarrhea and dysentery; also as a folk cancer remedy for leukemia. Flowers edible.

Chamaecyparis thyoides, Atlantic Whitecedar

We only have one variety of Chamaecyparis in my region. It grows down in the coastal swamps and up into the sandhills. It is not a common tree, but it was one with which I became familiar in Bladen County, NC, where my grandparents, great grandparents (etc) lived and farmed. Interestingly, "Whitecedar" is not really a cedar; it is a cypress. Although it was very likely used medicinally by Native American tribes in the area, I have not found any documentation.

Chamaecyparis has been used medicinally in other regions. Plants for A Future lists Chamaecyparis thyoides, or White Cypress as, "A decoction of the leaves has been used as a herbal steam for treating headaches and backaches. A poultice made from the crushed leaves and bark has been applied to the head to treat headaches." It also states that a decoction of the sap from the Lawson Cypress is a powerful diuretic. Of the Nootka Cypress: *The plant has been used in sweat baths for treating rheumatism and arthritis. An infusion of the branch tips has been used as a wash for sores and swellings. A poultice of the crushed leaves has been applied to sores. The soft bark has been used as a cover for poultices.*

Chionanthus virginicus, Fringetree, Old Man's Beard

Fringetree is another of our unique trees. It is native to my region and very pretty. The medicinal use of this one, fortunately, has been documented.

Mrs. Grieves lists its use as, "Aperient, diuretic. Some authorities regard it as tonic and slightly narcotic. It is used in typhoid, intermittent, or bilious fevers, and externally, as a poultice, for inflammations or wounds. Is useful in liver complaints."

King's American Dispensatory, 1898 tells us of Fringe Tree:

Action, Medical Uses, and Dosage.—Chionanthus acts principally upon the abdominal glandular organs, and to some extent upon the venous system, relieving congestion. It is an alterative in the Eclectic meaning of that term. While its main action is upon the visceral glands, especially the blood-making organs, its influence is also quite marked in other secretive structures. Besides its pronounced catalytic properties, it is diuretic, tonic, and is said to be aperient and narcotic. It is exceedingly doubtful if the latter statement be true and its aperient property, if it possesses such, is the result of its cholagogue action.

Prof. King, in former editions of the American Dispensatory, states that in bilious and typhoid fevers, as well as in obstinate intermittents, the infusion of the bark of the root is efficient. While the remedy is now but very little used for these conditions, still some "old school" authors, as well as some trade catalogues, seem to have appropriated the above statements in regard to its use. Prof. King further states that it is an excellent tonic in "convalescence from exhaustive diseases," and that it also proves a good local application in external inflammations, ulcers and wounds. The use of an infusion of the bark of the root is directed, still it is doubtful whether such a preparation would be as efficient as an alcoholic form, for the resin, or the resinoid, the active constituent of the drug, is insoluble in water. Goss states that the infusion is wholly inert. Chionanthus improves the appetite, aids digestion, promotes assimilation, and is a tonic to the whole system. It never produces catharsis, but ptyalism has resulted from its use.

Chionanthus has been successfully used in mercurial cachexia, scrofula, and syphilis, though we possess better agents for these classes of disease. Yet, if the patient be sallow, or yellow, and has hepatic pains, the remedy will prove a valuable accessory agent in hastening the cure.

It is for its prompt and efficient action in hepatic derangements that we most value fringe-tree preparations. If there is any one thing true in specific medicine, it is that chionanthus has a decidedly specific action in jaundice. The credit of having brought this remedy before the profession, for the purposes for which it is now used, belongs to the late Prof. I. J. M. Goss, of Georgia, who, in 1843, tested it on himself while suffering from an attack of jaundice, and reported the result in an eastern journal. Since then it has come to be the first remedy thought of for this complaint. Goss considered it the best remedy for all cases of jaundice, not dependent on gall stones. On the contrary, Prof. Scudder was high in his praise of it, even when calculi are present. He recommended it in 10 or 15-drop doses during the paroxysm, and also gave it to prevent a recurrence. Nux or dioscorea may be associated with it when called for, the former in atonic conditions, with broad, expressionless tongue, the latter in irritative states, the tongue being red, pointed, and elongated, with prominent papillae. Hypertrophy of the liver, chronic hepatic inflammation, and portal congestion are speedily relieved by chionanthus. The remedy acts quickly, often removing in from 1 to 2 weeks, an icteric hue that has existed for months, and even years. Jaundice once cured by it is not apt to recur. There are two direct indications for the drug—jaundice, as evidenced by the yellowness of skin and conjunctiva; and soreness and pain, "hepatic colic," as pointed out by Prof. Scudder. The latter is by far the most direct indication. There is the dull, heavy pain in right hypochondrium, with a feeling of fullness and weight, deep-seated tenderness ad soreness on pressure, occasional hectic flushes, light colored feces, sometimes diarrhoea with frothy, yeasty stools, and urine scanty and high colored.

These conditions, with the icteric hue of skin and conjunctiva, call for chionanthus. Sometimes the patient writhes in pain, can not find rest in any position. Rx Specific chionanthus, gtt. x, every half hour, and apply a cloth wrung out of hot water. In dyspepsia, with hepatic complications; in irritative states of the stomach from "high living," and the use of alcoholic stimulants; and in general chronic inflammatory conditions of the duodenum, and ductus communis choledochus, chionanthus serves a useful purpose. It is also a good remedy in infantile dyspepsia. Rheumatic affections, with soreness in the region of the liver, and a jaundiced condition, are ameliorated by this drug. Its tonic effects on the chylopoietic viscera render it a good agent in general debility. In intestinal dyspepsia, with jaundice, thin, watery, yeasty alvine discharges, with previous abdominal distension: Rx Specific chionanthus, gtt. v, every 2 hours.

Chronic splenitis and nephritis are conditions in which fringe-tree often proves a good remedy; also in pancreatic disease, inflammatory or otherwise. Glandular diseases, with evidence of imperfect waste, often call for its administration. Chionanthus is of utility in uterine and ovarian congestion, when the usual hepatic symptoms calling for it are present. If there be fullness and bearing down in the pelvic viscera, especially a desire to frequently evacuate the rectum, combine it with specific helonias. Rx Specific chionanthus, specific helonias, aa flʒi; aqua q. s., ʒiv. Mix. Sig. Teaspoonful every 2 hours.

In female disorders it may also be combined with gelsemium, macrotys, or pulsatilla, when indications for these drugs are present. Some cases of uterine leucorrhoea are promptly benefited by it. Cleansing injections should be employed at the same time. As a poultice it will be found an excellent local application in external inflammations, ulcers, and wounds.

Dose, from ½ fluid ounce of the infusion to 2 fluid ounces, repeated several times a day, according to its influence upon the system.

The usual dose of specific chionanthus (the best preparation), is 10 drops in water every 3 hours. Chionanthin, the so-called concentration, is of little value and is but seldom used. It was first prepared by Prof. Goss.

Specific Indications and Uses.—Dirty, sallow skin, with expressionless eyes and hepatic tenderness; an icteric hue, with or without pain; hepatic colic; intense pain from liver to umbilicus, attended with nausea and vomiting and great prostration; pain in epigastrium and right hypochondrium, simulating colic, sometimes extending to the abdomen; jaundice, with itching skin and thin, light-colored, watery stools; tympanites; colic, with green alvine discharges; urine stains the clothing yellow.

Plants for A Future states:

The fringe tree was commonly used by the North American Indians and European settlers alike to treat inflammations of the eye, mouth ulcers and spongy gums. In modern herbalism it is considered to be one of the most reliable remedies for disorders of the liver and gall bladder. The dried root bark is alterative, aperient, cholagogue, diuretic, febrifuge and tonic. It is used in the treatment of gallbladder pain, gallstones, jaundice and chronic weakness. A tincture of the bark was once widely used internally in the treatment of hypertrophy of the liver, jaundice, bilious headache, gallstones, rheumatism etc. The root bark also appears to strengthen function in the pancreas and spleen whilst anecdotal evidence indicates that it may substantially reduce sugar levels in the urine. Fringe tree also stimulates the appetite and digestion and is an excellent remedy for chronic illness, especially where the liver has been affected. A tea or a poultice can be made from the root bark for external use as a wash for wounds, inflammations, sores, infections etc. The roots can be harvested at any time of the year, the bark is peeled from them and is then dried for later use.

Peterson Field Guides Eastern and Central Medicinal Plants tells us:

Physicians formally used 10 drops every three hours of tincture for jaundice. The tincture was one part bark by weight in five parts 50% grain alcohol and water. In the late 19th century Fringe tree bark tincture was widely employed by physicians who thought it relieve congestion of glandular organs and the venous system. It was employed for hypertrophy of the liver, wounds, nephritis, and rheumatism. Once considered diuretic, alternative, cholagogue, and tonic. American Indians use the root bark tea to wash inflammations, sores, cuts, and infections. Warning: overdose causes vomiting, frontal headaches, slow poults, etc

The Physicians' Desk Reference for Herbal Medicine tells us:

Fringe tree, because of its saponin content, is said to have hepatic, cholagogue, diuretic and tonic effects. Unproven uses: French tree is used in the treatment of the liver and gallbladder conditions (including gallstones). North American folk uses include jaundice, hepatatrophy, wounds, and ulcers. No health hazards or side effects are known in conjunction with the proper administration of designated therapeutic doses.

Cladrastis kentukea, Yellowwood

As attractive as Fringetree is, it meets its match in Yellowwood. Unique to my region, this tree blooms with long trails of cascading flowers. I can find no documented medicinal use of this tree. It is in the legume family though and would be a beautiful addition to any landscape.

Clerodendrum trichotomum

Clerodendrum is another tree that has been naturalized in my region. Common names include Harlequin Glorybower and Chou Wu Tong.

Plants for A Future states:

Medicinal use of Chou Wu Tong: The leaves are mildly analgesic, antipruritic, hypotensive and sedative. They are used externally in

the treatment of dermatitis and internally for the treatment of hypertension, rheumatoid arthritis, joint pain, numbness and paralysis. When used in a clinical trial of 171 people, the blood pressure of 81% of the people dropped significantly - this effect was reversed when the treatment was stopped. The plant is normally used in conjunction with Bidens bipinnata. When used with the herb Siegesbeckia pubescens it is anti-inflammatory. The roots and leaves are antirheumatic and hypotensive. A decoction is used in the treatment of rheumatoid arthritis and hypertension. The pounded seed is used to kill lice.

Cornus, Dogwood

Twenty-eight Dogwoods are used medicinally: Cornus alternifolia - Green Osier, Cornus amomum - Silky Dogwood, Cornus asperifolia drummondii - Roughleaf Dogwood, Cornus australis, Cornus canadensis - Creeping Dogwood, Cornus capitata - Bentham's Cornel, Cornus controversa - Giant Dogwood, Cornus coreana, Cornus florida - Flowering Dogwood, Cornus hongkongensis, Cornus chinensis, Cornus iberica, Cornus kousa - Japanese Dogwood, Cornus kousa chinensis - Japanese Dogwood, Cornus macrophylla - Large-Leaf Dogwood, Cornus mas - Cornelian Cherry, Cornus monbeigii, Cornus nuttallii - Mountain Dogwood, Cornus occidentalis - Western Dogwood, Cornus officinalis - Shan Zhu Yu, Cornus poliophylla, Cornus quinquenervis, Cornus rugosa - Round-Leaved Dogwood, Cornus sanguinea, Cornus sericea - Red Osier Dogwood, Cornus sessilis, Cornus suecica - Dwarf Cornel, Cornus x unalaschkensis – Bunchberry

Only three dogwood varieties are native to my region, though many have been introduced: Cornus alternifolia (Alternate-leaved Dogwood, Pagoda Dogwood), Cornus asperifolia (Roughleaf Dogwood), Cornus florida (Flowering Dogwood)

The dogwoods were once widely more used in herbal medicine (especially by Native Americans). All are nice landscaping tees. Its main herbal value is as an astringent. A decoction of the bark is useful for mouth sores, sore throats, diarrhea and skin inflammations. It is good for swellings and blisters. It has also been used for colds and to lower fevers. A poultice of the leaves is good for wounds, being anesthetic and analgesic. Adding dogwood leaves and bark to a bath is good for sore joints and muscles.

Of special interest is the Cornelian Cherry. Cornelian Cherry or Cornus monbeigii produces a tasty fruit. The fruit is somewhat sour. It can be made into jam or used in pies like sour cherry. It is also said to be a good substitute for cranberry as a sauce to compliment meats. The herbalist and plant collector, Gerard, said it was to be found in the gardens "of such as love rare and dainty plants". In recent years, Cornelian Cherry has become popular with Permaculture and other folks who are interested in edible landscapes.

Brother Aloysius wrote of Cornelian Cherry:

The bark and fruit are used medicinally. The bark is astringent and febrifugal; the fruit is astringent and desiccant. Application of fresh, bruised leaves stanches bleeding. The fruit decoction is used for feverish burning and dysentery; it also stimulates appetite.

Resources of the Southern Fields and Forests states:

Dogwood {Cormis Florida').—During the late war, the bark has been employed with great advantage in place of quinine in fevers— particularly in cases of low forms of fever, and in dysentery, on the river courses, of a typhoid character. It is given as a substitute for Peruvian barks. In fact, in almost any case where the Cinchona bark was used.

This well known plant possesses tonic and anti-intermittent properties, very nearly allied to those of cinchona; in periodic fevers, one of the most valuable of our indigenous plants. "Dr. Gregg states that, after employing it for twenty-three years in the treatment of intermittent fevers, he was satisfied that it was not inferior to Peruvian bark.'" Generally given in con- junction with laudanum. It also possesses antiseptic powers. In the recent state, it is leas stimulating than the cinchona bark, but it affects the bowels more; the dried bark is the preferable form. The fresh bark will sometimes act as a cathartic. It is more stimulating than thoroughwort (Eupatorium,) and, therefore, is less applicable during the hot stages of fever. According to Dr. Walker's examination, the bark contains extractive matter, gum, resin, tannin and gallic acid;

and Dr. Carpenter announces in it a new principal, cornine. Dr. Jackson also, from experiment, is satisfied that it contains a principle analogous to quinia. It has been exhibited by Dr. S. G. Morton in intermittent fever, with success. Griffith, in his Med. Bot. 347, mentions that the infusion of the flowers is useful as a substitute for chamomile tea; for analysis, see Am. Journ. Pharm. i, 114; and Phil. Journal Med. and Phys. Sci. xl. Dose of the dried bark in powder, is twenty to sixty grains; the decoction is made with one ounce of the root to one pint of water, or the extract may be employed ; alcohol also extracts its virtues. The ripe fruit, infused in brandy, makes an agreeable and useful bitter, which may be a convenient substitute for the article prepared in the shops. Dr. D. C. O'Keeffe, of Georgia, published an article on the C. Florida in the So. Med. and Surg. Journal, January, 1849. He gave the extract in doses of ten grains to two drachms, without its producing any disturbance of the stomach, as alleged by some writers. Barton says, in his Collections, that the bark is valuable in a malignant disorder of horses called yellow water. From the gallic acid it contains, a good writing ink may be made, and from the bark of the fibrous roots the Indians extracted a scarlet color. Lindley mentions that the young branches, stripped of their bark;" and rubbed against the teeth, render them extremely white. It is often employed for this purpose by persons living in the country. Where there is need of astringent anti-periodics and tonics, the dogwood bark powdered will be found the best substitute for the Peruvian. Internally and externally, it can be applied in wherever the cinchona barks were found serviceable. The dogwood bark and root, in decoction, or in form of cold infusion, is believed by many to be the most efficient substitute for quinine, also in treating malarial fevers; certainly, it might be used in the cases occurring in camp, to prevent the waste of quinine, as it can be easily and abundantly procured. Dr. Richard Moore, of Sumter County, informs me that he not only finds it efficient in fevers, but particularly useful, with whiskey or alcohol, in low forms of fevers, and dysentery occurring near our river swamps. During convalescence also, where an astringent tonic is re- quired, this plant meets our requirements. See Enpatorium (boneset) and Liriodendron (Poplar.) These, with the black- berry and chinquapin as astringents, the gentians and pipsissewa as tonics and tonic diuretics, the sweet gum, sassafras, and bene for their mucilaginous and aromatic properties, and the wild jalap (Podophyllum) as a cathartic, supply the surgeon in camp -during a blockade with easily procurable medicinal plants, which are sufficient for almost every purpose. Nitrate and bi-carbonate of potash are most wanted, and with calomel may be procured from abroad. Our supply of opium can be easily reached by planting the poppy, and incising the capsules. Every planter could raise a full supply of opium, mustard and flaxseed. A tonic compound, as advised by the herbalists, is made with the bark of the root of dogwood, Colombo (Frasera,) poplar, each six ounces; bark of Avild cherry, six ounces ; leaves of thoroughwort, four ounces; cayenne popper, four ounces— sifted and mixed. Dose, a teaspoonful, in warm or cold water, repeated. The berries of the dogwood have also been highly recommended—given as a remedy for fever in place of quinine (1862.)

RED WILLOW; SWAMP DOGWOOD, (Cornus sericea, Ph.) Elliott says it grows in the mountains of South Carolina; sent to me from Abbeville District, by Mr. Reed ; North Carolina. Fl. June. Griffith, Med. Bot. 349. It possesses properties quite similar to those of the C. Florida, but it is more bitter and astringent. Mr. E. informs me that it is employed to a great extent in domestic practice in Abbeville. According to B. S. Barton, the bark was considered by the Indians a favorite combination with tobacco for smoking. The young shoots were used to make coarse baskets; and they extracted a scarlet dye from these and the roots.

BLOOD RED DOGWOOD, (Cornus sanguinea, Jj.) Grows, according to Elliott, in the valleys among the mountains. Fl. May. Diet, de Med. de Ferus. ii, 737; Mathiole, Comment, ii, 119;

Journal de Chim. xxxviii, 174, and xl, 107. See, also, Journal de Pharm. for an account of the oil extracted from it. M. Murion says they afford one-third of their weight of a pure and limpid oil, used for the table and for burning. A case of hydrophobia was said to have been cured by it. Griffith, Med. Bot. 349. There also exists in this, as in the others, a red coloring principle, soluble in water alone. Gornus stricta. Growls in swamps near Charleston; Newbern. Shec. Flora Carol. 44. C. Circinata is not included by Chap- man among the Southern species, though Dr. Wood says that it grows in Virginia. See U. S. Disp.

King's American Dispensatory, 1898 tells us:

Action, Medical Uses, and Dosage.—Dogwood bark is tonic, astringent, and slightly stimulant. It forms an excellent substitute for

Peruvian bark, having frequently proved efficient in periodic attacks when the foreign drug failed. It may be used in many cases where quinine is indicated and can not be administered, owing to idiosyncrasy, etc. It may be used with advantage in cases where tonics are required, in periodical fevers, typhoid fevers, etc. Its internal employment increases the strength and frequency of the pulse, and elevates the temperature of the body. It should be used in the dried state, as the recent bark is apt to derange the stomach, and cause more or less pain in the abdomen, but which may be removed by 10 or 15 drops of laudanum. It is useful in headaches from quinine, in general exhaustion and pyrosis. An extract of the bark prepared by boiling it in water, and evaporating to the proper consistence, will be found one of the best forms in which to administer it. Dose of the powdered bark, from 20 to 60 grains, as often as required; of the extract, from 5 to 10 grains. The ripe berries formed into a tincture with brandy or whiskey, are a popular bitters among some country people; the flowers are occasionally used in the place of chamomile. Specific cornus, 1 to 20 drops.

Specific Indications and Uses.—"Tonic and antiperiodic; intermittent or miasmatic fevers; headache from quinine; general exhaustion" (Scudder); feeble, relaxed tissues; pulse feeble and temperature subnormal; quinism.

The Rodale Herb Book states:

The Indians were the first to use this American native for healing, and the white settlers were quick to add it to their folk medicine. Although the bark was the principal part used, the flowers, leaves and fruit have also been used. The Delawares, Alabamas and Houmas of Louisiana all used the inner bark to make a febrifuge tea. "It is good in low continued forms of fever, where the patient is greatly exhausted,: reported one nineteenth-century Indian folk. Herbal.

During the Civil War, dogwood was one of several native plants which provided a substitute for quinine, which was obtained from the bark of the chinchona tree, a Peruvian native, when the South was cut off from outside supply sources."

Botany In a Day states:

The Dogwood contains varying amounts of cornic acid an the alkaloid cornine, mostly in the bark and or the inner bark. It has a mildly narcotic and analgesic effect, especially helpful for individuals who have negative reactions to Southside lights like Willow or aspirin. The bark is also quite astringent, which further helps draw down inflamed tissue.

The Physicians Desk Reference for Herbal Medicine tells us:

Cardiac effect: heart activity, at different levels up to the cessation of heartbeat, is examined depending on the concentration of the menthol extract. Antispasmodic effect: induced malaria in chicks in Peking ducks was treated for five days with the water insoluble fraction. As a result, antiplasmodic activity toward P cathemerium could be observed, similar to that deployed by quinine and sulfadiazine. To date, the results cannot be sufficiently assessed. The bark works as a tonic, an astringent and a stimulant. Unproven uses: in North America, the dried bark was used in folk medicine for strength, to stimulate appetite, for fever, and chronic diarrhea. It is used externally as an astringent for wounds and boils. Formally, it was used as a replacement for quinine. It is still used for headaches and fatigue. Health risks or side effects: following the proper administration of designated therapeutic dosages are not recorded.

Crataegus, Hawthorn

…. This is a big one!

There are seventy-eight varieties of Hawthorn used in herbal medicine: Crataegus acclivis, Crataegus aestivalis - Eastern Mayhaw, Crataegus altaica - Altai Mountain Thorn, Crataegus anomala, Crataegus apiifolia - Parsley-Leaved Hawthorn, Crataegus aprica, Crataegus armena, Crataegus arnoldiana, Crataegus atrosanguinea, Crataegus azarolus – Azarole, Crataegus baroussana, Crataegus caesa, Crataegus calpodendron – Pear Hawthorn, Crataegus canadensis, Crataegus canbyi, Crataegus coccinoides - Kansas Hawthorn, Crataegus columbiana - Columbian Hawthorn, Crataegus crus-galli - Cockspur Thorn, Crataegus cuneata – Sanzashi, Crataegus dilatate, Crataegus dispessa, Crataegus douglasii - Black Hawthorn, Crataegus durobrivensis, Crataegus ellwangeriana, Crataegus elongate, Crataegus festiva, Crataegus flabellate, Crataegus flava - Summer Haw, Crataegus gemosa, Crataegus heterophylla, Crataegus holmesiana, Crataegus hupehensis, Crataegus champlainensis, Crataegus chlorosarca, Crataegus chrysocarpa - Fireberry Hawthorn, Crataegus illinoiensis, Crataegus intricate, Crataegus jackii, Crataegus jonesiae, Crataegus laciniata, Crataegus laevigata - Midland Hawthorn, Crataegus lobulata - Red Haw, Crataegus macrosperma - Big-Fruit Hawthorn, Crataegus maximowiczii, Crataegus meyeri, Crataegus missouriensis, Crataegus monogyna, Crataegus nigra - Hungarian Hawthorn, Crataegus opaca - Western Mayhaw, Crataegus parvifolia, Crataegus pedicellata - Scarlet Haw, Crataegus pedicellata gloriosa - Scarlet Haw, Crataegus pensylvanica, Crataegus phaenopyrum - Washington Thorn, Crataegus pinnatifida - Chinese Haw, Crataegus pinnatifida major - Chinese Haw, Crataegus pontica, Crataegus pringlei, Crataegus pruinosa - Frosted Hawthorn, Crataegus pubescens – Manzanilla, Crataegus pubescens stipulacea – Manzanilla, Crataegus punctata - Dotted Hawthorn, Crataegus reverchonii - Reverchon's Hawthorn, Crataegus rivularis - River Hawthorn, Crataegus rotundifolia, Crataegus sanguinea, Crataegus schraderiana, Crataegus songorica, Crataegus stipulosa, Crataegus submollis - Quebec Hawthorn, Crataegus subvillosa, Crataegus succulenta, Crataegus szovitskii, Crataegus tanacetifolia - Tansy-Leaved Thorn, Crataegus uniflora, Crataegus x grignonensis

Native to my region are: Crataegus aestivalis (May Hawthorn, Mayhaw), Crataegus alabamensis (Alabama Hawthorn) , Crataegus alleghaniensis (Alleghany Hawthorn), Crataegus aprica (Sunny Hawthorn), Crataegus berberifolia var. berberifolia (Barberry Hawthorn), Crataegus berberifolia var. engelmannii (Barberry Hawthorn), Crataegus boyntonii (Boynton Hawthorn), Crataegus buckleyi (Buckley Hawthorn), Crataegus calpodendron (Pear Hawthorn), Crataegus coccinea (Scarlet Hawthorn), Crataegus collina (Chapman's Hill-thorn), Crataegus colonica, Crataegus craytonii (Crayton Hawthorn), Crataegus crus-galli var. crus-galli (Cockspur Hawthorn), Crataegus crus-galli var. pyracanthifolia, Crataegus dodgei (Dodge Hawthorn), Crataegus flabellata (Fanleaf Hawthorn), Crataegus intricata var. boyntonii (Boynton Hawthorn), Crataegus intricata var. intricata (Entangled Hawthorn), Crataegus intricata var. biltmoreana (Entangled Hawthorn), Crataegus iracunda (Red Hawthorn), Crataegus lassa (Sandhill Hawthorn),

Crataegus macrosperma (Bigfruit Hawthorn), Crataegus marshallii (Parsley Hawthorn), Crataegus munda, Crataegus pallens, Crataegus phaenopyrum (Washington Hawthorn), Crataegus pruinosa (Frosted Hawthorn), Crataegus punctata (Dotted Hawthorn), Crataegus schuettei (Schuette's Hawthorn), Crataegus senta, Crataegus spathulata (Littlehip Hawthorn), Crataegus succulenta (Fleshy Hawthorn), Crataegus viridis (Green Hawthorn), Crataegus visenda

As you can see, we have a LOT of Hawthorns! Although, these days, Hawthorn is often relegated to being a landscaping plant useful in keeping out intruders, or used for its fruit to make a rustic jam by too few people, Hawthorn is one of the most storied and useful plants used in herbal medicine.

Said to be both the wood that made the staff of Saint Joseph, and the thorns from Which the crown of Jesus was woven, Hawthorn has become a symbol of the Catholic Church. Early Christians decorated with Hawthorn as a type of Christmas tree.

In Culpepper's time, the Hawthorn was so commonly planted and used that he states:

It is not my intention to trouble you with a description of this tree, which is so well known that it needs none. It is ordinarily but a hedge bush, although being pruned and dressed, it grows to a tree of a reasonable height.

As for the Hawthorn Tree at Glastonbury, which is said to flower yearly on Christmas-day, it rather shews the superstition of those that observe it for the time of its flowering, than any great wonder, since the like may be found in divers other places of this land; as in Whey-street in Romney Marsh, and near unto Nantwich in Cheshire, by a place called White Green, where it flowers about Christmas and May. If the weather be frosty, it flowers not until January, or that the hard weather be over.

Government and virtues. It is a tree of Mars. The seeds in the berries beaten to powder being drank in wine, are held singularly good against the stone, and are good for the dropsy. The distilled water of the flowers stay the lask. The seed cleared from the down, bruised and boiled in wine, and drank, is good for inward tormenting pains. If cloths or sponges be wet in the distilled water, and applied to any place wherein thorns and splinters, or the like, do abide in the flesh, it will notably draw them forth.

And thus you see the thorn gives a medicine for its own pricking, and so doth almost every thing else.

Galen wrote:

The fruit of the Hawthorn tree is very astringent.

The haws or berries of the Hawthorn tree, as Dioscorides writeth, do both stay the lask, the menses, and all other fluxes of blood: some authors write, that the stones beaten to powder, and given to drink are good against the stone.

Dioscorides did, in fact, include Hawthorn in de Materia Medica, but his recommendation must be taken with a grain of salt as he said that Hawthorn consumed by a potential mother would ensure male children.

Mrs. Grieves listed the medicinal value of Hawthorn as:

Cardiac, diuretic, astringent, tonic. Mainly used as a cardiac tonic in organic and functional heart troubles. Both flowers and berries are astringent and useful in decoction to cure sore throats. A useful diuretic in dropsy and kidney troubles.

An Irish Herbal states:

The fruit is dry and astringent. It stops flows of extensive menstruation. The flowers are very good for breaking up stone in the kidneys and bladder.

Plants for A Future states:

The fruits and flowers of hawthorns are well-known in herbal folk medicine as a heart tonic and modern research has borne out this use. The fruits and flowers have a hypotensive effect as well as acting as a direct and mild heart tonic. They are especially indicated in the treatment of weak heart combined with high blood pressure. Prolonged use is necessary for it to be efficacious. It is normally used either as a tea or a tincture. The fruit is anodyne, anticholesterolemic, antidiarrhetic, antidysenteric, astringent, blood tonic, cardiotonic, haemostatic and stomachic. It is used in the treatment of dyspepsia, stagnation of fatty food, abdominal fullness, retention of lochia, amenorrhoea, postpartum abdominal pain, hypertension and coronary heart disease.

All varieties of hawthorn can be used. It may be harvested twice in a season - fresh, flowing tips, then ripe berries. Hawthorn is recognized as being good for irregularities of the heart. It dilates, strengthens and improves coronary arteries. It is good for over-exertion when we surpass the imitations of our age or fitness. Hawthorn is good for arrhythmia and good for angina. Hawthorn is especially good for the middle aged. Many herbalists believe that Hawthorn may be used as alternative to digitalis, or even used together, so one can use less digitalis.

The Rodale Herb Book states:

Aside from ornamental uses, hawthorn has been valued as a heart tonic, and this value has been increasingly studied in recent years. Promising results have been reported in connection with a variety of heart ailments, including angina pectoris and abnormal heart action. It is also said to be effective in stemming arteriosclerosis, commonly known as hardening of the arteries. Doses range from 3 to 15 grains, 3 to 4 times daily. But, the powder may also be made into a tincture by combining a pint of grain alcohol land an ounce of hawthorn berry powder. The tincture is given in doses ranging from 1 to 15 drop. Though non-toxic, hawthorn can produce dizziness if taken in large doses.

Hawthorne has also been used in treating arthritis and rheumatism, and for emotional stress in nervous conditions.

The Physicians' Desk Reference for Herbal Medicine tells us:

Crataegus is a well-studied herb for use in cardiovascular disease. Historically, it has been used for congestive heart failure, commonly in combination with cardiac glycosides as it may potentiate their effects, thereby reducing the dose of cardiac glycoside drugs. The use of Crataegus in hypertension, arterial sclerosis, and hyperlipidemia is well documented. The active principles are procyanidins in flavonoids, which cause an increase in coronary blood flow due to dilatory effects, resulting in an improvement of myocardial blood flow. The drug is positively inotropic and positively chronotropic. The cardiac effect of contagious is said to be caused by the increased membrane permeability for calcium as well as the inhibition phosphodiesterase with an increase of intracellular cyclo-AMP concentrations. Increased coronary and myocardial circulatory perfusion and reduction in peripheral vascular resistance were observed. High dose may cause sedation. This effect has been attributed to the old oligomeric procyanidins. Cretaceous extract has been found to prolong the refractory period and increase the action potential duration in Guinea pig papillary muscle. One study demonstrated that a Crataegus extract blocked the repolarizing potassium currents in ventricular myocytes of Guinea pigs. This effect is similar to that of class 3 antiarrhythmic drugs and may explain the antiarrhythmic effect of Hawthorne. Crataegus, due to its high flavonoid content may also be used to decrease inflammation, decrease capillary fragility, and prevent collagen destruction of the joints._

Cunninghamia lanceolata

This tree is naturalized in my region, and is commonly known as Chinese Fir.

Plants for A Future states:

Medicinal use of Chinese Fir: Antidote, carminative. A decoction of the wood is used in the treatment of varnish poisoning (from species of Rhus), chronic ulcers, hernia etc. An essential oil from the plant is used to treat bruises, pain, rheumatism and wounds. The ash of the bark is used to treat burns, scalds and wounds. A decoction of the cone is used in the treatment of coughs.

Cyrilla racemiflora, Swamp Titi

In stark contrast to the Hawthorn discussed above is the Swamp Titi. This is the one and only species of the genus Cyrilla, and its range is limited to the Americas. Here, it grows in the coastal swamps, extending about as far as the piedmont, or center of the state. It is an attractive plant, with white flowers and shiny, evergreen leaves.

The medicinal use of Cyrilla racemiflora is limited but important. The bark is both absorbent and astringent. It may be used as a styptic to stop bleeding.

Diospyros virginiana, common persimmon

Persimmon is found in various forms and places, but this is out native variety. It is quite different from the Asian Persimmons one may find in a grocery store. Our persimmons are an excellent fruit, mild and sugary sweet….when ripe! Ripe persimmons are delicious eaten fresh, out of hand, or baked into a fruit bread or cake. When baked, they taste a bit like sweet potato, with a bit of berry acidity and a mild bitter background that really makes such desserts special. A beer or cider made from Persimmons was very popular in early America, and the fruits of these scrubby trees kept many from starving, especially in the Revolutionary and Civil War.

The American Persimmon is a small tree, about the size of a dogwood. It likes the edges of woods and can often be found around old fields or roadsides.   It grows crooked and nobly and is considered almost a weed in our modern ignorance. An unripe Persimmon fruit may be the most puckeringly bitter substance known in nature. Perhaps the reason why native Persimmon is so lowly regarded, is because so many rural children have been tricked into eating the unripe fruit. An unripe persimmon not only puckers the mouth, it buckles the knees, takes away all sense of taste for up to a half hour and is the flavor equivalent of a punch in the mouth.

Persimmons ripen later than any fruit of which I am aware. Traditional lore is that Persimmons should not be harvested until after the first frost. Granted, many will be lost to deer, raccoons and opossums by, that time, but waiting until that kiss of frost does ensure sweet, ripe fruit. Persimmons turn from a powdery pink/orange to a purplish color when ripe. They are then soft, mushy… a texture and taste reminiscent of ripe figs. They will then pull easily from the stems, often falling off as you collect them. I generally eat almost as many as I bring home, just spitting out the seeds. They are perfect on a chilly October afternoon, when the smell of dry hardwood leaves fills the nose.

The secret to cooking with Persimmons is to not only remove all of the seeds, but to mash them through a fruit cone, colander or even a tea strainer or window screen. Persimmons contain little black flecks that even in very ripe fruit, will turn the pulp unbelievably bitter if not removed before cooking. You merely need to mash them through a screen or something similar, to produce a thick, orange fruit pulp, leaving the skins, seeds and black bits behind. Persimmons processed this way make the finest fruit breads, cakes and cookies. They combine very well with pumpkin, sweet potatoes, raisins, dried cranberries... the fruits of the season.

However, the fruit is not the only reason rural Southerners have traditionally seen the Persimmon tree as a major food source... perhaps the main asset of this tree is game. Cooking the game meat with the Persimmons on which it fed is a grand tradition. A cherished southern recipe that was widely beloved just a few generations ago, was "possum" roasted with persimmons and sweet potatoes. Occasionally, one still finds this beloved dish in Appalachia. Unfortunately, many modern people will not eat possum, considering it a "trash animal". Yes, this ancient animal, a remnant of a time long before people, is an omnivore that will scavenge anything edible it can find. Especially in our modern times, that can include roadkill or raiding garbage cans. But a possum that lives in a clean wilderness environment should not be viewed negatively. That possum will have fed on persimmons, apples and hickory nuts, and will be a gourmet treat for the adventurous and non-arrogant palate. The same is true of raccoons. I know of many African American communities in the rural South, where folks care nothing for turkey at Thanksgiving dinner. They want a big, fat coon that has been feeding on the fruits of the season... and, I've known several country boys who make some good holiday spending money illegally selling that very meat to the folks who desire it. It is a joy for them to hunt, and an obsession for the hounds they raise... a wonderful tradition that crosses racial boundaries and should not be prohibited by laws written by those who don't understand such things. Deer, turkey and bear also enjoy Persimmon. Along with the Hickories and Oaks, Persimmon is a tree any good hunter will scout for game.

King's American Dispensatory, 1898 tells us:

Action, Medical Uses, and Dosage.—Tonic and astringent. The bark has been used in intermittents, and both it and the unripe fruit have been beneficial in various forms of disease of the bowels, chronic dysentery, and uterine hemorrhage; used in infusion, syrup, or vinous tincture, in the proportion of 1 ounce of the bruised fruit to 2 fluid ounces of the vehicle, and ½ fluid ounce or more given to adults, and a fluid drachm or more to infants. The infusion may be used as a gargle in ulcerated sore throat. When ripe the fruit is very palatable, and as it matures at a time when fruits are generally departing for the season, the cultivation of the tree would undoubtedly be a valuable accession to our autumnal fruits. A kind of brandy is obtained by distillation of the fermented infusion.

According to Plants for A Future, Persimmon is:

Appetizer, sialagogue. The stem bark is astringent and styptic. The fruit is said to have different properties depending on its stage of ripeness, though it is generally antitussive, astringent, laxative, nutritive and stomachic. The fresh fully ripe fruit is used raw in the treatment of constipation and haemorrhoids and when cooked is used to treat diarrhoea. The dried ripe fruit is used in the treatment of bronchial complaints, whilst when ground into a powder it is used to treat dry coughs. Juice from the unripe fruit is used in the treatment of hypertension. The fruits, picked green and ripened in containers with the leaves, become very sweet and are considered to be antifebrile, antivinous and demulcent. The fruits are also peeled and then exposed to sunlight by day and dew by night. They become encrusted with a white powder and are then considered to be anthelmintic, antihaemorrhagic, antivinous, expectorant, febrifuge and restorative. The peduncle is used to treat coughs and hiccups. The calyx is used to treat hiccups.

Peterson Field Guides Eastern and Central Medicinal Plants tells us:

Inner bark tea highly astringent. In folk use, gargle for sore throats and thrush. Bark tea once used as a folk remedy for stomach aches, heartburn, diarrhea, dysentery, and uterine hemorrhage. The bark tea was used as a wash or poultice for warts and cancers.

Fruits edible, but astringent before ripening; Best after frost. Seed oil is suggestive of peanut oil in flavor. Warning: contains tannins; Potentially toxic in large amounts.

Euonymus atropurpureus, Wahoo or Burning Bush

Of this species, we only have one, as well. However, a couple of shrubs are called "Burning Bush", as well, so it can be confusing, so I find it best to use the common name of Wahoo for this one… Euonymus… besides, it is a fun name!

This tree goes by many names. The English variety is called "Spindle Tree". Mrs. Grieves attempts to unravel the mystery of the names in her comprehensive, A Modern Herbal, written in the 1930's:

Spindle Tree

Botanical: Euonymus atropurpureus, Euonymus Europoeus

The Latin name for Spindle is Fusus, and by some of the old writers this plant is called Fusanum and the Fusoria. By the Italians it is still called Fusano. The fruit is given three or four as a dose, as a purgative in rural districts; and the decoction, adding some vinegar, is used as a lotion for mange in horses and cattle. In allusion to the actively irritating properties of the shrub, its name Euonymus is associated with that of Euonyme, the mother of the Furies. In old herbals it is called Skewerwood or prickwood (the latter from its employment as toothpicks), and gatter, gatten, or gadrose. Chaucer, in one of his poems, calls it gaitre.

Prior says:

Gatter is from the Anglo-Saxon words, gad (a goad) and treow (a tree); gatten is made up of gad again and tan (a twig); and gadrise is from gad and hris (a rod).'

The same hardness that fitted it for skewers, spindles, etc., made it useful for the ox-goad.

Turner apparently christened the tree Spindle Tree. He says:

'I coulde never learne an Englishe name for it. The Duche men call it in Netherlande, spilboome, that is, spindel-tree, because they use

to make spindels of it in that country, and me thynke it may be as well named in English seying we have no other name. . . . I know no goode propertie that this tree hath, saving only it is good to make spindels and brid of cages (bird-cages).

The variety of Spindle Tree (Euonymus atropurpureus), common in the eastern United States, is known there as Wahoo, Burning Bush, or Indian Arrowwood. This is the kind generally used in medicine.

---Medicinal Action and Uses---Tonic, alterative, cholagogue, laxative and hepatic stimulant.

In small doses, Euonymin stimulates the appetite and the flow of the gastric juice. In larger doses, it is irritant to the intestine and is cathartic. It has slight diuretic and expectorant effects, but its only use is as a purgative in cases of constipation in which the liver is disordered, and for which it is particularly efficacious. It is specially valuable in liver disorders which follow or accompany fever. It is mildly aperient and causes no nausea, at the same time stimulating the liver somewhat freely, and promoting a free flow of bile.

To make the decoction, add an ounce to a pint of water and boil together slowly. A small wineglassful to be given, when cold, for a dose, two or three times a day.

Of the tincture made with spirit from the bark, 5 to 10 drops may be taken in water or on sugar.

Euonymin is generally given in pill form and in combination with other tonics, laxatives, etc.

Resources of the Southern Fields and Forests states:

CELASTRACEAE

DeCand. says an acrid principle has been detected among the species.

BURNINGBUSH; STRAWBERRY TEEE; FISHWOOD; SPINDLE TREE, (Euonymus Aynericanus.') Rare; grows in swamps; collected in St. John's Berkeley. N. C. Fl. May.

Griffith's Med. Bot. 220. Emetic, discutient and anti-syphilitic. It is also thought to be narcotic. The seeds are said to be nauseous, *purgative and emetic, and are used in some places to destroy vermin in the hair. The leaves are poisonous to cattle.*

WAHOO, (Euonymus atropurpureus.) Possesses properties similar to the above. Dr. Wood, in the 12th Ed. Of the U. S. Disp., slates that Mr. G. W. Carpenter had introduced a bark some twenty years since as a remedy for dropsy, under the name Wahoo, he having obtained a knowledge of its virtues in the Western States. Dr. W. ascertained that it was derived from this plant, which must be distinguished from the Elm of the Southern States, which is also called Wahoo. The bark imparts its virtues to water and alcohol. By analysis of Mr. W. T. Wenzel, it was found to contain a bitter principle, which he named euonymin, asparagin, resin, fixed oil, wax, starch, albumen, glucose, pectin and salts. (Am. J. Ph., Sept., 1862.) Mr. W. P. Clothier found the substance, which is the euonymine of the Eclectics, to purge actively without griping. Dr. Twyman, of Mo., informed Dr. Wood that he had found the bark, as a cathartic, rather to resemble rhubarb than to possess hydragogue properties, and he thought that he had obtained from it good results as an alterative to the hepatic functions. The decoction or infusion is used in dropsy, made in the proportion of an ounce to a pint of water, and given in the dose of a wineglassful several times a day. TJ. S. Disp. See a paper by C A. Santos, upon the Am. Species; Am. J. Pharm. Xx, 80

King's American Dispensatory, 1898 tells us:

Action, Medical Uses, and Dosage.—Euonymus has been in use among physicians for a long time. The bark is tonic, laxative, alterative, diuretic, and expectorant; the seeds are cathartic and emetic. In infusion, syrup, or extract, it has been successfully used in intermittents, dyspepsia, torpid liver, constipation, dropsy, and pulmonary affections. Prof. Locke states" there are but few good stomach tonics, and this agent is one of them." It stimulates the biliary flow, and has considerable anti-malarial influence, and may be used in intermittents after the chill has been broken with quinine. It stimulates the nutritive processes and improves the appetite. It may be used with advantage in atonic dyspepsia, and in indigestion due to hepatic topor or following malarial fevers. It is a remedy for chronic ague, and the consequent obstinate constipation and gastric debility accompanying or following it. A gin tincture (root ℥j to gin fl℥viij), is not without value in some cases of dropsy, particularly when associated with hepatic and renal inactivity. Dose of the tincture (℥viij to alcohol 76 per cent Oj), from 1 to 4 fluid drachms; of the syrup, from 1 to 2 fluid ounces; of the hydro-alcoholic extract, from 5 to 15 grains; of the powder, from 20 to 30 grains; of specific euonymus, 1 to 30 drops.

Specific Indications and Uses.—Prostration with irritation of the nerve centers; periodical diseases, to supplement the action of quinine; anorexia, indigestion, and constipation, due to hepatic torpor.

Plants for a future gives the following uses for out native Wahoo:

Wahoo was used in various ways by the North American Indians, for example as an eye lotion, as a poultice for facial sores and for gynaecological conditions. In current herbalism it is considered to be a gallbladder remedy with laxative and diuretic properties. The bark, however, is toxic and should only be used under professional supervision, it should not be given to pregnant women or nursing mothers. The stem and root bark is alterative, cardiac, cathartic, cholagogue, diuretic, expectorant, hepatic, laxative, stimulant and tonic. The root bark is the part normally used, though bark from the stems is sometimes employed as a substitute. In small doses it stimulates the appetite, in larger doses it irritates the intestines. The bark is especially useful in the treatment of biliousness and liver disorders which follow or accompany fevers and for treating various skin disorders such as eczema which could arise from poor liver and gallbladder function. It is also used as a tea in the treatment of malaria, liver congestion, constipation etc. The powdered bark, applied to the scalp, was believed to eliminate dandruff. The bark and the root contain digitoxin and have a digitalis-like effect on the heart. They have been used in the treatment of heart conditions. The bark, which has a sweetish taste, is gathered in the autumn and can be dried for later use. A tea made from the roots is used in cases of uterine prolapse, vomiting of blood, painful urination and stomach-aches. The seed is emetic

The positions desk reference for herbal medicine tells us:

The drug is reported to be a laxative and choleretic. Larger doses have an effect on the heart. Unproven uses: in the past, the drug was used as a cholagogue, laxative, diuretic and tonic, and for dyspepsia. Today it is used in homeopathy. Precautions and adverse reactions: poisoning caused by the berries have been recorded. A fatal dose is said to be 36 berries .... Wahoo root bark and fruit are not recommended for use, as the drug is considered too dangerous.

Fagus, Beech

Eight varieties of Fagus are used in herbal medicine, but another nine members of the Beech family are also used, falling under the closely related Nothofagus. Fagus crenata - Japanese Beech, Fagus grandifolia - American Beech, Fagus japonica - Japanese Beech, Fagus longipetiolata, Fagus lucida, Fagus orientalis - Oriental Beech, Fagus sylvatica, NothoFagus betuloides, NothoFagus cunninghamii - Myrtle Beech, NothoFagus fusca - Red Beech, NothoFagus menziesii - Silver Beech, NothoFagus obliqua – Robl, NothoFagus procera – Rauli, Notho, NothoFagus solanderi - Black Beech, Nothofagus solanderi cliffortioides - Mountain Beech

Only two Beeches are native to my region, Fagus grandifolia var. caroliniana (American Beech), Fagus grandifolia var. grandifolia (American Beech)

That we have only two native Beeches certainly does not mean that we have few Beech trees. Quite the contrary! In fact, just two peaks over from where I live now is Beech Mountain, NC. Beech mountain, known for ski slopes and The Land Of Oz amusement park (that closed in the 1980s), was also home to the folks who taught me herbs and Appalachian folktales. That was the "back side of Beech Mountain", away from the tourists and summer homes, down ten miles of dirt road. The Hicks family lived in a centuries old cabin, with no indoor plumbing, one electric light, a wood stove, a spring house, a view of Tennessee on clear, stary nights... far away from noise or most any trace of modernity. Peace and quiet, nature and the old ways.

Dioscorides included Beech in de Materia Medica:

… and the bark of the root of prinus boiled in water until it becomes tender and rotten and applied for a whole night dyes the hair black. It is first made clean with Cimolian earth. The leaves of all of them bruised and pounded into small pieces help oedema, and strengthen feeble parts.

Saint Hildegard von Bingen included a lengthy entry on Beech in her Physica, written around 1100:

The beech tree has correct balance, with equal heat and cold, both of which are good. It demotes discipline. When the leaves of the beech begin to come out, but do not yet fully show, go to this tree and take a branch of it in your left hand, say, "I cut your natural vigor from you, because you correct all a person's humors which have been turned the wrong path by the yellow bule, by the living Word, which makes a person without contrition." Hold the branch in your left hand while you say these words. Then cut the branch off with a steel knife. Save that branch for a year and repeat this each year. If anyone in that year has jaundice, cut a small piece from that branch. Place it in a metallic jar, and pour over it a moderate amount of wine. Whenever you pour the wine over these bits, say these words, " By the holy spark of thy holy incarnation, by which God became human, draw from this person (Name) the sickness of jaundice. " Then heat the wine, with the bits of wood which you had cut off, in a small crucible. For three day, give it as a warm drink to the one with jaundice. He will be cured unless God forbids it

If someone has ague, take some of the fruit of the beech tree when it forsts comes out and mix it with pure spring water. Say these words, "By the holy spark of the holy incarnation by which God became human, you ague, and you fevers, forsake this person, (Name) with your heat and cold. Then give him this water to drink. Offer it for five days, and he will be quickly healed from the quartan fevers, unless God does not wish to free him.

Also, when the root of the beech tree appears above the earth, take away its outer bark. Take as much as you can cut with one incision and say, By the first vision, when God saw a human being at the root of Mamre, break the waves of this person's poison, without his death." Again, cut as much as you can from the second incision and say the same words. In a similar way, cut a third incision in the root, so that you cut the root three times, lest it run short during the year. During the year, whenever anyone has freislich on his body, cut off a bit from one of these cuttings of wood, place it in a metallic jar, and pour over it pure spring water, saying these words each time, " By the first vision, when God was baptized in the Jordan, through this poison, without the death of the person (Name), carry from him every snare of disease, so that he be with pure life, just as Jesus was given." Give him this water to drink, while fasting, for three days. On each day offer it to him to drink in this way. He will be freed from the freislich, unless God prohibits it.

Anyone who prepares and eats a puree from the leaves of the beech, when they are new and fresh, will not be harmed by it. If someone eats its fruit, he will not be harmed, but will become fat.

To put it mildly, Saint Hildegard's remedies may seem esoteric to modern readers. It must be mentioned though, that she is not only a canonized saint, but a Doctor of the Church. Saint Hildegard received her knowledge of herbs and healing from "The voice of the living Light" and angelic visions. She was a mystic who was blessed with something akin to the Wisdom of Solomon, having little formal education due to extreme illness in her youth. She reluctantly shared her visions through several books, art and the largest body recorded religious music from the Middle Ages. She was celebrated by the Pope and bishops of her day, and was encouraged to travel as much as possible, preaching and teaching in Catholic churches throughout central Europe. Popularly, she was known as the "Sybil of the Rhine" and all who were able, including the crowned heads of Europe, flocked to her Abbey, to gain insight from her wisdom, insight and God-given knowledge.

Gerard, writing in 1597 says:

The leaves of Beech do cool: the kernel of the nut is somewhat moist.

A. The leaves of Beech are very profitably applied unto hot swellings, blisters, and excoriations; and being chewed they are good for chapped lips, and pain of the gums.

B. The kernels or mast within are reported to ease the pain of the kidneys proceeding of the stone, if they be eaten, and to cause the gravel and sand the easier to come forth. With these, mice and squirrels are greatly delighted, who do mightily increase by feeding thereon: swine also be fattened herewith, and certain other beasts also. Deer do feed thereon very greedily: they be likewise pleasant to thrushes and pigeons.

C. Petrus Crescentius writeth, That the ashes of the wood is good to make glass with.

D. The water that is found in the hollowness of Beeches cureth the naughty scurf, tetters, and scabs of men, horses, kine, and sheep, if they be wasled therewith.

Culpepper wrote of Beech, "It is a plant of Saturn, and therefore performs his qualities and proportion in these operations. The leaves of the beech-tree are cooling and binding, and therefore good to be applied to hot swellings to discuss them; the nuts do much nourish such beasts as feed thereon. The water that is found in the hollow places of decaying beeches will cure both man and beast of any scurf, scab, or running tetters, if they be washed therewith; you may boil the leaves into a poultice, or make an ointment of them when time of year serves."

Mrs. Grieves writes only of Beech, "The tar is stimulating and antiseptic, used internally as a stimulating expectorant in chronic bronchitis, or externally as an application in various skin diseases."

Fr. Johannes Künzle wrote of Beech in his Spring Cure:

There are many people who, without being bedridden, are almost always unwell, they have no appetite and dislike the best St. Gallen sausages, are clogged up like the gates of hell, they feel pressure on their chests and in their stomachs and there is heat and pain in the head. They can not sleep well and when they do sleep then restlessly and they have bad dreams; they run after all doctors and are a nuisance to them, write to all quacks as far as to London and New York, swing like party leaders after an election victory, and are like complaining organs with 365 stops, often with an accompaniment of an orchestra.

If such people have the serious will to get well, they should take one of the so-called spring cures for 8-14 days.

Unripe Blackberries

You send Tony or Jacob into the nearest bushes with a basket and a knife. There he cuts many shoots from all types of thorny bushes: dog rose (Rosa cantina), blackthorn (Prunus spinosa), hawthorn (Crataegus), raspberry (rubus idaeus), and blackberry (rubus fruticosus) and shoots from fir trees, beeches (fagus), hazel trees, cherry trees, oaks, larches, ash trees, poplars. Furthermore you can also take shoots from currants, from gooseberries, from fruit trees.

A handful of this mixture is then thrown into a pan, one to two liters of water are poured in, and the mixture is heated until it simmers. The sick person should drink one to two liters of this liquid daily with sugar. This tea cleanses the whole body. It has already turned very sick people into healthy and flourishing ones again. However, if the effect is to be lasting, this cure must be continued for eight days. The lost appetite returns, the headache and pressure in the abdomen are gone, the pale color vanishes, the grave digger can put his shovel back in his shed. And this poor creature, previously so pale and shaky, can again rule in the kitchen with power and dignity.

If she takes five or seven good fir tree twigs baths, she is fresh and sunny again like a bride! It is   known that mustard has extracting qualities, that is why mustard plasters are often used for painful rheumatic areas. The well-known, expensive American plasters contain extracting substances.

Jolanta WIttib writes of Beech:

I admire these mighty trees. They are so majestic, and they have very cute offsprings. Have you ever seen the young shoots of a beech? No? Look out for these. You will definitely enjoy the look of them. And have you ever eaten the nuts of a beech? My grandson introduced me to these. We do not have beeches in the Alps, but he lives next to huge beech forests. In autumn the paths are strewn with burrs - those tiny boxes with beech nuts. My grandson showed me how to open them with scissors. Just cutting the pointed upper part and then peeling the seed.

Mmmmm delicious!

A beech gives not only nuts. I have read that one huge beech tree releases per hour enough oxygen for 50 people to breath during that hour. We do need such trees!

Herbal Remedies of the Lumbee Indians tells us:

The Lumbee made Beech tea from the bark taken from the trunk. This tea was drunk to treat weak back and back aches. The same liquid was mixed with hog lard to form a slave rubbed on the affected area to treat bone rheumatism. The salve was also used to nurse pain from a sprain or broken bone. ... The Rappahannock soaked beech bark in salt water to produce a substance to be rubbed on the skin to treat poison ivy. The Iroquois League... used beech nut oil mixed with bear grease as a hair treatment and mosquito repellant.

Resources of the Southern Fields and Forests states:

The bark is astringent, and has been used, according to Dr. Farnham, in intermittent fever; but it is not possessed of any decided powers. The fruit pro-duces vertigo and headache in the human species. It is observed, in the Fl. Scotica, that "the fat of hogs, which feed on them, is soft, and will boil away." The seeds yield an oil little inferior to olive oil, and fit, also, for burning. The pulp remaining after expression may be converted into flour, similar in taste and color to wheat, but sweeter. A narcotic principle, called fagine, has been found in the husks. The young leaves are sometimes used by the common people as a potherb.

Peterson Field Guides Eastern and Central Medicinal Plants tells us:

American beach, Fagus grandifolia: American Indians chewed nuts as a worm experiment. Bark tea used for long elements. Leaf tea a wash for burns, frostbite, Poison Ivy rash (1 ounce to 1 pint salt water).

Botany In a Day states:

Beech leaves are edible raw or cooked as a pot or early in the spring. The seeds are rich in oil and high in protein, edible raw or cooked, but should not be eaten in large quantities due to an alkaloid in the outer covering. The seeds may be dried and ground into a flour. The roasted seed is used as a coffee substitute. The sprouted seeds are also edible and reportedly delicious. Oil from the seeds may be used in cooking and salad dressing or in lamps.

Ficus, Fig (my favorite fruit)

Only one variety of Fig has been naturalized in my region, Ficus carica.

Dioscorides wrote of Fig under the names, Suka, Suke Agria, Olunthoi and Konia Sukes

SUKA - Ficus sativa, Ficus communis, Ficus carica — Fig

Ripe new syca are bad for the stomach and loosen the intestines but the looseness that comes from them is easily stopped. They bring out pimples and sweat, quench thirst, and extinguish heat. The dried ones are nourishing and warming, cause thirst, and are good for the bowels. They are useless for discharges of the stomach and intestines, but good for the throat, arteries, bladder and kidneys, those who have a poor colour from a long illness, as well as asthma, epilepsy and dropsy. Boiled with hyssop and taken as a drink they clean away things in the chest. They are good for old coughs and long-lasting disorders of the lungs; and pounded together with saltpetre and cnicus and eaten, they soften the bowels. A decoction of them is good for inflammation around the arteries and tonsils, used in a gargle. They are mixed in poultices with barley meal, fenugreek or barley water for women's warm packs. Boiled with rue they are a suppository for griping. Boiled and afterwards pounded into small pieces and applied, they dissolve hard lumps and soften parotid tumours, boils and inflammatory tumours. They ripen pannus [opaque thickening of cornea with veins] more effectively with iris, saltpetre [potassium nitrate] or quicklime [calcium oxide — lime which has been burned but not yet slaked with water]. Pounded raw with the things previously specified they do the same. With pomegranate rind they clean away pterygium [membrane on the eye], and with calcanthum [limestone] they cure difficult, curable and malignant discharges in the tibiae [hollow bones, marrow, not only the tibia]. Boiled in wine and mixed with wormwood and barley meal they are good for dropsy applied as a poultice. Burnt and put into a wax ointment they cure chilblains. The raw ones pounded into small pieces mixed with moist mustard and put into the ears, cure noises and ringing in them. The (milky) juice of both the wild and cultivated figs coagulates milk like rennet, and dissolves coagulated milk like vinegar. Taken as a drink with almonds that have been pounded into small pieces it is able to make bodies break out into boils, to open pores, loosen the bowels and relax the womb. It expels the menstrual flow applied with the yolk of an egg or Tyrrhenian [Etruscan] wax. It is good put into poultices made for gout together with fenugreek flowers and vinegar. With polenta it cleans leprosy, lichen [papular skin disease], spots made by the heat of the sun, vitiligines [form of leprosy], parasitical skin diseases, and running sores on the head. Dropped on the sores it helps those stung by scorpions, and strikes of poisonous beasts, and those bitten by dogs. Taken on wool and put into the cavities of teeth it helps toothache. It takes away formicosam [anthill-shaped] warts if it is rubbed on the flesh with animal fat.

SUKE AGRIA - Wild Fig Tree

The juice of the tender leaves of the wild syca tree does the same things. When they are great with child (not yet fruiting) and the eye (bud) has not put out, they are pounded and pressed out, and the juice is dried in the shade and stored. Both the liquid and juice are taken for the strength they have to raise [fill] ulcers. The sprigs of this tree boiled with beef makes it boil quicker. They make milk more loosening if they are used to stir it with during boiling instead of a spatha. Olyntha (some of which are called erinei) boiled and applied as a poultice soften all nodules, scrofulous tumours [glandular swelling] and goitres. Applied raw with saltpetre [potassium nitrate] and meal they take away formicosam [anthill-shaped] warts and warty abnormal growths. The leaves can do the same. Applied as a poultice with vinegar and salt they heal running ulcers on the head, dandruff and epinycti [pustules which appear only at night]. Fig-like scabrous cheeks are rubbed with these. Vitiliginous [form of leprosy] white areas are plastered with the leaves or branches of the black fig. They are good also with honey for the bites of dogs, and the ulcers called favi by the Latins but by the Greeks ceria [honeycombed ulcers]. Grossi [unripe figs] with the leaves of wild poppy draw out (broken) bones, and theydissolve boils [inflammatory tumours] with wax. Applied with ervum and wine they are good against the bites of rodents, spiders, centipedes and millipedes.

KONIA SUKES - Ficus carica var sylvestris, Ficus variegata, Ficus amboinensis, Ficus racemosa, Caprificus amboinensis, Ficus carica

Lye is made from ashes of the burnt branches of the wild and cultivated syca trees. You must steep the ashes long and often. It is good both for caustic medicines and gangrenous parts, for it cleans and removes things which are superfluous. It must be used by moistening a sponge in it often and immediately applying it. Give it to some as a suppository for dysentery, old discharges, and hollow, undermining, great ulcers. For it cleans, heals, covers in flesh and closes together, similar to plasters made for bloody wounds. It is given for clotting blood together and against dripping fluids, hernia and convulsions, newly strained-out with a wine cupful of water and a little oil mixed in. By itself it helps coeliac complaints and dysentery, the amount of a wine cupful given. It is a convenient ointment with oil for those troubled with sores of the tendons, and convulsions that cause sweats. It is taken as an antidote in a drink for those who have swallowed gypsum [hydrous calcium sulphate — plaster of Paris] and for the bites of harvest spiders. The other sorts of lye have the same effects (especially that of the oak) and they are all astringent.

Saint Hildegard von Bingen wrote of Fig:

The fig tree Is more hot than cold. It will always have heat, and its cold is not strong. It signifies fear. Take its leaves and bark, and pound them moderately. Cook this well in water, and then make an unguent with bear fat and a little less butter. If you have a pain in your head, anoint your head with it. If your eyes hurt, rub it on your temples and around your eyes, without letting it touch the inside of your eyes. If it is your chest that hurts, anoint it; if your kidneys, anoint them with it, and you will be better

However, if its wood is burned in a fire, and its smoke touches someone, it harms him a bit so that it weakens him. If someone carries in his hand a staff made from that wood, it diminishes his strength.

.. If a healthy person wishes to eat it (the fruit), he should first soak it in wine or vinegar, so that its inconsistency is tempered. He should then eat it, but in moderation. It is not necessary for a sick person to temper it in this way.

Gerard wrote of Fig:

The Virtues.

A. The dry figs do nourish better than the green or new figs; notwithstanding they engender not very good blood, for such people as do feed much thereon do become lousy.

B. Figs be good for the throat and lungs, they mitigate the cough, and are good for them that be short winded: they ripen phlegm, causing the same to be easily spat out, especially when they be sodden with Hyssop, and the decoction drunk.

C. Figs stamped with salt, Rue, and the kernels of nuts withstand all poison and corruption of the air. The King of Pontus, called Mithridates, used this preservative against all venom and poison.

D. Figs stamped and made into the form of a plaster with wheat meal, the powder of Fenugreek, and linseed, and the roots of Marsh Mallows, applied warm, do soften and ripen impostumes, phlegmons, all hot and angry swellings and tumors behind the ears: and if you add thereto the roots of Lilies, it ripeneth and breaketh venereous impostumes that come in the flank, which impostume is called Bubo, by reason of his lurking in such secret places: in plain English terms they are called botches.

E. Figs boiled in Wormwood wine with some barley meal are very good to be applied as an emplaster upon the bellies of such as have the dropsy.

F. Dry figs have power to soften, consume, and make thin, and may be used both outwardly and inwardly, whether it be to ripen or soften impostumes, or to scatter, dissolve, and consume them.

G. The leaves of the Fig tree do waste and consume the King's Evil, or swelling kernels in the throat, and do mollify, waste, and consume all other tumours, being finely pounded and laid thereon: but after my practise, being boiled with the roots of marsh Mallows until they be soft, and so incorporated together, and applied in form of a plaster.

H. The milky juice either of the figs or leaves is good against all roughness of the skin, lepries, spreading sores, tetters, smallpox, measles, pushes, wheals, freckles, lentils, and all other spots, scurviness, and deformity of the body and face, being mixed with barley meal and applied: it doth also take away warts and such like excrescences, if it be mingled with some fatty or greasy thing.

I. The milk doth also cure the toothache, if a little lint or cotton be wet therein, and put into the hollowness of the tooth.

K. It openeth the veins of the hemorrhoids, and looseneth the belly, being applied to the fundament.

L. Figs stamped with the powder of Fenugreek, and vinegar, and applied plasterwise, do ease the intolerable pain of the hot gout, especially the gout of the feet.

M. The milk thereof put into the wound proceeding of the biting of a mad dog, or any other venomous beast, preserveth the parts adjoining, taketh away the pain presently, and cureth the hurt.

N. The green and ripe figs are good for those that be troubled with the stone of the kidneys, for they make the conduits slippery, and open them, and do also somewhat cleanse: whereupon after the eating of the same, it happeneth that much gravel and sand is conveyed forth.

O. Dry or barrel figs, called in Latin Caricæ, are a remedy for the belly, the cough, and for old infirmities of the chest and lungs: they scour the kidneys, and cleanse forth the sand, they mitigate the pain of the bladder, and cause women with child to have the easier deliverance, if they feed thereof for certain days together before their time.

P. Dioscorides saith, that the white liquor of the Fig tree, and juice of the leaves, do curdle milk as rennet doth, and dissolve the milk that is cluttered in the stomach, as doth vinegar.

Q. It bringeth down the menses, if it be applied with the yolk of an egg, or with yellow wax.

Culpepper was somewhat less effusive:

The tree is under the dominion of Jupiter. The milk that issues out from the leaves or branches where they are broken off, being dropped upon warts, takes them away. The decoction of the leaves is excellent good to wash sore heads with: and there is scarcely a better remedy for the leprosy than it is. It clears the face also of morphew, and the body of white scurf, scabs, and running sores. If it be dropped into old fretting ulcers, it cleanses out the moisture, and brings up the flesh; because you cannot have the leaves green all the year, you may make an ointment of them while you can. A decoction of the leaves being drank inwardly, or rather a syrup made of them, dissolves congealed blood caused by bruises or falls, and helps the bloody flux. The ashes of the wood made into an ointment with hog's grease, helps kibes and chilblains. The juice being put into an hollow tooth, eases pain; as also deafness and pain and noise in the ears, being dropped into them. An ointment made of the juice and hog's grease, is as excellent a remedy for the biting of mad dogs, or other venomous beasts, as most are; a syrup made of the leaves, or green fruit, is excellent for coughs, hoarseness, or shortness of breath, and all diseases of the breast and lungs; it is very good for the dropsy and falling sickness.

Mrs. Grieves gives us a bit of history along with medical use:

The Common Fig-tree provides the succulent fruit that in its fresh and dried state has been valued from the earliest days. It is indigenous to Persia, Asia Minor and Syria, but now is wild in most of the Mediterranean countries. It is cultivated in most warm and temperate climates and has been celebrated from the earliest times for the beauty of its foliage and for its 'sweetness and good fruit' (Judges ix. 2), there being frequent allusions to it in the Scriptures. The Greeks are said to have received it from Caria in Asia Minor - hence the specific name. Under Hellenic culture it was improved and Attic figs became celebrated in the East. It was one of the principal articles of sustenance among the Greeks, being largely used by the Spartans at their public table; and athletes fed almost entirely on figs, considering that they increased their strength and swiftness. To such an extent, indeed, were figs a part of the staple food of the people in ancient Greece that there was a law forbidding the exportation of the best fruit from their trees.

Figs were early introduced into Italy. Pliny gives details of no less than twentynine kinds known in his day, and specially praises those of Tarant and Caria and also those of Herculaneum. Dried Figs have been found in Pompeii in our days and in the wall-paintings of the buried city Figs are represented together with other fruits. Pliny states that homegrown Figs formed a large portion of the food of slaves, especially in the fresh state for agricultural workers.

The Fig plays an important part in Latin mythology. It was dedicated to Bacchus and employed in religious ceremonies. The wolf that suckled Romulus and Remus rested under a Fig tree, which was therefore held sacred by the Romans, and Ovid states that among the celebrations of the first day of the year by Romans, Figs were offered as presents. The inhabitants of Cyrene crowned themselves with wreaths of Figs when sacrificing to Saturn, holding him to be the discoverer of the fruit. Pliny speaks also of the Wild Fig, which is mentioned also in Homer, and further classical references to the Fig are to be found in Theophrastus, Dioscorides, Varro and Columella.

Medicinal Action and Uses---Figs are used for their mild, laxative action, and are employed in the preparation of laxative confections and syrups, usually with senna and carminatives. It is considered that the laxative property resides in the saccharine juice of the fresh fruit and in the dried fruit is probably due to the indigestible seeds and skin. The three preparations of Fig of the British Pharmacopoeia are Syrup of Figs, a mild laxative, suitable for administration to children; Aromatie Syrup of Figs, Elixir of Figs, or Sweet Essence of Figs, an excellent laxative for children and delicate persons, is compounded of compound tincture of rhubarb, liquid extract of senna, compound spirit of orange, liquid extract of cascara and Syrup of Figs. The Compound Syrup of Figs is a stronger preparation, composed of liquid extract of senna, syrup of rhubarb and Syrup of Figs, and is more suitable for adults.

Figs are demulcent as well as nutritive. Demulcent decoctions are prepared from them and employed in the treatment of catarrhal affections of the nose and throat.

Roasted and split into two portions, the soft pulpy interior of Figs may be applied as emolient poultices to gumboils, dental abscesses and other circumscribed maturating tumours. They were used by Hezekiah as a remedy for boils 2,400 years ago (Isaiah xxxviii. 21).

The milky juice of the freshly-broken stalk of a Fig has been found to remove warts on the body. When applied, a slightly inflamed area appears round the wart, which then shrivels and falls off. The milky juice of the stems and leaves is very acrid and has been used in some countries for raising blisters.

The wood of the tree is porous and of little value, though a piece, saturated with oil and spread with emery, is in France a common substitute for a hone.

Green Fig Jam is excellent. Choose very juicy Figs. Take off the stalks, but do not peel them. Make a syrup of 1/2 lb. of sugar and a glass of water (1/2 pint) for each pound of fruit. Put the Figs into it and cook them till the syrup pearls. Boil a stick of cinnamon with them and remove it before pouring the jam into pots.

The Sycamore Fig (Ficus Sycamorus) is a tree of large size, with heart-shaped, somewhat mulberry-like leaves. It is a favourite tree in Egypt and Syria, being often planted along roads, deep shade being cast by its spreading branches. It bears a sweet, edible fruit, somewhat like that of the Common Fig, but produced in racemes, on the older branches. The Ancients, after soaking it in water, preserved it like the Common Fig. The porous wood is only fit for fuel.

Our northern Sycamore tree is in no way related to this Sycamore Fig, but has wrongly acquired its name, Prior says, through a mistake of the botanist Ruellius, who transferred the Greek name, Sycamoros, properly the name of the Wild Fig, to the great Maple.

'This mistake,' says Prior, 'arose perhaps from this tree, the great maple, being on account of the density of its foliage, used in the sacred dramas of the Middle Ages to represent the Fig tree into which Zaccheus climbed and that in which the Virgin Mary on her journey into Egypt had hidden herself and the infant Jesus to avoid the fury of Herod; a legend quoted by Stapel on Theophrastus and by Thevenot in his Voyage de Levant: "At Mathave is a large sycamore or Pharaoh's Fig, very old, but which bears fruit every year. They say that upon the Virgin passing that way with her son Jesus and being pursued by the people, this Fig tree opened to receive her and closed her in again, until the people had passed by and then opened again. The tree is still shown to travellers." ' (See Cowper's Apocryphal Gospels.)

King's American Dispensatory, 1898 tells us:

Action and Medical Uses.—*Figs are nutritive, emollient, demulcent, and aperient, and are used in costive habits, and to flavor gruels, decoctions, etc. Roasted or boiled, they may be applied as a suppurative poultice to gum-boils, buboes, carbuncles, etc. A poultice of dried figs and milk will remove the stench of cancerous and fetid ulcers (Billroth).*

Plants for A Future stares:

Medicinal use of Fig: A decoction of the leaves is stomachic. The leaves are also added to boiling water and used as a steam bath for painful or swollen piles. The latex from the stems is used to treat corns, warts and piles. It also has an analgesic effect against insect stings and bites. The fruit is mildly laxative, demulcent, digestive and pectoral. The unripe green fruits are cooked with other foods as a galactogogue and tonic. The roasted fruit is emollient and used as a poultice in the treatment of gumboils, dental abscesses etc. Syrup of figs, made from the fruit, is a well-known and effective gentle laxative that is also suitable for the young and very old. A decoction of the young branches is an excellent pectoral. The plant has anticancer properties.

The Physicians' Desk Reference for Herbal Medicine tells us:

Fig preparations are used as a laxative. In China, figs are used for dysentery and enteritis. No health hazards or side effects are known in conjunction with proper administration of designated therapeutic dosages.

Firmiana simplex

This naturalized tree is called, Chinese Parasol Tree. Plants for A Future states:

Medicinal use of Chinese Parasol Tree: Astringent, salve. The seed is antiphlogistic, expectorant and refrigerant. A decoction of the roots is used to reduce swellings. A lotion of the leaves is used in the treatment of carbuncles, haemorrhoids and sores.

Frangula alnus or Rhamnus frangula

This naturalized tree is known as Alder Buckthorn. We also have Rhamnus davurica (Dahurian Buckthorn)

Dioscorides wrote of the Buckthorns under the name Ramnos:

Rhamnus is a shrub (growing around hedges) with upright stems and sharp thorns like oxyacantha, and the leaves are small, somewhat long, thick and soft. There is another besides this that is paler, and a third having darker and broader leaves, a little inclined to red; with long stems of five feet and more, thorny, with its hairs less strong and stiff. The fruit of it is broad, white and thin, shaped like a little pouch or whorl. The leaves of all of them are effective rubbed on for erysipelas [inflammatory skin disease] and herpes [viral skin infection]. It is said that the branches laid in gates or windows drive away the enchantments of witches. [If anyone picks up rhamnus while the moon is decreasing and holds it, it is effective against poison and mischief; and it is good for beasts to carry it around them; and for it to be put around ships; and it is good against headaches; and against devils and their assaults.] It is also called persephonion, or leucacantha, the Romans call it spina alba, some, spina cerualis, and the Africans call it atadin.

Gerard was less concerned about "mischief":

A. The same do purge and void by the stool thick phlegm, and also choleric humours: they are given being beaten into powder from one dram to a dram and a half: divers do number the berries, who give to strong bodies from fifteen to twenty or more; but it is better to break them and boil them in fat flesh broth without salt, and to give the broth to drink: for so they purge with lesser trouble and fewer gripings.

B. There is pressed forth of the ripe berries a juice, which being boiled with a little alum is used of painters for a deep green, which they do call sap green.

C. The berries which be as yet unripe, being dried and infused or steeped in water, do make a fair yellow colour; but if they be ripe they make a green.

Mrs. Grieves wrote of several varieties of Buckthorn. Of the Common Buckthorn she wrote:

-Laxative and cathartic.

Buckthorn was well known to the AngloSaxons and is mentioned as Hartsthorn or Waythorn in their medical writings and glossaries dating before the Norman Conquest. The Welsh physicians of the thirteenth century prescribed the juice of the fruit of Buckthorn boiled with honey as an aperient drink.

The medicinal use of the berries was familiar to all the writers on botany and materia medica of the sixteenth century, though Dodoens in his Herbal wrote: 'They be not meat to be administered but to the young and lusty people of the country which do set more store of their money than their lives.'

Until late in the nineteenth century, syrup of Buckthorn ranked, however, among favourite rustic remedies as a purgative for children, prepared by boiling the juice with pimento and ginger and adding sugar, but its action was so severe that, as time went on, the medicine was discarded. It first appeared in the London Pharmacopceia of 1650, where, to disguise the bitter taste of the raw juice, it was aromatized by means of aniseed, cinnamon, mastic and nutmeg. It was still official in the British Pharmacopoeia of 1867, but is no longer so, being regarded as a medicine more fit for animals than human beings, and it is now employed almost exclusively in veterinary practice, being commonly prescribed for dogs, with equal parts of castor oil as an occasional purgative.

The flesh of birds eating the berries is stated to be purgative.

There used to be a superstition that the Crown of Thorns was made of Buckthorn.

Of Alder-Buckthorn, she wrote:

Tonic, laxative, cathartic.

Dried seasoned bark from one to two years old alone should be used, as the freshly stripped bark acts as an irritant poison on the gastro-intestinal canal. The action of the bark becomes gradually less violent when kept for a length of time and more like that of rhubarb.

It is used as a gentle purgative in cases of chronic constipation and is principally given in the form of the fluid extract, in small doses, repeated three or four times daily, a decoction of 1 OZ. of the bark in 1 quart of water boiled down to a pint, may also be taken in tablespoonful doses.

Resources of the Southern Fields and Forests states:

RHAMNACEAE. (The Buckthorn Tribe.)

NEW JERSEY TEA TRKE; RED-HOOT, (Ceanothus Americanus, L.) Two varieties exist in the Southern States. Diffused in dry pine barrens; Richland; collected in St. John's; vicinity of Charleston ; Newbern. Fl. July. Lind. Nat. Syst. Bot. 108; Ferrein, Mat. Med. iii, 338; U. S. Disp. 1240; Ell. Bot. Med. Notes, 291; Mer. and de L. Diet, de M. Med. ii, 165; Boston Med. and Surg. Journal, 1835. See, also, the supplement to Mer. de L. Diet, de M. Med. 1846, 155. This plant possesses a considerable degree of astringency, and has been used in gonorrheal discharges. It is applied by the Cherokee doctors as a wash in cancer, and may be used wherever an astringent is likely to be useful. The Indians employed it in lues venerea, preferring it to lobelia; if the case was violent, the root of the blackberry (Rtibus villosiis) was mixed with it. Stearns' Am. Herbal, 97. Referring to its anti-syphilitie powers, Ferrein says : "Eue guerit aussi en moins de quinze jours, les veneriens los plus inveteres." It is not now supposed to be endowed with any very decided virtue in this respect. Dr.Hubbard prescribes it with advantage in the aphthous affections of infants, in malignant dysentery and in other maladies dependent upon debility; he usually combines with it a little borax. See Journal de Pharm. xxiii, 354. Mr. Tuomey, State Geologist, informs me that much use is made of it in domestic practice in Chesterfield District. An infusion of the leaves was employed during the war of independence as a substitute for tea. I have experimented with the leaves, and obtained a liquor somewhat resembling common tea, both in color and taste. It imparts to wool a fine, persistent, cinnamon, nankeen color. The above was included in my report on the Medical Botany of South Carolina, published in 1849. Since the beginning of the recent war I called the attention of our citizens to this plant as a substitute for foreign tea, in a brief communication, having again collected and used it, and induced others to do the same. I quote from this article: "Without any desire to exaggerate, I commend the substitute. It grows abundantly in our high pine ridges. The tea, prepared from this shrub, drawn as common tea, is certainly a good substitute for indifferent black tea. Properly dried and prepared, it is aromatic and not unpleasant. I am glad to report it as an article to be used in war times in place of a high-priced commodity, which, in every respect, it resembles, if it does not equal." Dr. John Bachman, also, at a later period (1802) directed attention to the plant, stating that he had used it for two months in his own family. The leaves should be carefully dried in the shade.

CAROLINA BUCJKTH0RN, (Frangola Caroliniana, Gray.) Mills, in his Statistics of South Carolina, states of Rhammus Carolinianus, that a purgative syrup is prepared from the berries; and of R. frangula, (Blackberry bearing alder,) that the bark dyes a yellow color, and that from a quarter to half an ounce of the inner bark boiled in small beer is a sharp purge; used as a certain purgative in constipation of the bowels of cattle.

King's American Dispensatory, 1898 tells us:

Action, Medical Uses, and Dosage.—Nausea, colicky pain, and violent emeto-catharsis are the effects produced by fresh frangula bark. When dried, however, it loses some of its acridity, and then acts as a purgative only. Both the alvine and renal discharges are colored dark-yellow by it. Narcotic symptoms have been produced by eating the berries and seeds, the toxic effects having been probably produced by the prussic acid contained in the seeds. The decoction has been administered in dropsies, and the same preparation as well as an ointment of the recent bark, has been used for the cure of itch. Its chief value, however, is as a laxative and cathartic, being quite popular for these effects with the Germans. It resembles senna and rhubarb in action, according to some, being harsher, but is regarded by Squibb as milder than either. It is a remedy for chronic constipation, from 1 to 3 doses of 20 minims of the fluid extract being administered in water in the course of a day. If desirable to evacuate the bowels at once, a fluid drachm may be given at bedtime. An elixir (4 parts of fluid extract to 12 parts of elixir of orange) may be given in from 1 to 2 fluid drachm doses; of the decoction (½ ounce of bark to ½ pint of water) the dose is a tablespoonful.

Plants for A Future states:

Medicinal use of Alder Buckthorn: Alder buckthorn has been used medicinally as a gentle laxative since at least the Middle Ages. The bark contains 3 - 7% anthraquinones, these act on the wall of the colon stimulating a bowel movement approximately 8 - 12 hours after ingestion. It is so gentle and effective a treatment when prescribed in the correct dosages that it is completely safe to use for children and pregnant women. The bark also contains anthrones and anthranols, these induce vomiting but the severity of their effect is greatly reduced after the bark has been dried and stored for a long time. The bark is harvested in early summer from the young trunk and moderately sized branches, it must then be dried and stored for at least 12 months before being used The inner bark is cathartic, cholagogue, laxative (the fresh bark is violently purgative), tonic, vermifuge. It is taken internally as a laxative for chronic atonic constipation and is also used to treat abdominal bloating, hepatitis, cirrhosis, jaundice, and liver and gall bladder complaints. It should be used with caution since excess doses or using the bark before it is cured can cause violent purging. Externally, the bark is used to treat gum diseases and scalp infestations, or as a lotion for minor skin irritations. The fruit is occasionally used, it is aperient without being irritating.

Peterson Field Guides Eastern and Central Medicinal Plants tells us of Carolina buckthorn, Rhamnus caroliniana:

American Indians used bark tea to induce vomiting; Also a strong laxative. Still used for constipation with nervous or muscular atony of intestines.

The Physicians Desk Reference for Herbal Medicine tells us:

Buckthorn: Buckthorn is used internally for Constipation and for bowel movement relief in cases of an anal fissures and hemorrhoids. It is used after recto-anal surgery and in preparation for diagnostic intervention in the gastrointestinal tract and to achieve a softer stool. Unproven uses: in folk medicine it is used as a diuretic in "blood purifying" remedies. Contraindications: Contraindicated in a intestinal obstruction, acute inflammatory intestinal diseases, appendicitis, and abdominal pain of unknown origin. Use during pregnancy or while nursing only after consulting a physician. The drug is not to be administered to children under 12 years of age

Fraxinus, Ash

Seventeen varieties of Ash are used medicinally: Fraxinus americana - White Ash, Fraxinus angustifolia - Narrow-Leaved Ash, Fraxinus bungeana - Xiao Ye Qin, Fraxinus excelsior, Fraxinus floribunda - Himalayan Ash, Fraxinus hookeri, Fraxinus chinensis, Fraxinus latifolia - Oregon Ash, Fraxinus longicuspis, Fraxinus nigra - Black Ash, Fraxinus sambucifolia, raxinus ornus - Manna Ash, Fraxinus pennsylvanica - Red Ash, Fraxinus quadrangulata - Blue Ash, Fraxinus texensis - Texas White Ash, Fraxinus velutina - Arizona Ash, Fraxinus xanthoxyloides

Only four Ashes grow in my region: Fraxinus americana (White Ash), Fraxinus caroliniana (Carolina Ash), Fraxinus pennsylvanica (Green Ash), Fraxinus profunda (Pumpkin Ash)

The bark of the ashes is astringent, like many trees. Taken as a decoction, it also has the effect of encouraging or increasing menstrual flow. Ash is also good for the liver and stomach, being a good bitter tonic for digestion. This bitter tonic is particularly good for stomach cramps. A soak in the infusion/tea made from Ash bark is good for cuts, scrapes and skin inflammations It has also been useful in getting rid of lice. The inner bark is a laxative. The leaves may be used as a poultice for sores and stings. Ash also has use in reducing fevers. Oddly enough, according to Plants for A Future, the seeds are thought to be an aphrodisiac. Ash may also help with painful urination and several women's issues, according to folk use.

Saint Hildegard von Bingen gave the following entry on Ash in Physica:

The Ash Tree is more hot than cold. It denoted counsel. If anyone is troubled by gitcht in his side or other part of his body, as if all his limbs were broken and bruised, cook the leaves of ash tree in water. Place the sick person, nude, in a linen cloth. Having poured off the water, place the warm, cooked leaves all around him, particularly on the place where he is ailing. Do this often, and he will be better.

If you want to prepare beer from oats, without hops, cook it only with groats, with many ash leaves added. The beer, when drunk, will purge the stomach and make the chest light and pleasant.

Saint Hildegard, it should be remembered, introduced hops to beer brewing. The next time you drink a beer, toast Saint Hildegard, without whom we would not have our ale and lager as we know it!

Gerard included Ash in his Herbal:

This tree is called in Greek, Melia, and of divers, Milea: in Latin, Fraxinus: in High Dutch, Eschernbaum, Eschernholtz, and Steynschern: in Low Dutch, Esschen, and Esschenboom: in Italian, Frassino: in French, Fresne: in Spanish, Fresno, Fraxino, and Freixo: in English, Ash tree.

The fruit like unto cods is called of the apothecaries, Lingua Avis, ["Bird's tongue"] and Lingua Passerina["Sparrow's tongue"]: it may be named in Greek, Ornithoglosson: yet some would have it called Orneoglossum; others make Ornus or the wild Ash to be called Orneoglossum: it is termed in English, Ash keys, and of some, Kite keys.

The Temperature and Virtues.

A. The leaves and bark of the Ash tree are dry and moderately hot: the seed is hot and dry in the second degree.

B. The juice of the leaves or the leaves themselves being applied, or taken with wine, cure the bitings of vipers, as Dioscorides saith.

C. The leaves of this tree are of so great virtue against serpents, as that they dare not so much as touch the morning and evening shadows of the tree, but shun them afar off, as Pliny reports, lib. 16. cap. 13. He also affirmeth, that the serpent being penned in with boughs laid round about, will sooner run into the fire, if any be there, than come near the boughs of the Ash: and that the Ash doth flower before the serpents appear, and doth not cast his leaves before they be gone again.

D. We write (saith he) upon experience, that if the serpent be set within the circle of a fire and the boughs, the serpent will sooner run into the fire than into the boughs. It is a wonderful courtesy in nature, that the Ash should flower before these serpents appear, and not cast his leaves before they be on again.

E. Both of them, that is to say the leaves and the bark, are reported to stop the belly: and being boiled with vinegar and water, do stay vomiting, if they be laid upon the stomach.

F. The leaves and bark of the Ash tree boiled in wine and drunk, do open the stoppings of the liver and spleen, and do greatly comfort them.

G. Three or four leaves of the Ash tree taken in wine each morning from time to time do make those lean that are fat, and keepeth them from feeding which do begin to wax fat.

H. The seed or kite-keys of the Ash tree provoke urine, increase natural seed, and stir up bodily lust, especially being powdered with nutmegs and drunk.

I. The wood is profitable for many things, being exalted by Homer's commendations, and Achilles' spear, as Pliny writeth. The shavings or small pieces thereof being drunk are said to be pernicious and deadly, as Dioscorides affirmeth.

K. The lye which is made with the ashes of the bark cureth the white scurf, and such other like roughness of the skin, as Pliny testifieth.

Culpepper said of Ash:

his is so well known, that time will be misspent in writing a description of it; and therefore I shall only insist upon the virtues of it.

Government and virtues. It is governed by the Sun; and the young tender tops, with the leaves, taken inwardly, and some of them outwardly applied, are singularly good against the biting of viper, adder, or any other venomous beast; and the water distilled therefrom being taken a small quantity every morning fasting, is a singular medicine for those that are subject to dropsy, or to abate the greatness of those that are too gross or fat. The decoction of the leaves in white wine helpeth to break the stone, and expel it, and cureth the jaundice. The ashes of the bark of the ash made into lee, and those heads bathed therewith, which are leprous, scabby, or scald, they are thereby cured. The kernals within the husks, commonly called ashen keys, prevail against stitches and pains in *the sides, proceeding of wind, and voideth away the stone by provoking urine.*

I can justly except against of all this, save only the first, viz. That ash-tree tops and leaves are good against the bitings of serpents and vipers. I suppose this had its rise from Gerrard or Pliny, both which hold, that there is such an antipathy between an adder and an ash-tree, that if an adder be encompassed round with ash-tree leaves, she will sooner run through the fire than through the leaves: The contrary to which is the truth, as both my eyes are witness. The rest are virtues something likely, only if it be in winter when you cannot get the leaves, you may safely use the bark instead of them. The keys you may easily keep all the year, gathering them when they are ripe.

Mrs. Grieves tells us:

The bark contains the bitter glucoside Fraxin, the bitter substance Fraxetin, tannin, quercetin, mannite, a little volatile oil, gum, malic acid, free and combined with calcium.

Ash bark has been employed as a bitter tonic and astringent, and is said to be valuable as an antiperiodic. On account of its astringency, it has been used, in decoction, extensively in the treatment of intermittent fever and ague, as a substitute for Peruvian bark. The decoction is odourless, though its taste is fairly bitter. It has been considered useful to remove obstructions of the liver and spleen, and in rheumatism of an arthritic nature.

A ley from the ashes of the bark was used formerly to cure scabby and leprous heads.

The leaves have diuretic, diaphoretic and purgative properties, and are employed in modern herbal medicine for their laxative action, especially in the treatment of gouty and rheumatic complaints, proving a useful substitute for Senna, having a less griping effect. The infusion of the leaves, 1 OZ. to the pint, may be given in frequent doses during the twenty-four hours.

The distilled water of the leaves, taken every morning, was considered good for dropsy and obesity.

A decoction of the leaves in white wine had the reputation of dissolving stone and curing jaundice.

The leaves should be gathered in June, well dried, powdered and kept in well corked bottles.

The leaves have been gathered to mix with tea and in some parts of the country are used to feed cattle, when grass is scarce in autumn, but when cows eat the leaves or shoots, the butter becomes rank.

The fruits of the different species of Ash are regarded as somewhat more active than the bark and leaves. Ash Keys were held in high reputation by the ancient physicians, being employed as a remedy for flatulence. They were also in more recent times preserved with salt and vinegar and sent to table as a pickle. Evelyn tells us: 'Ashen keys have the virtue of capers,' and they were often substituted for them in sauces and salads.

The keys will keep all the year round if gathered when ripe.

In Mexico, the bark and leaves of F. nigra (Marsh), the Black Swamp, Water Hoop or Basket Ash, are similarly employed to those of the Common Ash. In Mexico, also, the bark and leaves of F. lanceolata (Borch.), the Green or Blue Ash, are employed as a bitter tonic and the root as a diuretic.

In the United States, the bark of the American White Ash (F. Americana, Linn.) (F. acuminata, Lam.) finds similar employment. It has numerous small circular depressions externally and a slightly laminate structure.

There are many old superstitions concerning the tree. The ancient couplets connecting the flowering precedence of the Oak and Ash with the rainfall of the following summer, 'Oak choke, Ash splash,' etc., have no basis on fact.

According to another superstition, if the trunk of a sapling Ash were split and a ruptured child passed through, the sufferer would be cured.

The Ash had the reputation of magically curing warts: each wart must be pricked with a new pin that has been thrust into the tree, the pins are withdrawn and left in the tree, and the following charm is repeated:

'Ashen tree, ashen tree,

Pray buy these warts of me.'

And there was another superstition that if a live shrew mouse were buried in a hole bored in an Ash trunk and then plugged up a sprig of this Shrew Ash would cure the paralysis supposed to have been caused by a shrew creeping over the sick person's limbs.

Should one ever encounter a shrew creeping over one's body.. well, at least now, you know what to do about it!

An Irish Herbal states:

The leaves, bark and tender buds of the ash tree open up the liver, provoke urine and are useful against dropsy. The inward bark is given with success against fevers, and the wood, burnt into ashes, cures scabs and ringworm.

Brother Aloysius wrote of Ash:

Ash leaves are used medicinally. The infusion consists of 1 ½ to 2 ½ per 2 cups boiling water. Take two cups daily for gout or rheumatism. It also acts as a purgative. The decoction of the bark and the young wood, 2 to 3 tablespoons per 2 cups wine, is beneficial for blockages of the liver and spleen.

Resources of the Southern Fields and Forests states:

WHITE ASH, {Fraxinus Americana, L.) In the Southern States we have the white, red, green, blue and water ash. Wilson says that F. Americana differs in few respects from the English ash, F. excelsior, which in England is used for every conceivable purpose by the farmer, turner, cabinet-maker, wheelwright, and for firewood. " The bark of the tree is used for tanning calfskins, and for dyeing green, blue and black; the ashes of the trunk, root or branches are comparatively rich in potash." Coal was also made from it. The leaves of the F. Americana "are said to be so highly offensive to the rattlesnake that that formidable reptile is never found on land where it grows; and it is the practice of hunters and others having occasion to traverse the woods in the summer months to stuff their boots or shoes with white ash leaves as a preventative of the bite of the rattlesnake."

King's American Dispensatory, 1898 tells us:

Action, Medical Uses, and Dosage.—Tonic and astringent. An extract of the black ash used as a plaster is very valuable in salt-rheum and other cutaneous diseases. The infusion may be used internally as a tonic, and for all purposes where a combination of astringency with tonic influence is indicated. The white ash is also cathartic, and has been found beneficial in some cases of constipation, and also in dropsical affections. It may be used in the form of infusion or in bitters. The bark in white wine, is said to be efficient in curing ague-cake, or enlarged spleen. The seeds are said to prevent obesity. Dose of specific fraxinus, 10 to 60 drops.

Peterson Field Guides Eastern and Central Medicinal Plants tells us:

White or American ash Fraxinus americana: American Indians used inner bark tea as an emetic or strong laxative, to remove bile from intestines, as a tonic after childbirth, and to relieve stomach cramps, fevers; diuretic, promotes sweating, wash use for sores, itching, lice, snake bites. Inner bark chewed applied as a poultice to sores. Seeds thought to be aphrodisiac.

Botany In a Day states:

Ash is stimulating, diaphoretic, diuretic and laxative. Drink a tea of the inner bark for depression or tiredness; A strong tea for a laxative. A tea of the bark is used to reduce fever and to expel worms. A tea of the leaves is used as a laxative.

The Physicians Desk Reference for Herbal Medicines 3rd edition states of ash:

The main active principle is coumarin. Preparations of fresh ash bark showed an analgesic, antioxidative, and antiphlogistic action. Cyclo AMP phosphodiesterase is inhibited and antioxidative (radical trapping action) affect was proven for scopolotine, isofraxin, and fraxin. Preparations of ash leaf are used for arthritis, gout, bladder complaints, as well as, a laxative and diuretic. In folk medicine, ash leaf is internally used for fever, rheumatism, gout, edema, stones, constipation, stomach symptoms, and worm infestation; and for lower leg ulcers and wounds. Preparations of ash Barker used for fevers and as a tonic. Health risks or side effects following proper administration of design therapeutic dosages are not recorded.

Gleditsia triacanthos, Honey Locust

This tree is also mentioned under Black Locust, but is a different tree. Honey Locust is naturalized in my region. It is a tall and stately tree, that produces pods full of a sweet and nutritious pulp. It is very similar to carob, and these trees are the "pods" eaten by the prodigal son and the "wild locusts" that sustained John the Baptist in the Bible. Honey Locust is an extremely useful food tree and an often-overlooked source of natural sugar for beer brewing.

It is unknown whether Dioscorides wrote of Honey Locust or Carob under the name Keratia:

The pods (taken while they are fresh) are bad for the stomach and loosen the intestines, but dried they stop discharges of the bowels. They are also better for the stomach and diuretic, especially combined with the remains left after pressing out grapes.

Plants for A Future states:

Medicinal use of Honey Locust: The pods have been made into a tea for the treatment of indigestion, measles, catarrh etc. The juice of the pods is antiseptic. The pods have been seen as a good antidote for children's complaints. The alcoholic extract of the fruits of the honey locust, after elimination of tannin, considerably retarded the growth, up to 63% of Ehrlich mouse carcinoma. However, the cytotoxicity of the extract was quite high and the animals, besides losing weight, showed dystrophic changes in their liver and spleen. The alcoholic extract of the fruit exerted moderate oncostatic activity against sarcoma 180 and Ehrlich carcinoma at the total dose 350 mg/kg/body weight/mouse. Weight loss was considerable. An infusion of the bark has been drunk and used as a wash in the treatment of dyspepsia. It has also been used in the treatment of whooping cough, measles, smallpox etc. The twigs and the leaves contain the alkaloids gleditschine and stenocarpine. Stenocarpine has been used as a local anaesthetic whilst gleditschine causes stupor and loss of reflex activity. Current research is examining the leaves as a potential source of anticancer compounds.

Peterson Field Guides Eastern and Central Medicinal Plants states:

The seedpods of a Chinese species G sinensis are used in Chinese medicine for sore throats, asthmatic coughs, swelling, and stroke. Experimentally, seedpod causes the breakdown of red blood cells, is strongly antibacterial, antifungal, and acts as an expectorant, aiding in expelling phlegm and secretions of the respiratory tract. Minute amount of the seeds are taken in a powder for Constipation. The spines constitute another drug used in traditional Chinese medicine; they are users of wash to reduce swelling and disperse toxic matter, in the treatment of carbuncles and lesions. Early reports of cocaine in the plant have been discredited. Warning: all plant parts of both species contained potentially toxic compounds.

Gymnocladus dioica, Kentucky Coffee Tree

This naturalized tree is much like the locusts in bearing useful pods. It was an important tree in early America, for the "coffee" brewed from its seeds.

King's American Dispensatory, 1898 tells us:

Action, Medical Uses, and Dosage.—The tincture of the pulp and pods, and in some instances of the bark also, has been used with benefit in intermittent fever. More recently it has been tried, and with advantage, in cases of abnormal states of the nervous centers, as indicated, among other symptoms, by impaired sense of touch and vision, numbness, dull headache, apathy, and formication. In one case of locomotor ataxia it proved decidedly beneficial, and is valuable in some of the more serious symptoms resulting from excessive masturbation. Recent reports (Dr. N. G. Vassar) confirm its value as a remedy for spermatorrhoea. Prof. Roberts Bartholow,

M. D., investigated physiologically the purified tincture of the leaves as prepared for him by J. U. Lloyd and found it to be very marked in its qualities. It has likewise been recommended in laryngeal cough with chronic irritation of the mucous lining membrane of the air passages, in erysipelas, in all fevers presenting a typhoid condition, in puerperal peritonitis, and in the exanthematous affections. It is certainly deserving the attention of our practitioners. The tincture is best made by taking 2 ounces of the coarsely bruised seed and 1 ounce of the pulp, and adding to them 8 fluid ounces each of water and alcohol; let it macerate 12 or 14 days with frequent agitation, and then filter. One fluid drachm of this is to be added to 3 fluid ounces of water, of which the dose is a teaspoonful, to be repeated every 3 or 4 hours.

Plants for A Future States:

Medicinal use of Kentucky Coffee Tree: The pulverised root bark is used as an effective enema. A tea made from the bark is diuretic. It is used in the treatment of coughs due to inflamed mucous membranes and also to help speed up a protracted labour. A snuff made from the pulverized root bark has been used to cause sneezing in comatose patients. A tea made from the leaves and pulp from the pods is laxative and has also been used in the treatment of reflex troubles. A decoction of the fresh green pulp of the unripe fruit is used in homeopathic practice.

Peterson Field Guides Eastern and Central Medicinal Plants tells us:

Caramel like pod pulp used by American Indians to treat lunacy. Leaf and pulp tea formally employed for reflex troubles an as a laxative. Root bark tea used for coughs due to inflamed mucous membranes, diarrhetic, given to a childbirth in protracted labor, stops bleeding; Used in enemas for Constipation. Warning: toxic to grazing animals. Seeds contain toxic saponins.

Halesia, Silverbell

We have two Silverbells that are native to my region, but that is more than most folks have! Ours are Halesia tetraptera var. monticola (Mountain Silverbell) and Halesia tetraptera var. tetraptera (Common Silverbell).

I have not been able to find any historical info on their medicinal uses. However, the fruit is acidic and astringent. It is likely high in vitamin C, at the very least. The old timers used to pickle the fruit.

Hamamelis, Witch Hazel

Witch Hazel is one of our most important medicinal trees. Although it is still used commonly now, historically it was widely used. The Witch Hazel that grows in my region is simply, Hamamelis virginiana (American Witchhazel). This tree was widely used by Native Americans and was one of the first plants recognized by early settlers.

Mrs. Grieves was far more effusive in her description of the medicinal virtues of Witch Hazel:

The properties of the leaves and bark are similar, astringent, tonic, sedative, valuable in checking internal and external haemorrhage, most efficacious in the treatment of piles, a good pain-killer for the same, useful for bruises and inflammatory swellings, also for diarrhoea, dysentery and mucous discharges.

It has long been used by the North American Indians as poultices for painful swellings and tumours.

The decoction has been utilized for incipient phthisis, gleet, ophthalmia, menorrhagia and the debilitated state resultingfrom abortion.

A tea made of the leaves or bark may be taken freely with advantage, being good for bleeding of the stomach and in complaints of the bowels, and an injection of this tea is excellent for inwardly bleeding piles, the relief being marvellous and the cure speedy. An ointment made of 1 part fluid extract of bark to 9 parts simple ointment is also used as a local application, the concentration Hamamelin being also employed, mainly in the form of suppositories.

Witch Hazel has been supposed to owe its utility to an action on the muscular fibre of veins. The distilled extract from the fresh leaves and young twigs forms an excellent remedy for internal or external uses, being beneficial for bleeding from the lungs and nose, as well as from other internal organs. In the treatment of varicose veins, it should be applied on a lint bandage, which must be constantly kept moist: a pad of Witch Hazel applied to a burst varicose vein will stop the bleeding and often save life by its instant application.

Pond's Extract of Witch Hazel was much used in our grandmother's days as a general household remedy for burns, scalds, and inflammatory conditions of the skin generally and it is still in general use.

In cases of bites of insects and mosquitoes a pad of cotton-wool, moistened with the extract and applied to the spot will soon cause the pain and swelling to subside.

Diluted with warm water, the extract is used for inflammation of the eyelids.

Unfortunately, in modern times, Witch Hazel is seen as little more than a weedy shrub. That should certainly not be the case.

Resources of the Southern Fields and Forests tells us:

HAMAMELACE. {The Witch-Hazel Tribe)

This order, remarks Lindley, is found in the northern parts of North America, Japan and China. In my examination of the various authorities on the subject before me, I have frequently been struck with the correspondence prevailing between the species found in South Carolina and those of Japan, and this respects only the medical botany of the two; should the flora of each be compared, a still more universal relation might be established. Professor Agassiz has noticed something of the same kind existing between the fossil botany and the fauna of each. WITCH-HAZEL, {Hamamelis Virginica, L.) Grows along pine land bays; collected in St. John's, Charleston District ; vicinity of Charleston, Bach.; N. C.62 Mer. and de L. Diet, de M. Med. iii, 452; Coxo, Am. Disp. 310; U. S. Disp.

1258; Matson's Yeg. Pract. 201; Griffith's Med. Bot. 350 ; Eatinesque, Med. Flor. i, 227. It is said to be sedative, astringent, tonic and discutient. The bark was a remedy derived from the Indians, who applied it to painful tumors, using the decoction as a wash in inflammatory swellings, painful hemorrhoidal affections and ophthalmias. A cataplasm, and a tea of the leaves, as an astringent, were employed in hematemesis. The steam practitioners also administer it in irritable hemorrhoids, and during the bearing-down pains attending child-birth. No analysis has been made, but as it probably contains sedative and astringent principles, attention is directed to it. The curious reader may consult, besides the paper in Hutton's "Mathematics," on the wonderful properties of the witch-hazel in detecting water, a recent one in Patent Office Report on Agriculture, p. 16, 1851. This is from Prarie du Chien, by Mr. Alfred Burnson, and contains some remarkable statements of the certainty of finding water by divining rods. Some electrical and telluric influences are hinted at— Credat Judaeus! Persons living in the up-per districts of South Carolina assume to use the rod with success. Dr. James Fountain, of Peokskill, N, Y., speaks highly of the efficacy of the bark in hemorrhage of the lung and stomach, and also as one of the best applications for external piles, an ointment being prepared from lard, and a decoction of equal parts of this bark, white oak bark and that of the apple tree. He believes the witch-hazel to possess anodyne properties. (N. Y. J. Med. X, 208.) Dr. N. S. Davis in his report (Trans. Am. Med. Assoc, i, 350,) agrees with Dr. Fountain in his estimate of this remedy, which he has complied in the form of a decoction, made with one ounce to a pint of water; dose, a wine glass full every three to eight hours in incipient phthisis. U. S. Disp.,12th Ed. In the Eichmond Journal for January 1868, is an article from the Atlanta Med. and Surg. Journ. (1867,) in which Dr. W, W. Durham claims for this plant properties similar to those said by Dr. Phares to be those of the Viburnum prunifolium, and which tend to confirm opinions expressed above by Prof Davis and others. In reference to its power of preventing abortion or miscarriage, Dr. Durham says: "At one period of my practice the negroes used the cotton root so frequently to produce abortion, that my supply of black haw became exhausted, and having heard of this power of the hazel to affect the purpose for which I used the haw, I resorted to it (the hazel) with perfect success. Having only used it for the purpose of preventing abortion, from the effects of the cotton root, I cannot speak of it in other cases." He makes a decoction of one pint of the leaves to one pint of water, which is administered freely. See also Viburnum prunifolium. Dr. Joseph Bates, in an article on the Witch-hazel, published in Tilden's " Journ. of Mat. Med," February 1868, furnishes an analysis of this plant by Dr. A. Lee. (See J. of Mat. Med. 2, p. 200.) The bark contains organic and inorganic matter, allumen gum, extractive, tannin, a particular (bitter) principle, resin, starch, etc. Dr. Lee observes: " The great amount of tannin contained in this plant is worthy of notice; while the sumach contains three hundred and twenty-five and geranium one hundred and thirty-six parts in seven thousand, the hazel contains no less than four hundred." This is an important statement and deserves attention. In the Boston Med. J. Surg. J., v, 37, p. 348, is an account of the efficacy of this plant in arresting hemorrhages—the leaves being chewed and the juice swallowed. Tilden & (Co. prepare a fluid extract which may- be given in doses of one to two drachms. By means of this an infusion or a wash may be made by mixing with water in the proportion of one ounce to a pint.

*** Note: The mention of Cotton Root Bark as an abortifacient was once common folklore. According to the late herbalist, Michael Moore, this herb has since been discredited in use for such purpose, although it may enhance the potential of uterine contractions and should not be used during pregnancy. It is also noteworthy that this document contains an early description of "dowsing", a mysterious Appalachian tradition of finding water.

The Thomsonian System of Medicine states:

WITCH-HAZEL. Hamamelis Virginica. (Dr. Thomson.)

I found the use of this article as medicine when I was quite young, and have made much use of it in all my practice. It is too well known in the country to need any description; is a small tree or bush, and grows very common, especially in new lands. A tea made of the leaves is an excellent medicine in many complaints, and may be freely used to advantage. It is the best thing for bleeding at the stomach of any article I have ever found, either by giving the tea made of the dry leaves, or chewing them when green ; have cured several with it. This complaint is caused by canker eating off the small blood vessels, and this medicine will remove the canker and stop the bleeding. I have made much use of the tea, made strong for injection, and found it in all complaints of the bowels to be very serviceable. An injection made of this tea, with a little of No. 2, is good for the piles, and many complaints common to females ; and in bearing-down pains it will afford immediate relief, if properly administered. These leaves may be used in No. 3 to good advantage, as a substitute for either of the other articles, or alone for the same purpose.

The leaves and twigs are a pleasant, reliable, mild, soothing, diffusive, stimulating, astringent tonic. It chiefly influences the mucous membrane.

Locally it is used in gonorrhoea, and in gleet. The distilled, non-alcoholic extract is the best for this purpose. In the treatment of gonorrhoea it gives the best of results and no urethral contractions follow its use. In leucorrhoea it stimulates and tones the uterus and vagina. In dysentery and diarrhoea it may be used alone or in conjunction with other remedies as per Dr. Thomson's instructions.

It is a very good remedy in hemorrhages, either rectal, cystic or uterine.

It is valuable in the treatment of catarrh in any part of the system, whether vaginal or nasal. To the nose it can be applied with Nebulizer or anatomizer and to the womb on cotton.

It is of use in the treatment of prolapsus ani and in rectal hemorrhages. Is of use in sore eyes as a wash as it has no bad effect on the eyes. This remedy is indicated in all sores or bleeding surfaces, no matter what their nature may be. By bearing this in mind, the physician can make no mistake. It is also indicated in all irritations, but this comes properly under the heading of sores. The dose of the Tincture is from 30 to 60 minims. The use of this remedy leaves absolutely no ill effects.

King's American Dispensatory, 1898 tells us:

Action, Medical Uses, and Dosage.—Witch-hazel is tonic and astringent. Some have pronounced it sedative also. The decoction of the bark is very useful in hemoptysis, hematemesis, and other hemorrhages, as well as in diarrhoea, dysentery, and excessive mucous discharges, with full, pale, and relaxed tissues. It has been employed with advantage in incipient phthisis; in which it is supposed to unite anodyne influences with its others. It is useful in the form of poultice in swellings and tumors of a painful character, as well as in external inflammations. The American Indians used it for this purpose. The decoction maybe advantageously used as a wash or injection for sore mouth, painful tumors, external inflammations, bowel complaints, prolapsus ani and uteri, leucorrhoea, gleet, and ophthalmia.

Since the introduction of the distilled extract of witch-hazel and the specific hamamelis, the use of decoctions of the bark has been largely abandoned. The fluid extract has but little to recommend it. The articular field for hamamelis is in disorders involving the venous structures. Its most pronounced virtue is its stimulating and tonic action upon the venous coats, exhibited so markedly in its power over varicoses, hemorrhoids, hemorrhages, and other conditions due to relaxation of venous structures. The parts are usually pale and relaxed, though occasionally a deep redness, due to venous engorgement, is observed. Here, and especially as great pain is usually an accompaniment, belladonna may be associated with it. It is adapted to the whole venous system, overcoming debility, differing therein from such agents as act only upon localized vascular areas.

Prof. J. M. Scudder and others have found witch-hazel a valuable remedy in passive hemorrhages and congestion, especially in epistaxis, hemorrhoids, phlegmasia dolens (after acute phases have passed away), phlebitis, and varicose veins. He also found it valuable in diarrhoea, in chronic pharyngitis, and in chronic uterine congestion, where the cervix is enlarged without abnormal hardness, the os uteri being soft, open, and patulous, and perhaps leucorrhoea and some prolapsus present. It is specially adapted to diarrhoea with a tendency to or associated with passive hemorrhage. It also forms an excellent application to chronic vascular conditions of mucous tissues, and to old, flabby, fetid ulcers. Prof. A. J. Howe stated that in "several cases of uterine hemorrhage, all occurring within 2 years, he administered witch-hazel with success. In some instances, the cause of the flow, and the conditions upon which it depended, were unknown or rested on conjecture, yet the exhibition of the medicine was always followed by satisfactory results." Half-teaspoonful doses of specific hamamelis were mixed with water and repeated every few minutes while the flow lasted, and afterward every few hours to prevent a return of the hemorrhage. In menorrhagia and those wasting states so common after abortion, in the early months of pregnancy, he used no remedy that exerted such beneficial effects as witch-hazel. In uterine hemorrhage following delivery at full term, the remedy is *probably not equal to ergot, but in the kind of cases referred to it is a safer agent. In chronic diarrhoea and cholera infantum it is a valuable medicine. Hamamelis, both internally and topically, arrests oozing of blood from mucous surfaces. This action is well shown in non-inflammatory hematuria. It is not the remedy for active hemorrhage, but for passive bleeding, as from the lungs, stomach, bowels, renal or genital organs its action is satisfactory.*

Besides its control over actual hematuria hamamelis is often serviceable in renal affections due chiefly to vascular relaxation. Thus in diabetes insipidus it has been of some value, but it is of greater service in mucous profluvia of the urino-genital tract. It is of benefit in vesical catarrh, with tenesmus, and in irritation of the bladder, due to enlarged and relaxed scrotal veins. It should be used both internally and locally to the scrotum. While it relieves varicocele, too much must not be expected of it in the way of a cure. In female disorders it is indicated by venous fullness and relaxation. Dull, aching, ovarian pain is relieved by hamamelis, and in leucorrhoea, with fullness of the pelvic veins and relaxation of the uterine and vaginal walls, its internal and external exhibition is of marked benefit. It relieves ovarian and testicular congestion. Hamamelis is of pronounced value in hemorrhages into the eye ball, and locally relieves ecchymosis of the lids and conjunctiva.

Hamamelis is justly popular as a remedy for sprains, contusions, wounds, swellings, etc. A solution of a few grains of asepsin in distilled hamamelis forms an elegant and efficient dressing for burns, scalds, cuts, abrasions, crushed fingers, etc. Ten grains of menthol to 4 fluid ounces of distilled hamamelis are also efficient in burns and scalds (Ellingwood). Glycerin and hamamelis, or Lloyd's hydrastis and hamamelis, equal parts, has rendered us excellent service in irritated and inflammatory conditions of the external auditory meatus, especially when due to irritation from the presence of inspissated cerumen. Locally, hamamelis forms an excellent soothing application for chafing, due to excessive discharges; it is likewise useful in diffusive cutaneous inflammations. Few agents are more grateful in various subacute forms of sore throat, also in sore throat with deep redness and great pain, and it is particularly soothing in scarlatinal angina. It is a very valuable aid, locally, in the treatment of tonsilitis, phlegmonous ulceration of the throat, diphtheria, and acute catarrh. Chronic conjunctivitis, with vascularity of the palpebral and ocular conjunctiva, has yielded to a decoction of equal parts of hamamelis (bark), hydrastis, and lobelia, boiling the first two ingredients, and adding the lobelia to the hot liquid. Cover, allow to cool and strain. Hamamelis should not be neglected as a part of the treatment of inflamed breasts, and applied hot it gives great relief to the soreness of abdominal muscles and pelvic parts following childbirth. Muscular soreness and aching sensations, as of having been bruised, whether from colds, exposures, strains, bruises, or severe muscular action, are greatly relieved by the application of distilled hamamelis, either hot or cold, by means of compresses, while specific hamamelis may be given internally. It forms a good face wash for burning of the skin, for tan and freckles, for dilated facial capillaries, and a good application after shaving. Distilled hamamelis and Lloyd's colorless hydrastis form a safe and efficient injection for most cases of gonorrhoea. Witch-hazel enters into many of the ointments designed for application to piles. An ointment made with lard and a decoction of white oak bark, apple-tree bark, and witch-hazel has been successfully employed for this purpose. Dose of decoction of witch-hazel, from 2 to 4 fluid ounces, 3 or 4 times a day; of distilled hamamelis, 5 to 60 drops; of specific hamamelis, 1 to 30 drops.

Specific Indications and Uses.—Venous debility, with relaxation and fullness; pale mucous tissues (occasionally deep-red from venous engorgement, or deep-blue from venous stasis); mucous profluvia, with venous relaxation; passive hemorrhages; varicoses; capillary stasis; hemorrhoids, with full feeling; relaxed and painful sore throat; dull, aching pain in rectum, pelvis, or female organs; perineal relaxation, with fullness; muscular relaxation; muscular soreness and aching and bruised sensation, whether from cold, exposure, bruises, strains, or from physical exertion.

Plants for a Future states:

Witch hazel bark is a traditional herb of the North American Indians who used it to heal wounds, treat tumours, eye problems etc. A very astringent herb, it is commonly used in the West and is widely available from both herbalists and chemists. It is an important ingredient of proprietary eye drops, skin creams, ointments and skin tonics. It is widely used as an external application to bruises, sore muscles, varicose veins, haemorrhoids, sore nipples, inflammations etc. The bark is astringent, haemostatic, sedative and tonic. Tannins in the bark are believed to be responsible for its astringent and haemostatic properties. Bottled witch hazel water is a steam distillate that does not contain the tannins from the shrub, this is less effective in its action than a tincture. The bark is used internally in the treatment of diarrhoea, colitis, dysentery, haemorrhoids, vaginal discharge, excessive menstruation, internal bleeding and prolapsed organs. Branches and twigs are harvested for the bark in the spring. An infusion of the leaves is used to reduce inflammations, treat piles, internal haemorrhages and eye inflammations. The leaves are harvested in the summer and can be dried for later use. A homeopathic remedy is made from fresh bark. It is used in the treatment of nosebleeds, piles and varicose veins.

Botany In a Day states:

Hamamelis, witch Hazel: the seeds are reported to be addable, but there is some question about the validity of this claim. Medicinally, the leaves and bark contain tannic acid. Witch Hazel has long been used as an astringent in the typical ways, internally for sore throat and diarrhea, externally for stings, minor burns, and hemorrhoids. Native Americans used a tea of the leaves as a liniment for athletes.

The Physicians' Desk Reference for Herbal Medicine tells us:

The tannins and tannin elements have an astringent, anti-inflammatory and locally hemostatic effect. Indications and usage approved by Commission E: hemorrhoids, inflammation of the mouth and pharynx (leaf only), inflammation of the skin, venous conditions, wounds and burns. Unproven uses: witch hazel leaf and bark are used internally in folk medicine for nonspecific diarrhea such as inflammation of the mucous membrane of the large intestine and colon, hematemesis, hemoptysis and also for menstrual complaints. Efficacy in the treatment of diarrhea seems plausible because of the tannin content. Witch hazel is used externally for minor injuries the skin, localized inflamed swellings of the skin and mucous membranes, hemorrhoids and varicose veins. It is also used in folk medicine for inflammation of the mucosa of the colon. Precautions and adverse reactions: health risks following the proper administration of designated therapeutic dosages are not recorded if taken internally, the tannin content of the drug can lead to digestive complaints. Liver damage is conceivable following a long term administration, but rare.

Hibiscus syriacus, Rose of Sharon

Rose of Sharon is really more of a bush or shrub. It is a beautiful, old fashioned landscaping plant. Its scent and sight brings back childhood memories of my grandparent's and great grandparent's farms. This shrub is in the mallow family and is very useful.

Plants for A Future States;

Medicinal use of Rose of Sharon: The leaves are diuretic, expectorant and stomachic. A decoction of the flowers is diuretic, ophthalmic and stomachic. It is also used in the treatment of itch and other skin diseases, dizziness and bloody stools accompanied by much gas. The bark contains several medically active constituents, including mucilage, carotenoids, sesquiterpenes and anthocyanidins. A decoction of the root bark is antiphlogistic, demulcent, emollient, febrifuge, haemostatic and vermifuge. It is used in the treatment of diarrhoea, dysentery, abdominal pain, leucorrhoea, dysmenorrhoea and dermaphytosis.

Hovenia dulcis, Japanese Raisin Tree

This oddly named tree is naturalized in my region. It is so called, because of its fruit. The fruit is rarely eaten in our country, but there is no reason why this should be, other than ignorance.. the Latin name, "dulcis" indicates that the fruit is sweet..

Plants for A Future states:

Medicinal use of Japanese Raisin Tree: Antispasmodic, febrifuge, laxative. The fruit is antispasmodic, febrifuge, laxative and diuretic. The seeds are diuretic and are used in the treatment of alcohol overdose. The seeds are used to relieve intoxication due to wine. The stem bark is used in the treatment of rectal diseases.

Edible parts of Japanese Raisin Tree: Fruit - raw or cooked. They can be dried when they have the sweet flavour and texture of raisins and can be used similarly. The fruit is sweet and fragrant with a pear-like flavour. Dry and sub-acid. It is not a true fruit but a swollen receptacle. The fruit is up to 3cm long, it contains 11.4% glucose, 4.7% fructose and 12.6% sucrose. A sweet extract of the seed, boughs and young leaves is used as a substitute for honey. The seed contains 15% protein and 7.8% fat.

Ilex, Holly

Twenty-one varieties of Holly have been used medicinally: Ilex aculeolate, Ilex aquifolium, Ilex asprolla, Ilex cassine – Cassine, Ilex coriacea - Large Gallberry, Ilex cornuta - Horned Holly, Ilex crenata - Japanese Holly, Ilex glabra – Inkberry, Ilex chapaensis, Ilex integra - Mochi Tree, Ilex latifolia – Tarajo, Ilex macropoda, Ilex opaca - American Holly, Ilex pedunculosa, Ilex pubescens, Ilex purpurea, Ilex rotunda, Ilex verticillata - Winterberry Synonym: Prinos verticillatus, Ilex vomitoria - Yaupon Holly, Ilex x altaclerensis, Ilex yunnanensis

Eleven Hollys grow in my region: Ilex ambigua (Carolina Holly), Ilex amelanchier (Sarvis Holly), Ilex cassine var. cassine (Dahoon), Ilex collina (Long-stalked Holly), Ilex coriacea (Large Gallberry, Big Gallberry), Ilex decidua (Possumhaw, Deciduous Holly), Ilex longipes (Georgia Holly), Ilex montana (Mountain Holly, Mountain Winterberry), Ilex myrtifolia (Myrtle Dahoon), Ilex opaca var. opaca (American Holly), Ilex vomitoria (Yaupon)

Although rarely used now, Holly was once a much more popular medicinal.

Gerard described the virtues of Holly as:

A. They are good against the colic: for ten or twelve being inwardly taken bring away by the stool thick phlegmatic humours, as we have learned of them who oftentimes made trial thereof,

B. The birdlime which is made of the bark hereof is no less hurtful than that of Mistletoe, for it is marvellous clammy, it glueth up all the entrails, it shutteth and draweth together the guts and passages of the excrements, and by this means it bringeth destruction to man, not by any quality, but by his glueing substance.

C. Holly beaten to powder and drunk is an experimented medicine against all the fluxes of the belly, as the dysentery and such like.

Culpepper wrote of Holly:

For to describe a tree so well known is needless.

Government and virtues. The tree is Saturnine. The berries expel wind, and therefore are held to be profitable in the cholic. The berries have a strong faculty with them; for if you eat a dozen of them in the morning fasting when they are ripe and not dried, they purge the body of gross and clammy phlegm: but if you dry the berries, and beat them into powder, they bind the body, and stop fluxes, bloody-fluxes, and the terms in women. The bark of the tree, and also the leaves, are excellently good, being used in fomentations for broken bones, and such members as are out of joint. Pliny saith, the branches of the tree defend houses from lightning, and men from witchcraft.

Mrs. Grieves includes much on the traditional use of Holly in England in her Modern Herbal:

Holly, the most important of the English evergreens, forming one of the most striking objects in the wintry woodland, with its glossy leaves and clusters of brilliant scarlet berries, is in the general mind closely connected with the festivities of Christmas, having been from very early days in the history of these islands gathered in great quantities for Yuletide decorations, both of the Church and of the home. The old Christmas Carols are full of allusions to Holly:

.......'Christmastide

Comes in like a bride,

With Holly and Ivy clad.'

Christmas decorations are said to be derived from a custom observed by the Romans of sending boughs, accompanied by other gifts, to their friends during the festival of the Saturnalia, a custom the early Christians adopted. In confirmation of this opinion, a subsequent edict of the Church of Bracara has been quoted, forbidding Christians to decorate their houses at Christmas with green boughs at the same time as the pagans, the Saturnalia commencing about a week before Christmas. The origin has also been traced to the Druids, who decorated their huts with evergreens during winter as an abode for the sylvan spirits. In old church calendars we find Christmas Eve marked *templa exornantur* (churches are decked), and the custom is as deeply rooted in modern times as in either pagan or early Christian days.

An old legend declares that the Holly first sprang up under the footsteps of Christ, when He trod the earth, and its thorny leaves and scarlet berries, like drops of blood, have been thought symbolical of the Saviour's sufferings, for which reason the tree is called 'Christ's Thorn' in the languages of the northern countries of Europe. It is, perhaps, in connexion with these legends that the tree was called the Holy Tree, as it is generally named by our older writers. Turner, for instance, refers to it by this name in his Herbal published in 1568. Other popular names for it are Hulver and Holme, and it is still called Hulver in Norfolk, and Holme in Devon, and Holme Chase in one part of Dartmoor.

Pliny describes the Holly under the name of Aquifolius, needle leaf, and adds that it was the same tree called by Theophrastus Crataegus, but later commentators deny this. Pliny tells us that Holly if planted near a house or farm, repelled poison, and defended it from lightning and witchcraft, that the flowers cause water to freeze, and that the wood, if thrown at any animal, even without touching it, had the property of compelling the animal to return and lie down by it.

Holly leaves were formerly used as a diaphoretic and an infusion of them was given in catarrh, pleurisy and smallpox. They have also been used in intermittent fevers and rheumatism for their febrifugal and tonic properties, and powdered, or taken in infusion or decoction, have been employed with success where Cinchona has failed, their virtue being said to depend on a bitter principle, an alkaloid named Ilicin. The juice of the fresh leaves has been employed with advantage in jaundice.

The berries possess totally different qualities to the leaves, being violently emetic and purgative, a very few occasioning excessive vomiting soon after they are swallowed, though thrushes and blackbirds eat them with impunity. They have been employed in dropsy; also, in powder, as an astringent to check bleeding.

From the bark, stripped from the young shoots and suffered to ferment, birdlime is made. The bark is stripped off about midsummer and steeped in clean water; then boiled till it separates into layers, when the inner green portion is laid up in small heaps till *fermentation ensues. After about a fortnight has elapsed, it becomes converted into a sticky, mucilaginous substance, and is pounded into a paste, washed and laid by again to ferment. It is then mixed with some oily matter, goosefat being preferred, and is ready for use. Very little, however, is now made in this country. In the north of England, Holly was formerly so abundant in the Lake District, that birdlime was made from it in large quantities and shipped to the East Indies for destroying insects.*

The leaves of Holly have been employed in the Black Forest as a substitute for tea. Paraguay Tea, so extensively used in Brazil, is made from the dried leaves and young shoots of another species of Holly (Ilex Paraguayensis), growing in South America, an instance of the fact that similar properties are often found in more than one species of the same genus.

An Irish Herbal states:

The berries have a hot nature and it is believed that five of them when eaten relieve cholic and act as a purgative.

Resources of the Southern Fields and Forests states:

Holly (Ilex Opaca').—The bark of the holly root chewed, or a tea made with it, yields an excellent bitter demulcent, very useful in coughs, colds, etc. The bitter principle is also tonic. The Holly contains bird-lime.

King's American Dispensatory, 1898 tells us:

Action, Medical Uses, and Dosage.—Holly leaves are tonic and febrifuge; said to be very efficient in the treatment of intermittent fevers, in doses of 60 grains of their powder administered 1 or 2 hours previous to the chill. The infusion has also proved beneficial in icterus, pleuritis, catarrh, variola, arthritis, etc. The berries are said to be emeto-cathartic and cholagogue; from 8 to 15 of them will act as a hydragogue. According to Dr. Rousseau, ilicin acts decidedly upon the spleen, liver, and pancreas, producing a sedative effect, and is a cheap substitute for quinine. Its dose is 10 grains in pill form, gradually increased to 30 grains.

Brother Aloysius wrote of Holly:

The white flowers grow in racemes along the stems, they are followed by the red berries, with a strongly purgative effect. The leaves are used medicinally. The decoction of holly, consisting of 1/3rd to ½ cup per 2 cups water, is used for gout, colic and fever. Take 1 cup daily. The fruit also has medicinal use. If 10 to 12 berries are taken, they will have a very purgative effect and are a very powerful remedy for colic. The leaves should be gathered at the beginning of the flowering period.

The Rodale Herb book states, "The leaves and berries are used for medicinal purposes. The leaves are astringent and are used in fevers and rheumatism. The berries are used in dropsy."

Plants for A Future says of American Holly:

The berries are laxative, emetic and diuretic. They are used in the treatment of children's diarrhoea, colic and indigestion. A tea made from the leaves has been used as a treatment for measles, colds etc. The leaves have also been used externally in the treatment of sore eyes, sore and itchy skin. A tea made from the bark was once used in the treatment of malaria and epilepsy. It has also been used as a wash for sore eyes and itchy skin.

Of particular interest is the unfortunately named Ilex vomitoria, which fortunately is more commonly called Yaupon Holly. Yaupon received its Latin name due to the practice of some Native American tribes, who made a strong tea of the leaves and drank it ceremonially until they vomited. The leaves of Yaupon contain caffeine. In fact, Yaupon Holly is North America's only native caffeinated "tea". Yaupon tea is very similar to imported black tea (Camellia sinensis) and is considered to be of superior flavor by many of its adherents. To many Americans, Yaupon Holly is merely a weedy shrub, and often a nuisance. Were more to know its value as a tea, it might be seen as a valuable crop, especially in light of costs and concerns over chemical use in the growing and production of imported tea.

Ilex cornuta (Horned Holly) has been widely naturalized in my region. Plants for A Future States:

Medicinal use of Horned Holly: The whole plant is abortifacient, carminative, contraceptive, febrifuge and tonic. It particularly strengthens the back and knees. The leaf is made into a tea which is said to be contraceptive if used by women and is also used for termination pregnancies. The stem bark is tonic. The whole plant is used in the treatment of arthritis, recurring fever in pulmonary tuberculosis, tubercular lymph nodes, joint pained and lumbago.

Peterson Field Guides Eastern and Central Medicinal Plants tells us,

American Indians chewed berries for colic, indigestion. Leaf tea for measles, colds, flu, pneumonia; drops for sore eyes; Externally, for sores, itching. Thick syrup of berries formerly used to treat children's diarrhea. Chewing only 10 to 12 berries acts as a strong laxative, emetic, and diuretic. Bark tea once used in malaria and epilepsy. Warning: fruits considered poisonous, induced violent vomiting.

Juglans, Walnut

Sixteen varieties of Walnut have been noted for their medicinal value: Juglans ailanthifolia - Japanese Walnut, Juglans ailanthifolia cordiformis - Heartseed Walnut, Juglans californica - California Walnut, Juglans cathayensis - Chinese Walnut, Juglans cinerea, Juglans hindsii - Hind's Black Walnut, Juglans intermedia, Juglans major - Arizona Walnut, Juglans mandschurica - Manchurian Walnut, Juglans microcarpa - Texas Walnut, Juglans nigra - Black Walnut, Juglans regia, Juglans regia fallax, Juglans regia kamaonia, Juglans sinensis, Juglans x bisbyi – Buartnut

Only two Walnuts are native to my region: Juglans cinerea (Butternut) and Juglans nigra (Black Walnut)

Among the most regal and historied of these medicinal trees is the Juglandaceae, the Walnut family…. Walnuts, black walnuts, pecans and hickories. Although some members of the family have more specific actions or are stronger in one regard than another, I will generalize these under "Walnuts".

The properties of Walnuts are many, and not the least of these are the delicious and nutritious nuts. Walnuts are rich in protein, omega 3 and omega 6 fatty acids, ALA, copper, folic acid, manganese, B-6, vitamin E and a variety of other antioxidants and useful substances. Our herbalist ancestors, though, who subscribed to "The Doctrine of Signatures" (a school of thought that an herb's usefulness may be indicated by the similarity of its appearance to a corresponding body part or visible illness) would certainly have noticed the similarity between the nut and the human brain. William Cole, an exponent of the doctrine of signatures, says in Adam in Eden, 1657:

Wall-nuts have the perfect Signature of the Head: The outer husk or green Covering, represent the Pericranium, or outward skin of the skull, whereon the hair groweth, and therefore salt made of those husks or barks, are exceeding good for wounds in the head. The inner wooddy shell hath the Signature of the Skull, and the little yellow skin, or Peel, that covereth the Kernell, of the hard Meninga and Pia-mater, which are the thin scarfes that envelope the brain. The Kernel hath the very figure of the Brain, and therefore it is very profitable for the Brain, and resists poysons; For if the Kernel be bruised, and moystned with the quintessence of Wine, and laid upon the Crown of the Head, it comforts the brain and head mightily.

The medicinal properties of the Walnut are not in the nut alone, however. The husk, shell, leaves and bark all have their uses. The Lost Book of Herbal Remedies states, "Black walnut is an anti-inflammatory, anti-fungal, antiviral, astringent, emetic, laxative, painkiller, and vermifuge. The green hulls are more potent than the mature black hulls...."

Saint Hildegard, von Bingen recommend:

...take the leaves of this tree while they are fresh. Squeeze the juice from them onto the place where maggots are eating a person, or where maggots or other worms are growing on him. Do this frequently, and they will die. But, if worms are originating in his stomach, he should take the leaves of the walnut tree, with equal amount of peach tree leaves, before their fruits are ripe, and pulverize them over a fiery hot stone. He should eat this powder

often, either with an egg , or in broth, or cooked in a bit of cereal. The worms in his stomach will die.

If leprosy has begun to grow on someone, squeeze the juice from these leaves and add old fat to it, making an ointment. When the leprosy is still new on him, he should anoint himself with this, near the fire. Without a doubt he will be healed, unless God does not wish it.

One who has much phlegm in him should take that which exudes from the walnut tree when its branches or rootstock are cut. He should cook it gently in wine with fennel and a little savory, strain it through a cloth, and often drink it warm. It will throw off phlegm, and he will be cleared out.

One who has bad scabies on his head should take the outer skin of the walnut, that is its shell, and squeeze its juice over the wounds, that is over the scabies on his head. When they have swollen up from the bitterness of the juice, he should anoint them with olive oil, which will check the bitterness. If he does this often, the scabies will be cured.

John Gerard, the great herbalist, was a collector and grower of most any plant he could acclimate to the English climate. His gardens may have provided inspiration for William Shakespeare (believed to be a neighbor and friend), and likely provided much inspiration for those wonderful plays and poems full of woodland scenes and plant lore. Surely, the two knew much of the grand English Walnut and its uses. Of Walnut, Gerard wrote:

Dry nuts taken fasting with a fig and a little Rue withstand poison, prevent and preserve the body from the infection of the plague, and being plentifully eaten they drive worms forth of the belly. The green and tender nuts boiled in sugar and eaten as succade, are a most pleasant and delectable meat, comfort the stomach, and expel poison. The oil of walnuts made in such manner as oil of almonds, maketh smooth the hands and face, and taketh away scales or scurf, black and blue marks that come of stripes or bruises. Milk made of the kernels, as almond milk is made, cooleth and pleaseth the appetite of the languishing sick body. With onions, salt, and honey, they are good against the biting of a mad dog or man, if they be laid upon the wound....The outward green husk of the nuts hath a notable binding faculty.... The leaves and

133

first buds have a certain binding quality, as the same author showeth; yet there doth abound in them an hot and dry temperature. Some of the later physicians use these for baths and lotions for the body, in which they have a force to digest and also to procute sweat.

Being an herbal historian, Gerard also included, "Being both eaten, and also applied, they heal in short time, as Dioscorides saith, gangrenes, carbuncles, ægilops, and the pilling away of the hair: this also is effectually done by the oil that is pressed out of them, which is of thin parts, digesting and heating. Galen devised and taught to make of the juice thereof a medicine for the mouth, singular good against all inflammations thereof."

Culpepper believed Walnuts to be useful for dog bites (although I would not suggest them for rabies, unless there was no other treatment available!), and for other venoms and poisons:

...if they' [the leaves] be taken with onions, salt, and honey, they help the biting of a mad dog, or the venom or infectious poison of any beast, etc. Caius Pompeius found in the treasury of Mithridates, King of Pontus, when he was overthrown, a scroll of his own handwriting, containing a medicine against any poison or infection; which is this: Take two dry walnuts, and as many good figs, and twenty leaves of rue, bruised and beaten together with two or three corns of salt and twenty juniper berries, which take every morning fasting, preserves from danger of poison, and infection that day it is taken. . . . The kernels, when they grow old, are more oily, and therefore not fit to be eaten, but are then used to heal the wounds of the sinews, gangrenes, and carbuncles. . . . The said kernels being burned, are very astringent . . . being taken in red wine, and stay the falling of the hair, and make it fair, being anointed with oil and wine. The green husks will do the like, being used in the same manner. . . . A piece of the green husks put into a hollow tooth, eases the pain.

As usual, Maude Grieves gives us the most complete explanation of how herbs were used in the British tradition, her book being published in the 1930s and summing up so many centuries of folk medicine:

The bark and leaves have alterative, laxative, astringent and detergent properties, and are used in the treatment of skin troubles.

They are of the highest value for curing scrofulous diseases, herpes, eczema, etc., and for healing indolent ulcers; an infusion of 1 OZ. of dried bark or leaves (slightly more of the fresh leaves) to the pint of boiling water, allowed to stand for six hours, and strained off is taken in wineglassful doses, three times a day, the same infusion being also employed at the same time for outward application. Obstinate ulcers may also be cured with sugar, well saturated with a strong decoction of Walnut leaves.

The bark, dried and powdered, and made into a strong infusion, is a useful purgative.

The husk, shell and peel are sudorific, especially if used when the Walnuts are green. Whilst unripe, the nut has worm destroying virtues.

The fruit, when young and unripe, makes a wholesome, anti-scorbutic pickle, the vinegar in which the green fruit has been pickled proving a capital gargle for sore and slightly ulcerated throats. Walnut catsup embodies the medicinal virtues of the unripe nuts.

The leaves have a very strong, characteristic smell, aromatic and not unpleasant, but said to be injurious to sensitive people. They have three, sometimes four pairs of leaflets and a terminal one, the leaflets varying in size on the same leaf, being 2 1/4 to 4 inches in length and 1 to 1 1/2 inch wide, entire, smooth, shining, and paler below.

Gather the leaves only in fine weather, in the morning, after the dew has been dried by the sun. The prevalence of an east wind is favourable, as the dry air facilitates the process of drying. Reject all stained leaves.

Drying may be done in warm, sunny weather, out-of-doors, but in half-shade as leaves dried in the shade retain their colour better than those dried in the sun and do not become so tindery. They may be placed on wire sieves, or frames covered with wire or garden netting - at a height of about 3 or 4 feet from the ground, to ensure a current of air - and must be taken indoors to a dry room or shed, before there is any chance of them becoming damp from dew or showers.

The juice of the green husks, boiled with honey, is also a good gargle for a sore mouth and inflamed throat, and the distilled water *of the green husks is good for quinsy and as an application for wounds and internally is a cooling drink in agues.*

The thin, yellow skin which clothes the inner nut is a notable remedy for colic, being first dried, and then rubbed into powder. It is administered in doses of 30 grains, with a tablespoonful of peppermint water.

The oil extracted from the ripe kernels, taken inwardly in 1/2 OZ. doses, has also proved good for colic and is efficacious, applied externally, for skin diseases of the leprous type and wounds and gangrenes.

An Irish Herbal states:

Two or three walnuts eaten with a fig and a little rue, on an empty stomach, provide prevention against infection. The kernel oil will heal bruises and scabby and itchy skin, and taken internally, will break up the stone in the bladder and urinary crystals. A decoction of the green peel or husk of the walnut is useful against tumors and ulcers of the mouth and throat. The bark of the tree, either green, dried or crushed, encourages vomiting.

Brother Aloysius wrote of Walnut:

The infusion of the leaves contains ½ to ¾ cup per 2 cups boiling water and is one of the best remedies for scrofulous constitutions. An infusion of flowers contains 2/3 to 1 cup per 2 cups boiling water and is used for leukorrhea. The green rind of the unripe fruit, prepared in gin, is a well known stomatic. The fruit septa, ground to a powder, is a commonly known remedy for fleshy excrescences: this powder should simply be sprinkled on the effected area. It can especially be used for gangrene: 1 sugar spoon of powder should be taken twice a day in wine, and a little powder should be sprinkled on the wound. The young buds can be used to prepare an excellent ointment to prevent hair from falling out and the prevention of dandruff; a handful of buds should be fried for about ½ hour in 1 ½ cups lard. Take 1 to 2 cups of the flower infusion daily for jaundice, heavy bleeding or lupus.

Maria Treben wrote:

A tea of walnut cleanses the blood and is an effective remedy for intestinal disorders, as well as for constipation and lack of appetite. It is used successfully for jaundice and diabetes.

A decoction of the leaves, added to bath water, is beneficial for scrofula, rickets, caries, and swellings of the bone, as well as, for festering toe and finger nails. An improvement is noted soon, if areas affected by cradle- cap, scabs and scurf are washed with a decoction of the green leaves. Baths and washings enriched with his decoction are used for acne, festering eczema, sweaty feat and leucorrhea. As a mouthwash, it is used for stomatitis, inflamed gums, throat and larynx.

A strong decoction of the leaves, added to bathwater is used for chilblains. It is also beneficial for hair loss, when massaged frequently into the scalp. This decoction is an excellent remedy for head lice. The fresh leaves are used to repel insects.

About the middle of June, the unripe nuts are picked (a pin should easily run through them) and used to prepare a delightful cordial, which cleanses the stomach, liver and blood, strengthens weak stomachs and improves foul intestines. It is an excellent remedy for thick blood.

Jolanta WIttib writes:

Walnut is valued not only for the delicious nuts. I collect the leaves, the green shell of the nuts and the nuts, of course. The leaves and green outer layer of the nuts have a lot of tannins which make them valuable as home medicine. I add them to my mixtures for stomach problems, spasms or light diarrhea. My favorite is the nut! I add them to my apple pie (apple strudel), or baked apples. Or have nuts as a snack while hiking. Have you tried to store nuts in honey? It's delicious.

Resources of the Southern Fields and Forests states:

JUGLANDACEAE. (The Walnut Tribe.)

BUTTERNUT; OIL-NUT, (Juglans cinerea,Jj.) Grows in the mountains of South and North Carolina. Fl. April.358 IT. S. Disj). 710 ; Archives Gen. 3c seric, x, 399, and xi, 40; Frost's Elems. Mul.

Med. 131. ' The inner bark of the root. affords one of the most mild and efficient laxatives we possess.

The extract was a favorite remedy in General Marion's camp during the Revolutionary war. It is very efficacious in habitual constipation, in doses often to thirty grains; the tirst acting as a laxative, the maximum purging. Big. Am. Med Bot. ii, 115; Mx. N. Am. Sylva, 160; where it is spoken of as a mild cathartic, operating without pain or irritation, and resembling rhubarb in its property of evacuating without debilitating the alimentary canal. Dr. Rush employed it during the war. Wood says it is highly esteemed in dysentery, Lind. Nat, Syst. 181. The rind of the fruit and the skin of the kernel are extremely astringent, anthelmintic and cathartic; the oil extracted from the fruit is of a very drying nature. Mer. and do L. Diet, de M. Med. iii, 687, (J. cathartica.') He remarks that the inner bark of the root is acrid and caustic, and purges, but occasions neither heat nor irritation; adapted to bilious constitutions and to dysentery; often combined with calomel. It is given to animals in a disease called "yellow water;" Bull, des Sci. Med. Fer. xii, 338. To extract the cathartic principle, the bark is boiled in water for several hours; remove the extraneous matter and boil down the decoction to the consistence of honey or molasses—pills may be made of this. A syrup may also be made. The bark is strongest in the early summer. The powdered leaves are rubefacient, and act as a substitute for cantharides. Coxe, Am. Disp. 365. The bark of the branches af- fords a large quantity of soluble matter, chiefly of the extractive kind, water seeming to be a solvent. Wetherill found in it fixed oil, resin, saccharine matter, lime, potash, a peculiar principle, and tannin. Dr. B. S. Barton, in his Collections, 23, 32, thinks it is possessed of some anodyne property. Dr. Gray ascertained that four trees, eight to ten inches in diameter, produced in one day nine quarts of sap, from which was made one pound and a quarter of sugar, equal, if not superior to that produced from the maple. This plant is always given in the form of extract or decoction. Griffith's Med. Bot. 589; Thacher's Disp. 245; Eush's Med. Obs. i, 112; Pe. Mat. Med. and Therap. ii, 767 ; Lind. Med. Fl. 387.

BLACK WALNUT, {Juglans nigra, L.) Diffused in lower and upper country of South and North Carolina; Newbern. Fl. June. Mer. and de L. Diet, de M. Med. iii, 687; Griffith, Med. Bot. vi, 89. The bark is styptic and acrid; the rind of the unripe fruit is said to remove ring-worms and tetter ; and the decoction is given with success as a vermifuge. " A kind of bread is obtained from the fruit." In a communication received from J. Douglas, M. D., of Chester District, South Carolina, his correspondent, Mr. McKeown, informs me that a bit of lint, dipped in the oil of the walnut kernel and applied to an aching tooth, is an effectual palliative; he has employed it for thirty years with great satisfaction. The following appeared in one of the journals during the year 1861: Walnut leaves in the treatment of Diseases.—Dr. Negries, physician at Anglers, France, has published a statement of his success in the treatment of scrofulous disease in different forms by preparations of walnut leaves. He has tried walnut leaves for ten years, and of fifty six patients, afflicted in different forms, thirty-one were completely cured, and there were only four who appeared to have obtained no advantage. The infusion of the walnut tree leaves is made by cutting them and infusing a good pinch between the thumb and forefinger in half a pint of boiling water, and then sweetening it with sugar. To a grown person, M. Negries prescribed from two to three teacupsful of this daily. This medicine is a slightly aromatic bitter its efficiency is nearly uniform in scrofulous disorders, and it is stated never to have caused any unpleasant effects. It augments the activity of the circulation and digestion, and to the functions imparts much energy. It is supposed to act upon the lymphatic system, as under its influence the muscles become firm, and the skin acquires a ruddier hue. Dry leaves may be used throughout the winter, but a syrup made of green leaves is more aromatic. A salve made of a strong extract of the leaves mixed alone with clean lard and a few drops of the oil of bergamot is most excellent for sores. A strong decoction of the leaves is excellent for washing them.

The salutary effects of this medicine do not appear on a sudden— no visible effect may be noticed for twenty days, but per-severance in it will effect a cure. As walnut tree leaves are abundant in America, and as the extract of them is not dangerous or unpleasant to use, and scrofula not uncommon, a trial of this simple medicine should be made. In directing attention to it good results may be expected.

The Thomsonian System of Medicine states:

BUTTERNUT. Juglans Cinerea. (Dr. Thomson.)

This tree grows common in this country, and is well known from the nut which it bears, of an oblong shape and nearly as large as an egg, in which is a meat containing much oil, and very good to eat. The inner bark of this tree is used by the country people to color with. The bark taken from the body of the tree or roots, and boiled down till thick, may be made into pills, and operate as a powerful emetic and cathartic; a syrup may be made by boiling the bark and adding one-third molasses and a little spirit, which is good to give children for worm complaints. The buds and twigs may also be used for the same purpose, and are more mild.

BUTTERNUT. *Juglans Cinerea. (Dr. Greer.)*

The inner bark of the white walnut tree has an important place in the Materia Medica. Its principal use is as a physic, and in that respect it is exceedingly valuable on account of its mild action and the tonic impression left upon the structures of the bowels. Its chief influence is exerted upon the lower bowels, and for that reason it cannot be excelled for prolapsus and constipation due to a sluggish condition of the large bowels. It is best administered in the form of syrup made by slowly boiling a pound of the bark in water and evaporating to one pint and adding two pounds of sugar; dose, a teaspoonful. Butternut syrup is a valuable physic for use in protracted febrile diseases.

Juglans Cinerea. (Dr. Lyle.)

The inner bark of the root is more active than that of the trunk, but both are used. It yields its properties to boiling water, except its astringency, which property is yielded when alcohol is the menstruum used instead of boiling water. Juglans is an active stimulating hepatic and cathartic. It relieves the portal system, disgorges the liver and cleanses the bowels. For catharsis it usually takes from four to eight hours, according to the dose given. Juglans Cinerea tones the entire alvine mucous membrane, but especially that of the lower bowels, influencing peristalcis. The alcoholic fluid extract may be used in diarrhoea and dysentery. It cleanses the surface and leaves the parts toned and astringed. The aqueous extract being free from this astringency may be used to relieve chronic constipation. It is in this sphere one of the most valuable preparations. In relieving the portal circulation it also relieves hemorrhoids and rectal hemorrhages. In dysentery, in small doses, it cleanses the bowels, relieves the portal circulation and tones the mucous membranes. To prepare the syrup of Juglans, gather your *bark from the fifth to the twentieth of April in the country. It is then strongest. Crush or chop fine. Then boil till quite strong and pour off and cover a second and third time to completely exhaust the strength of the drug. Then boil all together and evaporate to threefourth or equality of one pint per pound of bark. Then for each twelve ounces add alcohol, two ounces, and sugar, four ounces. It is well adapted to the treatment of skin eruptions. It is a tonic to both mucous membrane and dermoid tissue and slightly increases the action of the kidneys. It is one of the most valuable agents in the whole materia medica. It relieves the liver, proves gently cathartic and leaves the bowels soluble and toned. These are qualities that can be accorded to but few agents. By the use of this agent the faeces becomes more or less darkened.*

King's American Dispensatory, 1898 tells us:

Action, Medical Uses, and Dosage.—Butternut in small doses is a mild stimulant to the intestinal tract, proving laxative and in larger doses is a gentle and agreeable cathartic, causing no griping, nor subsequent weakness of the intestines. It resembles rhubarb in its effect, but without inducing constipation after its action. It is very valuable in cases of habitual constipation, colorectitis, and several other intestinal diseases. It is generally used in the form of an extract, in doses of 1 to 30 grains. An excellent combination for chronic constipation is the following: Rx Ext. butternut, ʒj; ext. nux vomica, grs. v. Mix. Ft. Pil. No. 40. Sig. Two pills, 3 times a day (Locke). The same pill is very efficient in deficient gastric secretion, in atonic dyspepsia, and in indigestion accompanied with gastric irritation, sour eructations, and flatulent distension of the stomach. Administer 1 pill a day. Juglans is useful in tenesmic, burning, fetid diarrhoea and dysentery, and should be remembered in intestinal dyspepsia with irritation. The specific juglans may be given in from 1 to 10-drop doses. The same doses of the same preparation act as an efficient alterative in chronic skin affections and scrofula, being particularly indicated in those skin affections exhibiting vesicles or pustules. Webster believes it effectual in all skin diseases except those presenting parasitic, scrofulous, or syphilitic manifestations. Juglans is an efficient cathartic to use when a free action of the bowels is demanded in rheumatism and chronic respiratory affections. A strong decoction of it is much employed in some sections of the country, as a domestic remedy in rheumatism affecting the muscles of the back, and in intermittent and remittent fevers, as well as in other diseases attended with congestion of the abdominal viscera; it is also reputed efficient in murrain of cattle, and yellow water in horses. It was used with great advantage in the treatment of dysentery and diarrhoea occurring among our soldiers in the Civil War. Dose of the extract, from 1 to 30 grains, usually from 1 to 5 grains; specific juglans, 1 to 20 drops, the smaller doses being preferred for its specific action.

Specific Indications and Uses.—Chronic constipation; gastro-intestinal irritability, with sour eructations, flatulence, and either diarrhoea or constipation dependent thereon; diarrhoea and dysentery with tenesmus and burning and fetid discharges; torpid liver; chronic skin affections of a pustular or vesicular character, discharging freely; eczematous affections.

According to Plants for a Future:

The walnut tree has a long history of medicinal use, being used in folk medicine to treat a wide range of complaints. The leaves are alterative, anthelmintic, anti-inflammatory, astringent and depurative. They are used internally the treatment of constipation, chronic coughs, asthma, diarrhoea, dyspepsia etc. The leaves are also used to treat skin ailments and purify the blood. They are considered to be specific in the treatment of strumous sores. Male inflorescences are made into a broth and used in the treatment of coughs and vertigo. The rind is anodyne and astringent. It is used in the treatment of diarrhoea and anaemia. The seeds are antilithic, diuretic and stimulant. They are used internally in the treatment of low back pain, frequent urination, weakness of both legs, chronic cough, asthma, constipation due to dryness or anaemia and stones in the urinary tract. Externally, they are made into a paste and applied as a poultice to areas of dermatitis and eczema. The oil from the seed is anthelmintic. It is also used in the treatment of menstrual problems and dry skin conditions. The cotyledons are used in the treatment of cancer. Walnut has a long history of folk use in the treatment of cancer, some extracts from the plant have shown anticancer activity. The bark and root bark are anthelmintic, astringent and detergent. The plant is used in Bach flower remedies - the keywords for prescribing it are "Oversensitive to ideas and influences" and "The link-breaker".

Peterson Field Guides Eastern and Central Medicinal Plants tells us about butternut and black walnut:

Butternut: Inner bark tea or extract a popular early American laxative, thought to be effective in small doses, without causing griping or cramps. American Indians use bark tea for rheumatism, headaches, toothaches; strong warm tea for wounds to stop bleeding, promote healing. Oil from nuts used for tape worms, fungal infections. Juglone, a component, is antiseptic and herbicidal, some anti-tumor activity has also been reported.

Black walnut: American Indians used inner bark tea as an emetic, laxative; bark chewed for toothaches. Fruit husk juiced used on ringworms; Husk chewed for colic, poultice for inflammation. Leaf tea astringent, insecticidal against bedbugs.

Botany In a Day states:

There are about 20 species of walnuts in the world. They all produce edible nuts, but of varying quality… Medicinally, the leaves, bark and husks are rich in tannic acid, with some bitter components; walnut is used mostly as an astringent but also as a vermifuge, internally to get rid of worms, externally for ringworm fungus. The green husk is rich in vitamin C. Butternut bark contains naphthoquinone laxative.

One has to wonder how our ancestors discovered the medicinal uses of the Walnut family. I would suggest that it came about through observation. Walnuts, as the Latin name suggests, produce a substance called juglone. Juglone prevents many trees and plants from growing near the walnut - this most unsociable quality prevents faster growing trees from competing with the Walnut for sunlight, water and other resources. Some trees and bushes though are "juglone tolerant", and if you wish to include Walnuts in your landscape, you will want to research such plants. But basically, Walnuts don't play well with others! Could our ancestors have noticed this trait and wondered if such a unique and powerful plant could have medicinal use against other creatures that may compete for our resources…. parasites, bacteria, etc?

Obviously, I can only speculate. But I recall the horses on our farm when I was a kid, eating the tender spring pecan and black walnut leaves that grew in and near the pasture. I was told not to let them eat too much, but that the horses somehow knew to eat those leaves to prevent worms. I also heard of folks feeding them to chickens for the same reason. I don't know if that is recommended, but the old folks would often say, "animals know what they need; they know what plants are medicine." Of course, that wasn't always true, but this was the folk knowledge our ancestors knew. It makes me wonder what other wisdom is to be found just over our heads and under our feet?

Juniperus, Juniper

Twenty-two varieties of Juniper have been noted for their medicinal value: Juniperus ashei - Ashe Juniper, Juniperus californica - Californian Juniper, Juniperus communis, Juniperus communis nana, Juniperus conferta - Shore Juniper, Juniperus deppeana - Aligator Juniper, Juniperus drupacea - Syrian Juniper, Juniperus excelsa - Grecian Juniper, Juniperus horizontalis - Creeping Juniper, Juniperus chinensis - Chinese Juniper, Juniperus monosperma - One-Seed Juniper, Juniperus occidentalis - Western Juniper, Juniperus osteosperma - Desert Juniper, Juniperus oxycedrus - Prickly Juniper, Juniperus recurva - Himalayan Juniper, Juniperus rigida - Temple Juniper, Juniperus sabina – Savine, Juniperus scopulorum - Rocky Mountain Juniper, Juniperus silicicola - Southern Redcedar, Juniperus squamata - Flaky Juniper, Juniperus tetragona, Juniperus virginiana - Pencil Cedar

Only two Junipers grow in my region, and both are virginiana: Juniperus virginiana var. virginiana (Eastern Redcedar), Juniperus virginiana var. silicicola (Southern Redcedar). These are generally referred to simply as cedar, although they are junipers.

Juniper has a long history as a medicinal herb. Galen stated that Juniper berries, "cleanse the liver and kidneys, and they evidently thin and thick and viscous juices, and for this reason they are mixed in health medicines."

Dioscorides wrote in de Materia Medica:

Some juniper is bigger, some smaller. Either of the junipers [the bigger and the smaller] are sharp, diuretic and warming, and when burned the fumes drive away snakes. One type of the fruit (called the juniperberry) is the size of a hazelnut, the other equal to a bean — both round and fragrant, sweet, and a little bitter to chew. It is mildly warming and astringent, good for the stomach, good taken in drink for infirmities of the chest, coughs, gaseousness, griping, and the poisons of venomous creatures. It is also diuretic; as a result it is good for convulsions and hernia, and those who have congested or blocked wombs. It has sharp leaves, as a result applied as a plaster and taken as a drink (or the juice taken with wine) they are good for those bitten by vipers. The bark (burned and rubbed on with water) removes leprosy, but the scraping dust of the wood (swallowed down) kills. There is a great juniper too, which some call cypressus sylvestris, some mnesitheus, some acatera, and the Romans juniperus, and it is known to most like cypress growing for the most part in rough places and near the sea. It has the same properties as the former. The lesser juniper some call archeuthis, some, mnesitheus, others, acatalis, the Africans zuorinsipet, the Egyptians libium, the Romans juniperus, and the Gauls jupicellusum.

Dioscorides also wrote of a Juniper wine:

Cedar, juniper, cypress, bay, pine or fir wines are made the same way. Separate the newly cut wood when it gives out fruit, lay it in a bath in the sun or near the fire so that it may sweat, and then mix one pound of this to four and a half litres of wine. Mix it and leave it alone for two months. Then put it in another jar, and having placed in the sun for a while, put it in smaller jars.

We must fill up the jars of wines made like this, for if we do not they grow sour. Nevertheless these medicinal wines are unfit for the healthy. They are all warming, urinary, and somewhat astringent. That of bay is the most warming. A wine is also made from the fruit of the bigger cedars. Mix half a pound of bruised cedar berries to four and a half litres of must and keep it in the sun for four days, and after all this strain it and pour it into another jar.

Wine is also made from the berries of juniper trees, as well as from the fruit of the cedar, which has the same effects.

A Juniper beer was very popular in Scandinavian countries before hops came into common use, and is still enjoyed by some craft brewers.

Saint Hildegard von Bingen wrote:

The juniper is more hot than cold, and signifies excess. Take its fruit, cook it in water, strain this water through a cloth. To this add honey and a bit of vinegar and licorice, and less ginger than licorice. Cook it again, and place it in a little bag, and make a spiced wine. Drink it often, whether fasting, or having eaten. It diminishes and mitigates pain in the chest, lungs or liver. Also, take the green twigs and cook them in water. Make a sauna bath with that water. Often bather in it, and it diminishes the bad fevers in you.

Juniper has also been widely used among British herbalists. Gerard state:

Juniper is hot and dry, and that in the third degree, as Galen teacheth; the berries are also hot but not altogether so dry: the gum is hot and dry in the first degree, as the Arabians write.

The Virtues.

A. The fruit of the Juniper tree doth cleanse the liver and kidneys, as Galen testifieth: it also maketh thin clammy and gross humours: it is used in counterpoisons and other wholesome medicines: being over-largely taken it causeth gripings and gnawings in the stomach, and maketh the head hot: it neither bindeth nor looseth the belly: it provoketh urine.

B. Dioscorides reporteth, that this being drunk is a remedy against the infirmity of the chest, coughs, windiness, gripings and poisons, and that the same is good for those that be troubled with cramps, burstings, and with the disease called the mother.

C. It is most certain that the decotion of these berries is singular good against an old cough, and against that with which children are now and then extremely troubled, called the chin cough, in which they use to rise up raw, tough and clammy humours, that have many times blood mixed with them.

D. Divers in Bohemia do take instead of other drink, the water wherein those berries have been steeped, who live in wonderful good health.

E. This is also drunk against poisons and pestilent fevers, and it is not unpleasant in the drinking: when the first water is almost spent, the vessel is again filled up with fresh.

F. The smoke of the leaves and wood driveth away serpents, and all infection and corruption of the air, which bring the plague, or such like contagious diseases: the juice of the leaves is laid on with wine, and also drunk against the bitings of the viper.

G. The ashes of the burned bark, being applied with water, take away scurf and filth of the skin.

H. The powder of the wood being inwardly taken, is pernicious and deadly, as Dioscorides' vulgar copies do affirm; but the true copies utterly deny it, neither do any of the old writers affirm it.

I. The fume and smoke of the gum doth stay phlegmatic humours that distil out of the head, and stoppeth the rheum: the gum doth stay raw and phlegmatic humours that stick in the stomach and guts, if it be inwardly taken, and also drunk.

K. It killeth all manner of worms in the belly, it stayeth the menses, and hæmorrhoids: it is commended also against spitting of blood; it dryeth hollow ulcers, and filleth them with flesh, if it be cast thereon: being mixed with oil of roses, it healeth chops in the hands and feet.

L. There is made of this and of oil of Linseed, mixed together, a liquor called varnish, which is used to beautify pictures and painted tables with, and to make iron glister, and to defend it from the rust.

Culpepper wrote:

This admirable solar shrub is scarce to be paralleled for its virtues. The berries are hot in the third degree, and dry but in the first, being a most admirable counter-poison, and as great a resister of the pestilence, as any growing: they are excellent good against the biting of venomous beasts, they provoke urine exceedingly, and therefore are very available to dysuries and stranguaries. It is so powerful a remedy against the dropsy, that the very lye made of the ashes of the herb being drank, cures the disease. It provokes the terms, helps the fits of the mother, strengthens the stomach exceedingly, and expels the wind. Indeed there is scarce a better remedy for wind in any part of the body, or the cholic, than the chymical oil drawn from the berries; such country people as know not how to draw the chymical oil, may content themselves by eating ten or a dozen of the ripe berries every morning fasting. They are admirably good for a cough, shortness of breath, and consumption, pains in the belly, ruptures, cramps, and convulsions. They give safe and speedy delivery to women with child, they strengthen the brain exceedingly, help the memory, and fortify the sight by strengthening the optic nerves; are excellently good in all sorts of agues; help the gout and sciatica, and strengthen the limbs of the body. The ashes of the wood is a speedy remedy to such as have the scurvy, to rub their gums with. The berries stay all fluxes, help the hæmorrhoids or piles, and kill worms in children. A lye made of the ashes of the wood, and the body bathed with it, cures the itch, scabs and leprosy. The berries break the stone, procure appetite when it is lost, and are excellently good for all palsies, and falling-sickness.

An Irish Herbal states:

The berries provoke urine and cure old coughs, flatulence and cholic pains. The gum of the tree expels worms from the body and stops excessive menstrual flow.

Juniper is also an excellent herb to stimulate appetite and to help the liver. It is a natural bitter, and just thoroughly chewing and eating a few berries before a meal can be among the best helps in digestion for elderly and chronically ill people. Care should be taken not to overuse them though, as in large amounts they can irritate the kidneys. Juniper is also good for the immune system and cleaning the blood – a good spring tonic.

Fr. Kneipp wrote of Juniper:

Juniper. (Juniperus communis L.)

Who does not know the Juniper-berry?

Juniper, when used for fumigation, spreads an agreeable odour through the rooms and passages, and improves the air. I am no friend of the so-called "fumigation" with sugar, vinegar, etc. for I do not see how one can speak of fresh air there. But if it is a question of disinfecting a room in which a patient with an infectious disease, or a corpse has been lying, or at the time of infections illnesses to purify the air by fumigating, then I al- ways like such juniper vapour. It thoroughly destroys all fungi, and whatever the volatile infection and disease- bringer may be called. Juniper works with similar effects upon the interior of the human organism. The berries fumigate, as it were, the mouth and stomach, and ward off contagion.

Those who are nursing patients with serious illnesses, as scarlet fever, smallpox, typhus, cholera, etc, and are exposed to contagion by raising, carrying, or serving the patient, or by speaking with him, should always chew a few juniper-berries (six to ten in a day). They give a pleasant taste in the mouth, and are of good ser- vice to the digestion. They burn up, as it were , the harmful miasms, exhalations, etc. when these seek to enter through the mouth or nostrils. Those who are suffering from a weak stomach, may try the following little course with juniper-berries.

The first day they should begin with 4 berries, the second day take 5 berries, the third day 6, the fourth 7, and so increase by one berry every day until the twelfth, on which they will take 15 berries ; then they may continue for five days longer taking each day one berry less.

I know many whose stomach, filled with gases and thereby weakened , has been purified and strengthened by this simple berry-cure. Juniper berries have been noted since olden times as a remedy for stone and gravel, and for complaints of the kidneys and liver ; also in all cases where foul gases, foul, watery and slimy matter are to be removed from the body. Not only the berries, but also the young shoots of the juniper bush are made use of for tea, in the first stages of dropsy, and also as purifying medicine.

The oil is best bought from the chemist. The tincture can be made at home with wine, brandy, or spirit.

I would not praise the father or mother of a family, who were certainly very careful and diligent in preserving their meat and vegetables with berries from the juniper bush, and were punctual and careful in fumigating their dwelling with the same, but who allow ed their body, the dwelling of their soul, to lie in dust and dirt. They ought to apply such a fumigator for this much more important dwelling, at least a few times in the year.

Brother Aloysius wrote of Juniper:

The berries and young twigs are used medicinally. The berries principally have diuretic, diaphoretic, warming and wind-breaking properties and promote digestion. They are especially used for ascites, gastric weakness accompanied by wind, accumulation of mucus, etc. They are also recommended as a protection from intermittent fever, rheumatism and gout pain. The young twigs, mixed with woodruff and wild strawberry leaves, make a delicious and healthy drink, which can take the place of Indian tea, and is certainly much healthier; milk and sugar can be added according to taste.

One of the preparations is juniper oil, which has excellent diuretic properties. The dose is 2 – 10 drops. You can use 10-15 berries for one cup of tea. …. Juniper berries strengthen the nerves, cleanse the blood and the stomach; are also used for kidney, lung and liver complaints, gravel, stones, bladder catarrh, diarrhea and migraines. The decoction of twigs and berries is ½ cup per 2 cups water. The decoction of young twigs and wood is 2/3 to 1 cup per 2 cups water, which can be taken for rheumatism, gout, syphilis, chronic cough and congestion in the chest.

Or, use 3 tablespoons of berries, ground to a powder, and cooked with 2 tablespoons of lard as an excellent remedy for scurf in children; the head should be smeared with it twice a day. A remedy fo phlegm in the chest and coughs, 3 tablespoons juniper berries should be boiled in 2 cups barley water and reduced by half, add a little sugar candy and drink this quantity throughout the day.

Fr. Johannes Kunzel wrote in Herbs and Weeds:

The juniper or Reckolder (Juniperus) is a medicinal plant of the first rank; everything about it is medicinal: wood, needles, berries, bark.

It has the power to warm up, relieve internal colds, cleans everything whatever it can reach, stomach, intestines, lungs, blood, and is therefore used in almost all herbal mixtures, except for hot diseases (such as fever etc.).

Even stronger than the common Juniper is the kind found on the high Alps that creeps along the ground.

Juniper baths are usually a good remedy for old rheumatisms; I have seen old people twisted by gout become straight and healthy again through continued use of such baths; and how people who stayed in bed stiff like a piece of wood for six months were healed by washings and later bathing in Juniper decoction.

Of course, the green Juniper twigs have to be boiled for three hours; the patient is washed with this (warm) water ten times a day all over his body until he is able to take a bath.

Because the bath is very sharp and aggressive, it is advisable to mix it with fir tree or green pine tree twigs' decoction. The baths must be warm and last for half an hour; At the end the whole body has to be poured over with cold water; if you fail to do this, it is better not to take the bath, otherwise the rheumatism will come back even more severely.

Jolanta Wittib writes:

Whenever I see a juniper with berries/cones on my walk in the forest, I collect a few junipers ripe - black or dark blue ones and chew them while walking.

I love them: they have a sweetish and a very aromatic taste and I know that they will strengthen my body and spirit.

Fr. Sebastian Kneipp, who has already been mentioned more than once in this book, suggested juniper cone therapy after a long illness, exhaustion, after cancer treatment, etc, because Juniper cones clean the body, clean the blood, improve metabolism. They are good for rheumatism, arthritis, they have an antibacterial effect. Besides, they are tasty, disinfect one's mouth and leave a nice flavor.

Resources of the Southern Fields and Forests states:

CEDAR, (Juniperus Virginiana, Linn.) Grows in upper and lower districts; Newbern. Fl. March. Big. Am. Med. Bot. iii, 49; Pe. Mat.

Med. ii, 184; Fr. Elems. 195; U. S. Disp. 413; Mer. and de L. Diet, de M. Med. iii, 698;589 Mich. N. Am. Sylva, iii, 221; Am. Journal Pharm. xiv, 23; Thacher's Disp. 247; Lind. Nat. Syst. Bot. 316; Griffith Med. Bot. 607; Supplem. to the Diet, de M.Med. 1846, 406; Bull, de l'Acad. Eoy. de Med. vi, 478; S. Cubieres' Mem. on the Eed Cedar of Virginia, in French, Paris, 1805; Nicolet's Essai on the Physiol, and Chemistry of genus Juniperus; see Journal de Pharm. xxvii, 309, and Bonastie's note on a volatile oil from the Virginia cedar, in Journal de Pharm. xxi, 177, 1834. The bark is employed in Abyssinia, under the name of Bisenna.

The expressed oil is very useful as an application to rheumatic pains and swellings of the joints. One bushel of the driednshavings, heated in an inverted iron vessel, will yield a half pint of oil. A decoction of the berries promotes diaphoresis, and is also beneficial in rheumatic pains, stiff joints, etc. The leaves act very much as shavings, being stimulant and emmenagogue, and are employed in catamenial obstructions. The cedar berry is used in a popular remedy for dropsy, which is claimed by some to be highly efficacious. We can readily understand the reason that it may prove useful when we remember its close alliance with the juniper berry. It is as follows: take one handful of the seed of the cedar, the same of mullein, the same of the root of dogwood; put into two quarts and a pint of water, boil down to one quart, and add one gill of whiskey. Dose, a wineglassful night and morning. A cerate is made for keeping up the irritation and discharge from blisters; this is quite serviceable, and is prepared by boiling the fresh leaves in twice their weight of lard, with the addition of a little wax. The fungoid excrescences on this tree are thought to be anthelmintic. The wood of the tree is well known. It is sometimes dug up in the mud of our swamps in a perfect state of preservation. It is aromatic, light, soft, bearing exposure to water and weather, and suitable for all kinds of cabinet work, in the construction of posts, staves, buckets, the inner work of houses, and particularly in the building of boats. Cedar boxes are not infested by insects, moths, etc., and are used for storing away woollens. The leaves also prevent the attacks of insects when spread over cloth. The roots make a beautiful purple dye.

King's American Dispensatory, 1898 tells us:

Action, Medical Uses, and Dosage.—Both the berries and oil are stimulating, carminative, and diuretic. The oil is said to act like copaiba in arresting mucous discharges, especially from the urethra. It is contained in the spiritous liquor called Hollands, one of its best forms as a diuretic. Five minims of the oil, with 1 fluid drachm of nitrous ether, given 3 times a day in any common vehicle, produces diuresis in dropsy when other means fail. Combined with an equal part of watermelon seeds, and made into an infusion, I have cured several cases of ascites occurring in children, having them to make free use of it (King). The berries are employed principally as an adjunct to other diuretics, and have been found efficient in gonorrhoea, gleet, leucorrhoea, cystirrhoea, affections of the skin, scorbutic diseases, etc. Pyelitis, pyelo-nephritis, and cystitis when chronic, and particularly when in old people, are relieved by juniper. Uncomplicated renal hyperemia a is cured by it. The indications are a persistent weight or dragging in lumbar region. Dose of the berries, from 1 to 2 drachms; of the oil, from 4 to 20 minims. The infusion (berries, ℥i; aqua, Oj), may be given in wineglassful doses, a pint being taken in a day. It is very useful in the dropsy following scarlatina, and other infectious diseases, and may be combined with acetate or bitartrate of potassium if desired. OIL OF CADE has been successfully employed in parasitic skin diseases, moist eczema, and psoriasis.

Preparation of Juniper.—HOWE'S JUNIPER POMADE. This preparation is a compound of lard, oil of juniper and Fowler's solution, the proportions of which have been published in the Eclectic Medical Journal. Much pharmaceutical skill is required to blend the ingredients so as to prevent subsequent separation. Juniper pomade is useful in "all forms of eczema or tetter. It allays the itching and destroys the vesicles and scales. The unguent may be used upon all parts of the body, though sparingly upon mucous surfaces. It is employed in the nasal cavities with a camel's hair brush to mitigate the symptoms of catarrh, to arrest hay-fever, to heal nasal ulcers, to arrest ringing in the ears, and to improve states of deafness depending upon thickening of the linings of the Eustachian tubes. Juniper pomade softens the scaly patches oil the face which are often epitheliomatous. It has proved an excellent dressing for tetter of the edges of the eyelids, which leads to 'wild hairs', and induration of the tarsal borders. The pomade is reliable in the treatment of sore nipples in nursing women. and it will cure chapped hands" (Prof. A. J. Howe, M. D.).

The Rodale Herb Book states:

Juniper is considered one of the most useful medicinal plants. Stimulating for appetite and digestion, helpful in coughs and to eliminate mucus, it has a diuretic effect, stimulating the function of kidneys and bladder. A strong tea of the berries is considered an excellent wash for bites and poisonous insects, snake bites, dog bites and bee stings.

Rodale's Illustrated Encyclopedia of Herbs states:

Rheumatism, arthritis, bruises, ulcers and wounds are said to be relieved by juniper poultices and rubs. Adding a handful of leaves to warm bathwater is said to sooth aching muscles. For poultices, berries can be simmered in olive oil or simply mashed and applied ot the sore area. American Indians simply tied bundles of the boughs to sore limbs. Juniper tincture has been used externally on painful swellings, bruises and sores.

Sacred and Healing Herbal Beers tells us that Juniper was once widely used in beer brewing. After discussing the various folk medicine and spiritual beliefs traditionally associated with Juniper, as well as its documented medicinal uses, Mr. Buhner leaves us with this very reasonable statement:

Generally, juniper is a marvelous herb to use in brewing, and the taste of juniper ale is good and very refreshing. Given the many benefits from the herb, as a preservative and a medicine, especially on nutrition and digestive health and as a potentially useful herb in the treatment of colds and flu, it seems and excellent herb to use in ales and beers.

Peterson Field Guides Eastern and Central Medicinal Plants tells us:

Eastern red cedar: American Indians used fruit tea for colds, worms, rheumatism, coughs, to induce sweating, Chewed fruit for canker sores. Leaf smoke or steam inhaled for colds, bronchitis, purification, rheumatism. Said to contain the anti-tumor compound podophyllotoxin, best known from mayapple

Botany In a Day states:

Cypress: A tea of the leaves is used internally or externally to stop bleeding and for colds.

Juniper, red cedar: juniper berries can be eaten raw or used in tea. The bitter berries are the main ingredient in gin. Most people would consider them unpalatable, but I have acquired a taste for them. Juniper berries contain volatile oils and resins; they are eaten as a carminative to expel gas and the distilled oil is rubbed on painful joints. Additionally, juniper berries are diuretic, but may irritate the kidneys with prolonged use. They are not recommended for pregnant women. A boiled tea of the fruits and leaves as a treatment for coughs. You may be able to decrease the risk of catching a virus by keeping juniper berries in the mouth while around others who are infected. Also, try chewing the berries when drinking unclean water. Juniper needles can be added to bathwater for a stimulating effect on rheumatism.

Cedar, Arbor vitae: cedar contains toxic volatile oils. It is used as a diaphoretic to promote sweating, emmenagogue to promote menstruation, and as an irritant poultice to stimulate healing for rheumatic pains. It should not be used without medical supervision. It is also expectorant.

The Physicians Desk Reference for Herbal Medicine tells us:

Juniper has been primarily noted for its anti-inflammatory, diuretic, and dyspeptic effects. Because of its ability to inhibit cyclooxygenase, it is useful in inflammatory conditions, such as arthritis. Juniper is used to treat chronic urinary tract, bladder and kidney infections as well as herpes and flu infections. The diuretic effect is probably primarily due to the volatile oil terpinene-4-ol. In addition to drug works to lower blood pressure and may regulate hyperglycemia. In animal experiments a hypertensive, an antiexudative effect was proved. In vitro, an antiviral effect was also demonstrated.

Kalmia latifolia, Mountain Laurel

This member of the Ericaceae family is not much used anymore due to its toxicity. According to Plants for A Future:

Mountain laurel is a very poisonous narcotic plant the leaves of which were at one time used by some native North American Indian tribes in order to commit suicide. Because of its toxicity, it is a remedy that is seldom used in modern herbalism, but the leaves have been used externally in herbal medicine and are a good remedy for many skin diseases and inflammation. The leaves are analgesic, astringent, disinfectant, narcotic, salve and sedative. An infusion of the leaves is used as a disinfectant wash and liniment to treat pain, scratches, rheumatism, inflammations and to get rid of body parasites. Used internally, the leaves have a splendid effect in the treatment of active haemorrhages, diarrhoea and flux. They are also used in the treatment of syphilis, inflammatory fevers, neuralgia, paralytic conditions, tinnitus and angina. The leaves should be used with great caution however, and only under the guidance of a qualified practitioner. Excess doses cause vertigo, headache, loss of sight, salivation, thirst, nausea, palpitations, slow pulse and difficulty in breathing.

Mrs. Grieves wrote similarly of Mountain Laurel:

A beautiful evergreen shrub from 4 to 20 feet. When in full flower it forms dense thickets, the stems are always crooked, the bark rough. It was called Kalmia by Linnaeus in honour of Peter Kalm, a Swedish professor. The hard wood is used in the manufacture of various useful articles. Leaves ovate, lanceolate, acute on each end, on petioles 2 to 3 inches long. Flowers numerous, delicately tinted a lovely shade of pink; these are very showy, clammy, interminal, viscid, pubescent, simple or compound heads, branches opposite, flowering in June and July. The flowers yield a honey said to be deleterious. The leaves, shoots and berries are dangerous to cattle, and when eaten by Canadian pheasants communicate the poison to those who feed on the birds. The fruit is a dry capsule, seeds minute and numerous.

Leaves possess narcotic poisoning properties and contain tannic acid, gum, fatty matter, chlorophyll, a substance resembling mannite, wax extractive, albumen, an acrid principle, Aglucosidearbutin, yellow calcium iron.

Medicinal Action and Uses---Indians are said to use the expressed juice of the leaves or a strong decoction of them to commit suicide. The leaves are the official part; powdered leaves are used as a local remedy in some forms of skin diseases, and are a most efficient agent in syphilis, fevers, jaundice, neuralgia and inflammation, but great care should be exercised in their use. Whisky is the best antidote to poisoning from this plant. An ointment for skin diseases is made by stewing the leaves in pure lard in an earthenware vessel in a hot oven. Taken internally it is a sedative and astringent in active haemorrhages, diarrhoea and flux. It has a splendid effect and will be found useful in overcoming obstinate chronic irritation of the mucous surface. In the lower animals an injection produces great salivation, lachrymation, emesis, convulsions and later paralysis of the extremities and laboured respiration. It is supposed, but not proved, that the poisonous principle of this plant is Andromedotoxin.

Preparations and Dosages---A saturated tincture of the leaves taken when plant is in flower, is the best form of administration, given in doses of 10 to 20 drops every two or three hours. Decoction, 1/2 to 1 fluid ounce of powdered leaves from 10 to 30 grains. Salve made from juice of the plant is an efficient local application for rheumatism.

King's American Dispensatory, 1898 tells us:

Action, Medical Uses, and Dosage.—In immoderate doses, sheep laurel is a poisonous narcotic, producing the symptoms above named, with diminished circulation. In medicinal doses, it is antisyphilitic, sedative to the heart, and somewhat astringent. Internally, either in powder, decoction, or tincture, it is an efficient remedy in primary or secondary syphilis, and will likewise be found invaluable in febrile and inflammatory diseases and hypertrophy of the heart, allaying all febrile and inflammatory action, and lessening the action of the heart. In active hemorrhages, diarrhoea, and flux, it has been employed with excellent effect, and will be found useful in overcoming obstinate chronic irritation of mucous surfaces. I have extensively used this agent, and regard it as one of our most efficient agents in syphilis; and have likewise found it very valuable in inflammatory fevers, jaundice, and ophthalmic neuralgia and inflammation. The remedy must always be used with prudence; and should any of the above mentioned symptoms appear, the dose must be diminished, or its use suspended for a few days. In cases of poisoning by this article, stimulants, as brandy, whiskey, etc., must be given, with counter-irritation to the spine and extremities. Sheep poisoned by eating the leaves, have been saved by administering 1 or 2 gills of whiskey to them (King). Scudder (Spec. Med.), states that he has employed it with marked advantage in secondary syphilis and atonic chronic inflammations. For the treatment of aching pains in the muscles of the face, muscular rheumatism with shifting pains, and in the early stage of rheumatism of the heart, success has been claimed for this drug, the specific medicine being used in from 1 to 5-drop doses. Bright's disease (?) is asserted to have been benefited by its use. Pain in the back during the menstrual period, and pain upon moving the eyes are said to be relieved by kalmia. Externally, the fresh leaves stewed in lard, or the dried leaves in powder mixed with lard to form an ointment, are said to be beneficial in tinea capitis, psora, and other cutaneous affections. "Some time since I treated a case of syphilis of five weeks' standing, which had not received any kind of treatment during that period. The patient, at the time I first saw him, had several chancres, the surface of the body and head was covered with small red pimples, elevated above a jaundiced skin, and he was in a very debilitated condition. I administered a saturated tincture of the leaves of kalmia, and touched the chancres with a tincture of chloride of iron, and effected a cure in 4 weeks, removing the jaundice at the same time" (King). The saturated tincture of the leaves or specific kalmia, are the best forms of administration; they may be given in doses of from 10 to 20 drops every 2 or 3 hours; the decoction may be given in doses of from ½ to 1 fluid ounce; and of the powdered leaves, from 10 to 30 grains. For acute disorders, particularly affections of the heart, from 5 to 20 drops of specific kalmia may be added to 4 fluid ounces of water, and the dilution administered in teaspoonful doses every hour. A salve made of the juice of the plant, forms an efficient local application for rheumatism. This remedy was a great favorite with Prof. King, especially for troubles depending primarily upon syphilitic infection.

Specific Indications and Uses.—Syphilis with excitation of the heart and circulation; rheumatism with shifting pains; cardiac excitation; cardiac palpitation excited reflexly from gastro-intestinal irritation; pain upon movement of the eyes.

Koelreuteria, Golden Rain Tree

Two varieties of Golden Rain Tree have been naturalized in my region, Koelreuteria bipinnata and Koelreuteria paniculate. This ornamental tree is not widely used in Herbal Medicine. However, Plants for A Future States:

Medicinal use of Golden Rain Tree: The flowers are ophthalmic. They are used in the treatment of conjunctivitis and epiphora.

Lagerstroemia indica, Crape-myrtle

Crape Myrtle is probably the most widely planted naturalized ornamental tree/shrub in my region. There is even an annual Crape Myrtle Festival in Scotland Neck, NC. I imagine it would surprise many native residents to find out that Crape Myrtle is not a native tree!

Plants for A Future states:

Medicinal use of Crepe Myrtle: The stem bark is febrifuge, stimulant and styptic. The bark, flowers and leaves are considered to be hydrogogue and a drastic purgative. A paste of the flowers is applied externally to cuts and wounds. The root is astringent, detoxicant and diuretic. A decoction of the flowers is used in the treatment of colds.

Ligustrum, Privet

Privet is another one that would surprise many to learn that it is not native to my region. Privet is so widespread as to be considered and "invasive weed" by many. Four varieties of Privet have been naturized here: Ligustrum lucidum (Glossy Privet), Ligustrum ovalifolium (California Privet), Ligustrum quihoui (Waxy-leaf Privet), Ligustrum sinense (Chinese Privet)

Brother Aloysius wrote of Privet (Ligustrum vulgare):

Leaves and flowers are used medicinally, but only externally, for inflammation, and as a gargle for an ulcerated throat and mouth, ulceration of the gums and scurvy.

Ligustrum lucidum (also called Chinese Privet, but not to be confused with Ligustrum sinese) is the only member of this olive family of shrubby trees to be widely used in Herbal Medicine.

Plants for A Future States:

Medicinal use of Chinese Privet: Chinese privet has been used in traditional Chinese medicine for over 1,000 years. The fruit is antibacterial, antiseptic, antitumour, cardiotonic, diuretic and tonic. It is taken internally in the treatment of complaints associated with weak kidney and liver energy such as menopausal problems (especially premature menopause), blurred vision, cataracts, tinnitus, rheumatic pains, palpitations, backache and insomnia. Modern research has shown that the plant increases the white blood cell count and is of value when used to prevent bone marrow loss in cancer chemotherapy patients, it also has potential in the treatment of AIDS. Extracts of the plant show antitumour activity. Good results have also been achieved when the fruit has been used in treating respiratory tract infections, hypertension, Parkinson's disease and hepatitis. The fruit is harvested when fully ripe and is dried for later use. It is often decocted with other herbs in the treatment of a wide variety of ailments and also as a general tonic. Some caution is advised in their use, since the fruits are toxic when eaten in quantity. The leaves are anodyne, diaphoretic, febrifuge, pectoral and vulnerary. The bark of the stems is diaphoretic.

Liquidambar, Sweet Gum

Three varieties of Sweet Gum have been found useful in herbal medicine: Liquidambar formosana - Formosan Gum, Liquidambar orientalis - Oriental Sweet Gum, Liquidambar styraciflua - Sweet Gum

Only Liquidambar styraciflua, Sweet Gum grows in my region.

For me, this tree brings memories of chickens pecking while my mother, grandmother and great aunt sat and talked, shelling beans with my great grandmother on my great grandparent's farm. I was a small child, playing with the "gumballs" and the dogs in the sandy soil of an old fashioned swept yard. These trees are in the hamamela family, along with Witch Hazel, but they are very different. It is the gum, the resinous sap that gives them their name.

Resources of the Southern Fields and Forests states:

Sweet Gum (Liquidamhar Styraciflua)—The inner bark contains an astringent, gummy substance. If it is boiled in milk, or a tea made with water, its astringency is so great that it will easily check diarrhea, and associated with the use of other remedies, dysentery also. The leaf of the gum, when green, I have also ascertained to be powerfully astringent, and to contain as large a proportion of tannin as that of any other tree. I believe that the Gum leaf and the leaf of the Myrtle and Blackberry can be used wherever an astringent is required; cold water takes it up. They can, I think, be also used for tanning leather, when green, in place of oak bark.

In former times the resin was used in scabie ; and it is said(Am. Herbal, by J. Stearns) to be useful in resolving hard tumors in the uterus. The Indians esteemed it an excellent febrifuge and employed it in healing wounds. Mer. and de L, Diet, de M. Med. iv, 128, and the Supplem. 1846; Ann. de Montpcllier, 1805, 327; Journal de Pharm. vii, 339, and vii, 568; Bull, de Therap., October, 1833, where I). L'lleritier proposes to treat blennorrhagias and leucorrhoeas with liquid styrax. A kind of oil, called copalm, is extracted from it in Mexico, which, when. solidified, is called copalm resin; this is an excitant of the mucous system, and it is given in chronic catarrhs, and in affections of the lungs, intestines and urinary passages. This is cordial and stomachic; it excites both perspiration and urine; it is also used in perfumery. In South Carolina and Georgia the temperature is not high enough for this tree to furnish much gum. Dr. Griffith experimented with it in the latitude of Baltimore, and obtained a small quantity by boiling the twigs and branches; he found that it exists in greatest abundance in the young trees just before the appearance of the leaves. It is about the consistence of honey, of a yellow color, and of a pleasant, balsamic odor and taste. The acid obtained from the gum is not benzoic, as the English assert, but cynamic. See Am. J. Pharm. The tree is of rapid growth, and is ornamental—frequently assuming the appearance of a sugar-loaf. The wood is soft, but not durable. A decoction of the inner bark of the gum in a quart of milk, or a tea made with boiling water is one of the most valuable and useful mucilaginous astringents that we possess. It can be employed with advantage in eases of diarrhea and dysentery'. Dr. C. W. Wright, of Louisville, Ky., states that the bark of the tree is used with great advantage in the Western States in the diarrhea and dysentery of summer, especially in children. A syrup from the bark is prepared in the same manner as the syrup of wild cherry bark. The dose is a fluid ounce for an adult, repeated after each stool. Am. J. Med. Sc. N. S. xxxii, 126. The editor of the Va. Med. J., August, 1856, says that the use of a decoction of the bark in milk is common in many parts of Virginia as a remedy in the diarrhea of children. U. S. Disp., 12th Ed. In Georgia, also, a common domestic remedy for diarrhoeas is made by boiling in water equal parts of the barks of the rod oak and sweet gum—a small proportion of spirits may often be added with advantage. Dr. Wright claims that the syrup is retained by an irritable stomach when almost every other form of astringent medicine is rejected. See, also, Parrish Pract. Pharm., p. 230.

King's American Dispensatory, 1898 tells us:

Action, Medical Uses, and Dosage.—Sweet-gum probably has virtues similar to the concrete juice of Styrax officinale, which see. It makes an excellent and agreeable ointment when melted with equal parts of lard or tallow, which I have found decidedly useful in hemorrhoids, psora, ringworm of the scalp, porrigo scutulata, and many other cutaneous affections; also in that indolent species of ulcer, known as "fever sores on the legs." In anal fistula, it maintains an increased discharge, softens the callosity of the walls of the sinus, and produces a normal result, and effects this without pain to the patient. If necessary, in fistula, a little creosote, or other stimulant may be added to it. This employment of sweet-gum is not generally known, and physicians would do well to avail themselves of its use in the above diseases. It is also used in chronic catarrh, coughs, and pulmonary affections. The dose internally is from 10 to 20 grains (J. King).

Plants for A future states:

A resin obtained from the trunk of the tree (see "Uses notes" below) is antiseptic, carminative, diuretic, expectorant, parasiticide, poultice, salve, sedative, stimulant, vulnerary. It is chewed in the treatment of sore throats, coughs, asthma, cystitis, dysentery etc. Externally, it is applied to sores, wounds, piles, ringworm, scabies etc. The resin is an ingredient of "Friar's Balsam", a commercial preparation based on Styrax benzoin that is used to treat colds and skin problems. The mildly astringent inner bark is used in the treatment of diarrhoea and childhood cholera.

The aromatic resin "Storax" is obtained from the trunk of this tree. It forms in cavities of the bark and also exudes naturally. It is harvested in autumn. Production can be stimulated by beating the trunk in the spring. The resin has a wide range of uses including medicinal, incense, perfumery, soap and as an adhesive. It is also chewed and used as a tooth cleaner. Wood - heavy, fairly hard, fine-grained, not strong, light, tough, resilient. It weighs about 37lb per cubic foot. The wood takes a high polish and can be stained then used as a cherry, mahogany or walnut substitute. It is also used for furniture, flooring, fruit dishes, veneer etc.

Peterson Field Guides Eastern and Central Medicinal Plants tells us:

Gum or balsam (resin) was traditionally chewed for sore throats, coughs, colds, diarrhea, dysentery, ringworm; used externally for sores, skin ailments, wounds, piles. Ingredient in "compound tincture of benzoin", available from pharmacies. Considered expectorant, antiseptic, antimicrobial, anti-inflammatory. Children sometimes chew the gum in lieu of commercial chewing gum. The mildly astringent inner bark was used as a folk remedy, boiled in milk for diarrhea and cholera infantum.

Botany In a Day states:

Liquidambar, sweet gum: the sap of the tree may be used as a chewing gum the gum is used medicinally as a drawing poultice also for sore throats. It is astringent and expectorant in effect.

Tuliptree (Liriodendron tulipifera), Tulip Poplar

Tuliptree is very common in my region.

Native Plants, Native Healing states of Tulip Poplar:

Tulip poplar, as a medicine, is particular to the heart. It has a tonic effect, cleaning plaque slowly, from the inside of the arteries, so it is useful for hardening of the arteries. A tincture is made by soaking strips of inner bark in strong alcohol. ... This is good for people recovering from stroke, people with pre-heart attack conditions, or those who have suffered several heart attacks and/or bypasses.

Resources of the Southern Fields and Forests states:

Tulip Bearing Poplar {Liriodendron) and the Willow bark supply remedies for the fevers met with in camp. The Cold infusion is given.

This plant is tonic, diuretic and diaphoretic, and is generally considered one of the most valuable of the substitutes for Peruvian bark. It has been employed as a warm sudorific in the treatment of chronic rheumatism and gout; and Bigelow thinks it valuable as a stomachic. It was administered by Dr. Young and himself, combined with laudanum, in hysteria, and the former says that in all the materia medica be does not know of a more certain, speedy, and effectual remedy for that disease. See his letter to Governor Clayton. He has never known it to fail in a single case of worms. Am. Museum, xii; Griffith, Med. Bot. 98. Eafinesque says the seeds are laxative, and the leaves are used as an external application for headache; they are washed and applied to the forehead. Merat states that it is useful in phthisis, and he also refers to its vermifuge properties; employed in relaxed states of the stomach (reldchemens) and in the advanced stages of dysentery; this is corroborated by Thacher. Anc. Journal de Med. lxx, 530 ; J. C. Mayer, Mem. on L. tulipifera, in the Mem de l'Acad. de Berlin, 1796; Euch. Mem. sur le tulipier, Tilloch's Magazine; Hildebrande, Essai sur un nouveau succedane du quinquina in Ann. de Chim. lxvi, 201; Carminati sur les proprietes medicinales de l'ecorce de tulipier. Its analysis, etc., in the Mem. of Eoy. Inst. Lombardy, iii, 4; in the Supplcm. to Mer. Diet. 1846, 436. M. Bouchardat advises, as the most preferable mode of exhibiting it in fevers, the wine made with the bark in equal parts of alcohol, to which he adds of white wine seven or eight times the amount of the alcohol infusion. Bull, de Therap. xix, 246; S. Cubicre's Hist. Tulip. Paris, 1800; see Tract, of Bouchardat in Ann. de Therap. 75, 1841. Dr. J. P.Emmet, in his Analysis in the Phil. J. Pharm. iii, 5, announced the discovery of a new principle in it— liriodendrine. This is solid, brittle and inodorous at 40°, fusible at 180°, and volatile at 270° It is soluble in alcohol, thought to be analogous to camphor, and to the principle found in the Magnolia grandifiora, and to consist of a resin and a volatile oil; hence the alcoholic tincture is preferable. The powdered bark in syrup is given to children who are liable to convulsions from worms, to promote their expulsion, and to strengthen the tone of the digestive organs. The bark should be pulverized and bottled. I have employed a strong infusion of the bark and root of this lant as an anti-intermittent, among a number of negroes, and am much pleased with its efficacy. See the wild Jalap {Podophyllum peltatiwi,) in conjunction with which it was usually given. In Virginia, the decoction of the bark, with that of the Cornus Florida (dogwood) and the Pmios verticillatus, is given to horses affected with the hots. The poplar bai-k powdered is a valuable remedy as a tonic for horses. An infusion may be given to a horse, or the bark placed in his trough to be chewed. It gives tone to the digestive organs when they are "off their feed," in veterinary or jockey parlance. This tree I notice in unusual abundance along the line of railroad from Kingville to Columbia, S. C; also in Spartanburg district, S. C, on the banks of streams. Dose of bark xx-xxx grs. It is a stimulant tonic, slightly, diaphoretic. The infusion or decoction is made in the proportion of an ounce to a pint of water; dose one or two fluid ounces. Dose of the saturated tincture a fluid drachm.

King's American Dispensatory, 1898 tells us

Action, Medical Uses, and Dosage.—Tulip-tree bark is an aromatic stimulant tonic, and has proved beneficial in intermittents, chronic rheumatism, chronic gastric and intestinal diseases, worms, and hysteria. In hysteria, combined with a small quantity of laudanum, it is said to be speedy, certain, and effectual, and also to abate the hectic fever, night-sweats, and colliquative diarrhoea of phthisis. The warm infusion is diaphoretic, and under certain states of the system has proven diuretic. It is now seldom used. Prof. Bartholow found the alkaloid tulipiferine to act energetically upon the nervous system of frogs and rabbits. Dose of the powdered bark, from 20 grains to 2 drachms; of the saturated tincture, which is the best form of administration, 1 fluid drachm; of the infusion, from 1 to 2 fluid ounces; of liriodendrin, from 5 to 10 grains.

Turning to Plants for A Future once more:

The intensely acrid bitter inner bark, especially of the roots, is used domestically as a diuretic, tonic and stimulant. The raw green bark is also chewed as an aphrodisiac. The bark contains "tulipiferine", which is said to exert powerful effects on the heart and nervous system. A tea is used in the treatment of indigestion, dysentery, rheumatism, coughs, fevers etc. Externally, the tea is used as a wash and a poultice on wounds and boils. The root bark and the seeds have both been used to expel worms from the body.

Peterson Field Guides Eastern and Central Medicinal Plants tells us:

American Indians used bark tea for indigestion, dysentery, rheumatism, pinworms, fevers, and in cough syrups; Externally, as a wash on fractured limbs, wounds, boils, snake bites. Green bark chewed as an aphrodisiac, stimulant. Bark tea a folk remedy for malaria, toothaches; Ointment from buds used for burns, inflammation. Crushed leaves poulticed for headaches.

Botany In A Day states:

Tulip tree: some Native Americans ate the bark to expel worms and gave the seeds to children for the same purpose. The Tulip tree has also been used to reduce fevers, as a diet diuretic for rheumatism. The root has been used in Canada to take away the bitterness in brewing alcohol.

The Physicians' Desk Reference for Herbal Medicine tells us:

The alkaloids contained in the drug are antimicrobial in effect, a positively entropic effect has been described. Its usefulness is a tonic and stimulant appears to be plausible, based upon its qualities as a bitter substance. Unproven uses: folk medicine indications have included fever, menstrual complaints, insomnia, and malaria. Precautions and adverse reactions: the drug is considered toxic, due to its alkaloid content.... No case of poisoning among humans has been recorded.

Maclura pomifera, Osage Orange

Osage Orange is not native to my region but has been naturalized. It was once widely used for hedges and the wood as fence posts.

Plants for A Future states:

Medicinal use of Osage Orange: A tea made from the roots has been used as a wash for sore eyes. The inedible fruits contain antioxidant and fungicidal compounds. A 10% aqueous infusion and an extract diluted 1:1 have cardiovascular potentialities.

Peterson Field Guides Eastern and Central Medicinal Plants tells us:

American Indians use root tea as a wash for sore eyes. Fruit sections used in Maryland and Pennsylvania as a cockroach repellent. Inedible fruits contain antioxidant and fungal compounds. Warning: milk (latex or sap(may cause dermatitis.

Magnoliaceae, Magnolia

Eleven varieties of Magnolia have been found useful in herbal medicine: Magnolia acuminata - Cucumber Tree, Magnolia campbellii, Magnolia denudata - Lily Tree, Magnolia grandiflora, Magnolia hypoleuca, Magnolia Kobus, Magnolia liliiflora - Mu-Lan, Magnolia macrophylla - Bigleaf Magnolia, Magnolia officinalis - Hou Po, Magnolia stellata - Star Magnolia, Magnolia virginiana - Laurel Magnolia

Six varieties of Magnolia are native to my region: Magnolia acuminata (Cucumber-Tree), Magnolia fraseri (Fraser Magnolia), Magnolia grandiflora (Southern Magnolia, Bull-bay), Magnolia macrophylla (Bigleaf Magnolia), Magnolia tripetala (Umbrella-Tree, Umbrella Magnolia), Magnolia virginiana (Sweetbay)

No tree is as emblematic of the American South as Magnolia grandiflora, and certainly no tree is as beautiful or fragrant. The large, strongly lemon scented and edible blossoms mix with the aroma of gardenia on those warm, sultry southern nights for which our region is known. This is an inseparable part of the magical charm of the South. But, in the mountains where I was born, the Cucumber Tree is far more common. And, in my childhood spent off the mountain, I well remember the Sweetbay in the eastern piedmont and coastal swamps.

Mrs Grieves wrote of Magnolia:

The genus is named in commemoration of Pierre Magnol, a famous professor of medicine and botany of Montpellier in the early eighteenth century. All its members are handsome, with luxuriant foliage and rich flowers. The leaves of Magnolia acuminata are oval, about 6 inches long by 3 broad, and slightly hairy below, with a diameter of 6 inches, and the fruit or cone, about 3 inches long, resembles a small cucumber.

It is a large tree, reaching a height of 80 or more feet and a diameter of 3 to 5 feet, but only grows to about 16 feet in England. The wood is finely grained, taking a brilliant polish, and in its colour resembles that of the tulip or poplar, but it is less durable. It is sometimes used for large canoes and house interiors.

The bark of the young wood is curved or quilled, fissured outside, with occasional warts, and orange-brown in colour, being whitish and smooth within and the fracture short except for inner fibres. The older bark without the corky layer is brownish or whitish and fibrous. Drying and age cause the loss of its volatile, aromatic property.

The bark has no astringency. The tonic properties are found in varying degree in several species.

Medicinal Action and Uses---A mild diaphoretic, tonic, and aromatic stimulant. It is used in rheumatism and malaria and is contra-indicated in inflammatory symptoms. In the Alleghany districts the cones are steeped in spirits to make a tonic tincture.

A warm infusion is laxative and sudorific, a cold one being antiperiodic and mildly tonic.

Dosage---Fluid Extract. Frequent doses of 1/2 to 1 drachm, or the infusion in wineglassful doses.

Other Species---

Both M. virginiana and M. tripetala were recognized as official with M. acuminata.

M. virginiana, or M. glauca, White Laurel, Beaver Tree, Swamp Sassafras, White Bay, Sweet Bay, Small or Laurel Magnolia, or Sweet Magnolia, is much used by beavers, who favour it both as food and building material. The light wood has no commercial use.

The bark and seed cones are bitter and aromatic, used as tonics, and in similar ways to M. acuminata. The leaves yield a green, volatile oil with a more pleasant odour than fennel or anise. There is probably also a bitter glucosidal principle.

M. tripetala, Umbrella Tree or Umbrella Magnolia. The fruit yields a neutral crystalline principle, Magnolin.

The bark, if chewed as a substitute for tobacco, is said to cure the habit.

Resources of the Southern Fields and Forests states:

MAGNOLIACEAE. {The Magnolia Tribe.)

This order is characterized by the possession of a bitter tonic taste, and fragrant flowers; the latter generally producing a decided action upon the nerves.

BAY; BEAYER TREE; SWAMP-LAUREL, (Magnoliaglauca, L.) - It is a stimulant, aromatic tonic, with considerable diaphoretic powers. The leaves, steeped in brandy, or a decoction of them, are valuable in pectoral affections, recent cold, etc. The tincture, made by macerating the fresh cones and seeds, or bark of root, in brandy, which best extracts its virtues, is much used as a popular remedy in rheumatism, and in intermittent fevers ; and, according to Barton, in inflammatory gout. Lindley refers to it as a valuable tonic, but it is said to be destitute of tannin or gallic acid. The bark of the root, according to Griffith, was employed by the Indians to fulfil a variety of indications; the warm decoction acts as a gentle laxative, and subsequently as a sudorific, whilst the cold decoction, powder of, or tincture, is tonic. These have proved very beneficial in the hands of regular practitioners in the treatment of remittents of a typhoid character. It is supposed by many residing in the lower portions of South Carolina that this tree prevents the water of bogs and galls from generating malaria. It certainly seems that the water is much clearer in which the bay tree grows.

MAGNOLIA, (Magnolia grandijlora, L.) - This magnificent tree grows beautifully along the seacoast, and in the streets of Charleston. Found sparingly in St. John's Berkley, forty-five miles from the ocean; grows in Georgia, also, in North Carolina. . The medicinal and chemical properties of these plants are supposed to be identical. See M. glauca. Mr. Proctor, in his analysis, Am. Journal Pharm. xiv. 95, and viii, 85, found iii this species volatile oil, resin, and a crystallizable principle analogous to the liriodendrine of Prof. Emmett, obtained from the L.tulipifer growing in the Southern States (vide L. tulip.) Merat says that in Mexico the seeds are employed with success in paralysis.

CUCUMBER TREE, {Magnolia acuminata, Linn. Mich.) - Mountainous districts; grows in Georgia, also, in North Carolina. Fl. Lindley speaks particularly of the cones of this species being employed in the form of a spirituous tincture in rheumatic affections. Mer. and de L. Diet, de M. Med. iv, 193 ; Griffith, Med. Bot. 98. Used as a prophylactic in autumnal fevers. The flowers of most magnolias exhale a strong aromatic fragrance; the bark of all possesses a combination of bitter and hotly aromatic properties, without astringency, and that of many acts as a powerful medicine, in a similar way to Peruvian bark and Winter's bark.

King's American Dispensatory, 1898 tells us:

Action, Medical Uses, and Dosage.—Magnolia bark is an aromatic tonic bitter, of reputed efficacy, and appears likewise to possess antiperiodic properties. Intermittent fevers have been cured by it after cinchona had failed. It is not so apt to disagree with the stomach and bowels, nor to induce fullness of the head as cinchona and can be continued a longer time with more safety in all respects. Its curative agency is said to be favored by the diaphoretic action which generally follows its administration. In dyspepsia, with loss of tone in the stomach, it is very useful as a tonic, and has also proved of much service in the treatment of remittents with typhoid symptoms. A warm infusion acts as a gentle laxative and sudorific; a cold one as a tonic and antiperiodic, as does also the tincture and powder. The powder is considered the preferable form of administration. The bark of the M. Umbrella, chewed as a substitute for tobacco, has cured an inveterate tobacco chewer of the filthy habit, and deserves a further trial among those who wish to break up the pernicious practice. The bark in powder may be administered in ½- drachm or drachm doses, to be repeated 5 or 6 times a day; the infusion may be taken in wineglassful doses, repeated 5 or 6 times a day. It is used in the above forms of disease, as well as in chronic rheumatism. The tincture, made by adding an ounce of the powder to a pint of brandy, and allowing it to macerate for 10 or 12 days, may be given in tablespoon doses 3 times a day, for the same purposes. A tincture made by adding 2 ounces of the cones to a pint of brandy, has long been used as a domestic remedy for dyspepsia and chronic rheumatism; it is given 3 or 4 times a day in doses of from 1 to 4 fluid drachms. Magnolia is contraindicated whenever inflammatory symptoms are present. Though possessing undoubted tonic properties, magnolia is now seldom employed.

Plants for A Future states::

(grandiflora) The bark is diaphoretic, stimulant, tonic. It is used in the treatment of malaria and rheumatism. A decoction has been used as a wash and a bath for prickly heat itching. The decoction has also been used as a wash for sores and as a steam bath for treating dropsy. An alcoholic extract of the plant reduces the blood pressure, produces a slight acceleration in respiration but has no action on the heart.

(acuminata, Cucumber Tree) A tea made from the bark is antiperiodic, aromatic, mildly diaphoretic, laxative, stimulant, tonic. It has historically been used as a substitute for quinine in the treatment of malaria. An infusion has been used in the treatment of stomach ache and cramps. The bark has been chewed by people trying to break the tobacco habit. A hot infusion of the bark has been snuffed to treat sinus problems and has also been held in the mouth to treat toothaches. The bark is harvested in the autumn and dried for later use. It does not store well so stocks should be renewed annually. A tea made from the fruit is a tonic, used in the treatment of general debility and was formerly esteemed in the treatment of stomach ailments.

(macrophylla) An infusion of the bark has been used in the treatment of stomach aches or cramps. A hot infusion of the bark has been snuffed for treating sinus problems and has been held in the mouth for treating toothache.

(virginiana) A tea made from the bark is antiperiodic, aromatic, diaphoretic, laxative, stimulant and tonic. It has historically been used as a substitute for quinine in the treatment of malaria and is also taken internally in the treatment of colds, bronchial diseases, upper respiratory tract infections, rheumatism and gout. The bark has been chewed by people trying to break the tobacco habit. The bark is harvested in the autumn and dried for later use. It does not store well so stocks should be renewed annually. A tea made from the fruit is a tonic, used in the treatment of general debility and was formerly esteemed in the treatment of stomach ailments. The leaves or bark have been placed in cupped hands over the nose and inhaled as a mild hallucinogen.

Peterson Field Guides Eastern and Central Medicinal Plants tells us:

Cucumber Magnolia: bark tea historically used in place of chinchona the source of quinine, for malarial and typhoid fevers; Also, for indigestion: rheumatism: worms: toothaches. Bark chewed to break tobacco habit. Fruit tea a tonic for general debility; formerly esteemed for stomach ailments.

Sweetbay: Magnolia virginiana. American Indians use leaf tea to "warm blood", cure colds. Traditionally bark used like that of M acuminata. Bark also used for rheumatism, malaria, epilepsy.

Botany In a Day states:

Magnolia: the bark of Magnolia is known for its aromatic and astringent properties. A tea of the bark is used as a diaphoretic, and for indigestion or diarrhea. Reportedly, drinking the tea can help break the tobacco habit.

Malus, Apple

Forty-one varieties of Malus have been found to be useful in herbal medicine: Malus angustifolia - Southern Crab, Malus baccata - Chinese Crab, Malus baccata mandschurica - Manchurian Apple, Malus bracteate, Malus brevipes, Malus coronaria - Garland Crab, Malus domestica – Apple, Malus Florentina, Malus floribunda - Japanese Crab, Malus fusca - Oregon Crab, Malus glabrata, Malus glaucescens, Malus halliana, Malus halliana spontaneae, Malus hupehensis - Chinese Crab, Malus ioensis - Prairie Crab, Malus ioensis palmeri - Prairie Crab, Malus kansuensis, Malus lancifolia, Malus praecox, Malus prattii, Malus prunifolia - Chinese Apple, Malus prunifolia rinkii - Chinese Apple, Malus pumila - Paradise Apple, Malus pumila nervosa - Crab Apple, Malus pumila paradisiaca - Paradise Apple, Malus sargentii, Malus sieversii, Malus sikkimensis, Malus spectabilis - Chinese Flowering Apple, Malus sylvestris - Crab Apple, Malus toringo, Malus toringoides, Malus transitoria, Malus trilobata, Malus tschonoskii, Malus x adstringens, Malus x astracanica, Malus x microMalus - Kaido Crab Apple, Malus x robusta, Malus x soulardii, Malus yunnanensis

Only two Crabapples are native to my region, though the number of "heirloom" apples that have become feral over the centuries is vast. Our natives are: Malus angustifolia (Southern Crabapple) and Malus coronaria (Sweet Crabapple). Innumerable heirloom varieties of sweet Apple have been grown in my region. Many homesteaders and longtime residents – descendants of those who won America's independence, were forced off of their family lands to create the Blue Ridge Parkway, the Tennessee Valley Authority, etc. Like the Cherokee before them, also forced from their homes, they left their food plants behind. Old apple trees can be found throughout my region, often near old stack stone chimneys and abandoned family cemeteries that are the only reminders that the "Land of the Free" ceased to be so early on in our history… as early as the Whisky Rebellion, and was surely lost but the 1940s.

Dioscorides wrote of Apples:

Melimela — Honey Apples, Must Apples, Cider Apples

Melimela soften the intestines and drive living creatures from there [worms]. They are bad for the stomach and cause a burning heat.

They are called glycymela by some — as we should say, sweet apples.

Pyrus malus var sylvestris — Crab Apples, Wild Apples

Wild apples are similar to spring apples and are astringent, but for those things which need an astringent you must use those which are least ripe.

Saint Hildegard wrote:

A person, whether young or old, who suffers from fogginess in his eyes for any reason should take the leaves of this tree in the springtime, before it produces its fruit for the year. When these first come out at the beginning of spring, they are tender and healthy, as young girls before they produce children. He should pound these leaves and express their sap, and to this add an equal measure of the drops that flow from the grapevine. He should place this in a metallic jar and, at night when he goes to bed, he should moisten his eyelids and eyes with a feather dipped in a bit of it. It should be like dew falling on grass, and care should be taken that it not enter the eyes. Then he should sprinkle the crushed leaves with a bit of the drops that flow from the grapevine, and place them over his eyes. He should hold this on with a cloth and sleep with it on. If he does this often, the fogginess will be driven from his eyes and he will see clearly.

When in springtime he first shoots of the apple tree burst forth, tear off one little branch, without cutting it with iron, and draw a strap of deer-hide back and forth over the break in the tree and the branch, so that it becomes damp with sap. When you sense that there is no more moisture, then hack, with very tiny blows, this broken spot with a small knife, so that more of the moisture flows out. By drawing the deer hide strap over the same place and on the same branch, drench it with as much sap as you can. Then, put it in a damp place so that it may absorb even more sap. Anyone who has pain in his kidneys or trouble urinating should gird himself with this strap, over his naked flesh, so that the sap which it drew from the apple tree might pass into his flesh, and he will become better.

Anyone who has pain from an illness of the liver or spleen, from bad humors of the belly or stomach, or from a migraine in his head should take the first shoots of the apple tree and place them in olive oil. He should warm them in a little jar in the sun. If he drinks this often when he goes to bed, his head will be better.

Also in the springtime, when the blossoms come out, take earth, which has been around the root of this tree, and heat it on the fire. Anyone who has pain in his shoulders, loins or stomach should place it, thus warmed, over the painful place, and he will be better. After the fruits of this tree have increased, so that they begin to enlarge, the earth is no longer powerful against these infirmities. The humor of this earth and the sap of the tree will have ascended to the fruits, leaving that in the earth and branches much weaker.

The fruit fo this tree is gentle and easily digested and, eaten raw, does not harm healthy people. Apples grow from dew when it is strong, namely from the first sleep of the night untilt he day is nearly breaking. They are good for healthy people to eat raw, since they are ripened by the strong dew. Raw apples are a bit harmful for sick people to eat, because of their weakness. But cooked or dried apples are good for both sick and healthy people. After apples have gotten old, and the skin has contracted as happens in winter, then they are good for both sick and healthy people to eat raw.

Gerard wrote of Apples:

A. Roasted apples are always better than the raw, the harm whereof is both mended by the fire, and may also be corrected by adding unto them seeds or spices.

B. Apples be good for an hot stomach: those that are austere or somewhat harsh do strengthen a weak and feeble stomach proceeding of heat.

C. Apples are also good for all inflammations or hot swellings, but especially for such as are in their beginning, if the same be outwardly applied.

D. The juice of apples which be sweet and of a middle taste, is mixed in compositions of divers medicines, and also for the tempering of melancholy humours, and likewise to mend the qualities of medicines that are dry: as are Serapium ex pomis Regis Saporis, Confectio Alkermes, and such like compositions

E. There is likewise made an ointment with the pulp of apples and swines' grease and Rose-water, which is used to beautify the face, and to take away the roughness of the skin, which is called in shops Pomatum: of the apples whereof it is made.

F. The pulp of the roasted apples, in number four or five, according to the greatness of the apples, especially of the Pome Water, mixed in a wine quart of fair water, laboured together until it come to be as apples and ale, which we call lambs' wool, and the whole quart drunk last at night within the space of an hour, doth in one night cure those that piss by drops with great anguish and dolour; the strangury, and all other diseases proceeding of the difficulty of making water; but in twice taking it, it never faileth in any: oftentimes there happeneth with the foresaid diseases the gonorrhæa, or running of the reins, which it likewise healeth in those persons, but not generally in all; which myself have often proved, and gained thereby both crowns and credit.

G. The leaves of the tree do cool and bind, and be also counted good for inflammations, in the beginning.

H. Apples cut in pieces, and distilled with a quantity of camphor and buttermilk, take away the marks and scars gotten by the smallpox, being washed therewith when they grow unto their state and ripeness: provided that you give unto the patient a little milk and saffron, or milk and mithridate to drink, to expel to the extreme parts that venom which may lie hid, and as yet not seen.

And, of Crabapples:

A. The juice of wild Apples or crabs taketh away the heat of burnings, scaldings, and all inflammations: and being laid on in short time after it is scalded, it keepeth it from blistering.

B. The juice of crabs or verjuice is astringent or binding, and hath withal an abstersive or cleansing quality, being mixed with hard yeast of ale or beer, and applied in manner of a cold ointment, that is, spread upon a cloth first wet in the verjuice and wrung out, and then laid to, taketh away the heat of Saint Anthony's fire, all inflammations whatsoever, healeth scabbed legs, burnings and scaldings wheresoever it be.

Culpepper states:

Apple-trees are all under the dominion of Venus. In general they are cold and windy, and the best are to be avoided, before they are thoroughly ripe; then to be roasted or scalded, and a little spice or warm seeds thrown on them, and then should only be eaten after or between meals, or for supper. They are very proper for hot and bilious stomachs, but not to the cold, moist, and flatulent. The more ripe ones eaten raw, move the belly a little; and unripe ones have the contrary effect. A poultice of roasted sweet apples, with powder of frankincense, removes pains of the side: and a poultice of the same apples boiled in plantain water to a pulp, then mixed with milk, and applied, take away fresh marks of gunpowder out of the skin. Boiled or roasted apples eaten with rose water and sugar, or with a little butter, is a pleasant cooling diet for feverish complaints. An infusion of sliced apples with their skins in boiling water, a crust of bread, some barley, and a little mace or all-spice, is a very proper cooling diet drink in fevers. Roasted apples are good for the asthmatic; either raw, roasted or boiled, are good for the consumptive, in inflammations of the breasts or lungs. Their syrup is a good cordial in faintings, palpitations, and melancholy: The pulp of boiled or rotten apples in a poultice, is good for inflamed eyes, either applied alone or with milk,or rose or fennel-waters. The pulp of five or six roasted apples, beaten up with a quart of water to lamb's wool, and the whole drank at night in an hour's space, speedily cures such as slip their water by drops, attended with heat and pain. Gerard observes, if it does not effectually remove the complaint the first night, it never yet failed the second. The sour provokes urine most; but the rough strengthens most the stomach and bowels.

Of Apples, Mrs. Grieves wrote:

The chief dietetic value of apples lies in the malic and tartaric acids. These acids are of signal benefit to persons of sedentary habits, who are liable to liver derangements, and they neutralize the acid products of gout and indigestion. 'An apple a day keeps the doctor away' is a respectable old rhyme that has some reason in it.

The acids of the Apple not only make the fruit itself digestible, but even make it helpful in digesting other foods. Popular instinct long ago led to the association of apple sauce with such rich foods as pork and goose, and the old English fancy for eating apple pie with cheese, an obsolete taste, nowadays, is another example of instinctive inclination, which science has approved.

The sugar of a sweet apple, like most fruit sugars, is practically a predigested food, and is soon ready to pass into the blood to provide energy and warmth for the body.

A ripe raw apple is one of the easiest vegetable substances for the stomach to deal with, the whole process of its digestion being completed in eighty-five minutes.

The juice of apples, without sugar, will often reduce acidity of the stomach; it becomes changed into alkaline carbonates, and thus corrects sour fermentation.

It is stated on medical authority that in countries where unsweetened cider is used as a common beverage, stone or calculus is unknown, and a series of inquiries made of doctors in Normandy, where cider is the principal drink, brought to light the fact that not a single case of stone had been met with during forty years.

Ripe, juicy apples eaten at bedtime every night will cure some of the worst forms of constipation. Sour apples are the best for this purpose. Some cases of sleeplessness have been cured in this manner. People much inclined to biliousness will find this practice very valuable. In some cases stewed apples will agree perfectly well, while raw ones prove disagreeable. There is a very old saying:

'To eat an apple going to bed

Will make the doctor beg his bread.'

The Apple will also act as an excellent dentifrice, being a food that is not only cleansing to the teeth on account of its juices, but just hard enough to mechanically push back the gums so that the borders are cleared of deposits.

Rotten apples used as a poultice is an old Lincolnshire remedy for sore eyes, that is still in use in some villages.

It is no exaggeration to say that the habitual use of apples will do much to prolong life and to ameliorate its conditions. In the Edda, the old Scandinavian saga, Iduna kept in a box, apples that she gave to the gods to eat, thereby to renew their youth.

A French physician has found that the bacillus of typhoid fever cannot live long in apple juice, and therefore recommends doubtful drinking water to be mixed with cider.

A glucoside in small crystals is obtainable from the bark and root of the apple, peach and plum, which is said to induce artificial diabetes in animals, and thus can be used in curing it in human beings.

The original pomatum seems to date from Gerard's days, when an ointment for roughness of the skin was made from apple pulp, swine's grease, and rosewater.

The astringent verjuice, rich in tannin, of the Crab, is helpful in chronic diarrhoea.

The bark may be used in decoction for intermittent and bilious fevers.

Cider in which horse-radish has been steeped has been found helpful in dropsy.

Cooked apples make a good local application for sore throat in fevers, inflammation of the eyes, erysipelas, etc.

Stewed apples are laxative; raw ones not invariably so.

An Irish Herbal states of Apple:

Apples comfort and cool the heat of the stomach, especially those that are somewhat sour. The leaves should be laid upon hot swellings, and they can also be applied to fresh wounds to prevent them from turning bad.

Of Crab Apple:

The juice of crabs is a useful astringent in gargles for ulcers of the mouth, throat and also for dropped uvulas. It is also good for burns, scalds and inflammations.

Of Quince (also in the Malus family):

Quince stops diarrhea, dysentery and hemorrhages of all kinds. They also strengthen the stomach, aid digestion and stop vomiting.

King's American Dispensatory, 1898 tells us of Apple:

Action, Medical Uses, and Dosage.—Apple tree bark is tonic and febrifuge, and a decoction of it has been used with advantage in intermittent, remittent, and bilious fevers, and in convalescence from exhausting diseases. It may be given in. doses of 1 to 4 fluid ounces, 3 times a day. A strong decoction or syrup of the sweet apple tree bark has been employed with success in some cases of gravel. The fruit, or apple, contains both malic and acetic acids, has a pleasant and refreshing flavor, and is a useful and healthy article of diet. However, it should not generally be eaten by dyspeptics or patients afflicted with gout, rheumatism, renal, and cutaneous diseases. If indications for an acid are present, however, it is not especially contraindicated by rheumatism and dyspepsia. When baked, stewed, or roasted, it becomes valuable as an agreeable and healthy diet in febrile diseases, exanthemata, etc., and is more easily digested than when raw; it is also slightly laxative, and is beneficial in cases of habitual constipation. Raw apples should always be well masticated before being swallowed, as otherwise, they may become a source of serious difficulties, especially with children. An apple tea may be made for fever patients, by boiling a tart apple in ½ pint of water, and sweetening with sugar.

Cider forms not only a refreshing and agreeable drink for patients with fever, but actually exerts a salutary medicinal influence, especially where the tongue is coated deep-red, brown, or black. I have used cider, in which horseradish has been steeped, as an efficient remedy in dropsy, for many years; and it is now used in the preparation of a valuable agent for this disease, the Compound Infusion of Parsley. Cooked apples form an excellent local application in ophthalmic inflammation, erysipelatous inflammations, sore and swelled throat in scarlatina, ulcers, etc. (J. King).

Phloridzin is tonic and antiperiodic, and has cured cases of intermittent fever, even where quinine has proved ineffectual; its dose is from 5 to 20 grains. Unlike quinine, it does not cause gastralgia.

Melia azedarach – Chinaberry

This naturalized tree is quite useful as a medicinal herb.

Plants for A Future states:

Used externally in the treatment of rheumatism. An aqueous extract reduces the intensity of asthmatic attacks. (This report does not specify the part of the plant that is used.) The leaf juice is anthelmintic, antilithic, diuretic and emmenagogue. A decoction is astringent and stomachic. The leaves are harvested during the growing season and can be used fresh or dried. The flowers and leaves are applied as a poultice in the treatment of neuralgia and nervous headache. The stem bark is anthelmintic, astringent and bitter tonic. It is used as a tonic in India. It can be harvested at any time of the year and is used fresh or dried. The fruit is antiseptic and febrifuge. The pulp is used as a vermifuge. The fruit is harvested in the autumn when it is fully ripe and can be used fresh or dried. The seed is antirheumatic. It is used externally. The root bark is emetic, emmenagogue, purgative and vermifuge. It is highly effective against ringworm and other parasitic skin diseases. It can be harvested at any time of the year and is used fresh or dried. A gum that exudes from the tree is considered by some to have aphrodisiac properties. This plant should be used with caution, preferably under the supervision of a qualified practitioner. Excess causes diarrhoea, vomiting and symptoms of narcotic poisoning.

Wax Myrtle, Morella cerifera or Myrica cerifera

Also called Bayberry.

Mrs. Grieves writes:

Astringent and stimulant. In large doses emetic. It is useful in diarrhoea, jaundice, scrofula, etc. Externally, the powdered bark is used as a stimulant to indolent ulcers, though in poultices it should be combined with elm. The decoction is good as a gargle and injection in chronic inflammation of the throat, leucorrhoea, uterine haemorrhage, etc. It is an excellent wash for the gums.

The powder is strongly sternutatory and excites coughing. Water in which the wax has been 'tried,' when boiled to an extract, is regarded as a certain cure for dysentery, and the wax itself, being astringent and slightly narcotic, is valuable in severe dysentery and internal ulcerations.

Resources of the Southern Fields and Forests states:

MYRICACEAE. {The Gale Tribe.)

Aromatic and sometimes astringent.

WAX MYRTLE; BAYBEEEY, (Myrica cerifera, L.) Grows abundantly in the swamps of the lower country; Newbern. Fl. May. Ell. Bot. .Med. Notes, ii, 27S; Matson's Yeg. Pract. 1118; U. S. Disp. 200; Pe. Mat. Med. and Therap, 78(5 ; Biir. Am. Med. Pot.iii, 32 ; Am. Journal Med. Sei. ii, 313; Bergii, Mat. Med. ii, 541 ; Nicholson's Journal, iv, 187 ; Kalnvs Travels, i, 120 ; Dana in Silliman's Journal 1; Thacher's U. S. Disp. 288; Mor. ami de L. Diet, de M. Med. iv, 531; Pe Cand. Kssai, 772; Pind. Nat. Syst. Bot. 180. The root is a powerful astringent, and a decoction is employed in diarrhea, dysentery, hemorrhage from the uterus, in dropsies which succeed fevers, and as a gargle in sore throat. It is also given to some extent by the vegetable practitioners. Griffith states (Med. Bot. 583) that the bark of the root is also stimulant and acrid, and in doses of a drachm causes a sensation of heat in the stomach followed by vomiting and sometimes diuresis. The powder is an active errhine,, and the leaves have some celebrity in domestic practice, as being anti- spasmodic, anti-scorbutic and astringent. Dr. Dana found the powdered root powerfully sternutatory, Bigelow says that the bark and leaves contain gallic acid, tannin, resin and a small quantity of mucilage. The berries afford a large amount of wax, which rises to the surface when they are boiled, not re- markable for adhesiveness or unetuosity. Dr. Bostock considers it a tixed, vegetable oil, rendered concrete by oxygen; and by the experiments of Dr. Dana, it constitutes one-third of the whole berry. It is employed for candles, emitting a fragrant odor, and it also forms the basis of a tine soap. It appears to possess some astringent and slightly narcotic properties, and has been administered by Dr. Fahnestock in an epidemic of typhoid dysentery. He gave it in doses of one to two drachms, and he is of opinion that its active principle resides in the green coloring matter. Am. Journal Med. Sci. ii, 313. Eatinesque states that a tincture of the berries, with heracleum, is beneficial in flatulent colic.

The Thomsonian System of Medicine states of Bayberry:

BAYBERRY. Myrica Cerifera. This is a species of the myrtle, from which wax is obtained from the berries, and grows common in many parts of this country. It is a shrub growing from two to four feet high, and is easily known by the berries which it produces annually, containing wax in abundance. These grow on the branches close to them similar to the juniper. The leaves are of a deep green. The bark of the roots is what is used for medicine, and should be collected in the spring, before it puts forth its leaves, or in the fall, after done growing, as then the sap is in the roots ; this should be attended to in gathering all kinds of medicinal roots; but those things that the tops are used should be collected in the summer when nearly full grown, as then the sap is on the top. The roots should be dug and cleaned from the dirt, and pounded with a mallet or club, when the bark is easily separated from the stalk, and may be obtained with little trouble. It should be dried in a chamber or loft, where it is not exposed to the weather; and, when perfectly dry, should be ground or pounded to a fine powder. It is an excellent medicine, either taken by itself or compounded with other articles ; and is the best thing for canker of any article to be found. In scrofulous diarrhoea and chronic cholera in- fantum and goitre it is one of the best agents. its influence on the uterus is very positive. In prolapsus uteri it is splendid, and in parturition it cannot be well excelled. It induces better contractions and when given near the end of the confinement it will anticipate flooding, and should there be excessive lochia it will assist in stopping the excess. Its in- fluence is also good in excessive menstruation or hemorrhages from other parts of the body and in female weakness. In hot infusion it gradually arouses the circulation and favors an outward flow of blood. A good free perspiration will follow, which will be more abundant if Zingiber be added. When the stomach is very foul, it will frequently operate as an emetic. In connection with lobelia it is used in producing emesis, which will be very valuable in the treatment of the conditions found in mercurial cachexia, scrofula and secondary syphilis. For emetic purposes it should be given with lobelia in hot infusion and is excellent to rid the system of impurities. The dose of the Fluid Ext. or Tincture is from one half to one drachm.

King's American Dispensatory, 1898 tells us:

Action, Medical Uses, and Dosage.—Bayberry bark is astringent and stimulant, and as such is valuable in debilitated conditions of the mucous membranes; in drachm doses, it is apt to occasion emesis. It was largely employed by the followers of Samuel Thomson, in catarrhal states of the alimentary tract. The bark has been successfully employed in scrofula, jaundice, diarrhoea, dysentery, aphthae, and other diseases where astringent stimulants were indicated. Specific myrica, in small doses (2 to 5 drops) will be found a good stimulant to the vegetative system of nerves, aiding the processes of digestion, blood making, and nutrition. In larger doses (5 to 20 drops) it is a decided gastric stimulant. In small doses it has been found advantageous in chronic gastritis, chronic catarrhal diarrhoea, muco-enteritis, and in dysentery having a typhoid character. It is said to restore arrested lochial discharges. Cases calling for myrica show feeble venous action, while the pulse is full and oppressed. It is not adapted to acute disorders of the alimentary tract, as a rule. A weak infusion used as an injection, is an admirable remedy in amenorrhoea and atonic leucorrhoea. Use the specific medicine or tincture internally also. In scarlatina in the latter stages, when the tissues are swollen and enfeebled, it may be used both for its antiseptic and stimulating effects (Locke).

The powdered bark, combined with bloodroot, forms an excellent application to indolent ulcers, and has likewise been employed as a snuff for the cure of some forms of nasal polypus. In the form of poultice, with elm or alone, it is a valuable application to scrofulous tumors or ulcers. The decoction is beneficial as a gargle in sore mouth and throat, and is of service in injection, in leucorrhoea and fistula, and also as a wash for ulcers, tinea capitis, etc. It also forms an excellent gum wash for tender, spongy, and bleeding gums. The leaves are reputed astringent, and useful in scurvy and spasmodic affections. Probably the M. pennsylvanica, M. carolinensis, and M. Gale, possess similar properties. Bayberry or myrtle wax, has been used by Dr. Fahnestock in epidemic dysentery with typhoid symptoms, with considerable success; it possesses mild astringent, with some narcotic properties. It is also used in the form of plaster, as an application to scrofulous and other ulcers. Dose of the powdered bark, from 20 to 30 grains; of the wax, 1 drachm; of the decoction of the leaves or bark, from 2 to 4 fluid ounces; specific myrica, 2 to 20 drops. Bayberry bark was a constituent of "Thomson's Composition Powder or No. 6."

Specific Indications and Uses.—Profuse mucous flows; catarrhal states of the gastro-intestinal tract; atonic diarrhoea, typhoid dysentery, atony of the cutaneous circulation; full oppressed pulse. Locally and internally—sore mouth; spongy, flabby, bleeding gums; sore throat of scarlet fever when enfeebled and swollen.

Plants for A Future States:

Wax myrtle is a popular herbal remedy in North America where it is employed to increase the circulation, stimulate perspiration and keep bacterial infections in check. The plant should not be used during pregnancy. The root bark is antibacterial, astringent, emetic (in large doses), sternutatory, stimulant and tonic. It is harvested in the autumn, thoroughly dried then powdered and kept in a dark place in an airtight container. It is used internally in the treatment of diarrhoea, irritable bowel syndrome, jaundice, fevers, colds, influenza, catarrh, excessive menstruation, vaginal discharge etc. Externally, it is applied to indolent ulcers, sore throats, spongy gums, sores, itching skin conditions, dandruff etc. The wax is astringent and slightly narcotic. It is regarded as a sure cure for dysentery and is also used to treat internal ulcers. A tea made from the leaves is used in the treatment of fevers and externally as a wash for itchy skin.

The Rodale Herb Book states:

The bark and roots are used medicinally as an astringent, tonic and stimulant. leaves are aromatic and stimulant. A tea is used as an excellent gargle for sore throats, catarrh and jaundice. The bark is used for diarrhea and dysentery, a decoction is made and injected as an enema. This is also used as a wash or poultice for sores, boils and carbuncles, or the powdered bark may be directly applied to wounds... The root bark is the official medicinal part.

Sacred and Healing Herbal Beers tells us about Gruit, the highly inebriating beer made, in part, with Myrica... by the way, Ledum palustre is not the herb we normally call rosemary (Rosmarinus officinalis, a member of the salvia family); this "wild rosemary" is relative to American Labrader Tea, a relative of the Myrica. It is interesting to note that Gruit was the primary beer consumed for around 700 years in Europe, until Hops was introduced, in large part due to the writings of Saint Hildegard von Bingen and her influence. The use of hops in beer though, became law in many nations due to political and economic interests... as well as a likely reasonable social concerns:

Gruit was, primarily, a combination of three mild to moderately narcotic herbs: sweet gale (Myrica gale), also called bog myrtle, yarrow (Achillea millefolium) and wild rosemary (Ledum palustre), also called marsh rosemary. Gruit varied somewhat, each gruit producer adding additional herbs to produce unique tastes, flavors and effects. ... It is important to keep in mind the properties of gruit ale; it is highly intoxicating – narcotic, aphrodisiacal and psychotropic when consumed in sufficient quantity.

Morus, Mulberry

Eleven varieties of Mulberry have been found useful in herbal medicine: Morus alba - White Mulberry, Morus alba multicaulis - White Mulberry, Morus australis - Korean Mulberry, Morus bombycis – Kuwa, Morus cathayana - Hua Sang, Morus macroura - Himalayan Mulberry, Morus microphylla - Texas Mulberry, Morus mongolica - Mongolian Mulberry, Morus nigra - Black Mulberry, Morus rubra - Red Mulberry, Morus serrata - Himalayan Mulberry, Morus tiliaefolia

Morus rubra, Red Mulberry, is the only Mulberry that is native to my region, but Morus alba, White Mulberry been naturalized. Red Mulberry can be found in the most unlikely places. It pops up in the understory, with usually just the shiny leaves giving it away. Deer love the leaves, and usually the birds and raccoons get most of the berries. Although the fruit is generally under-appreciated, Mulberry has a long use in haerbalism.

Dioscorides wrote:

Morus or sycaminus is a well-known tree. Its fruit makes the intestines soluble. It is easily spoiled and bad for the stomach and the juice is the same. Boiled in a brass jar or left in the sun it is made more astringent. A little honey mixed with it makes it good for

the discharge of fluids, for gangrenous ulceration of the cheeks, and for inflamed tonsils. The strength of it is increased if alumen in small pieces, galls [oak], myrrh and crocus are mixed with it as well as the fruit of myrica, iris and frankincense. Unripe mulberries dried and pounded are mixed with sauces or rhus and they help coeliac [intestinal complaints]. The bark from the root boiled in water and taken as a drink loosens the bowels, expels broadworms from the intestines, and is an antidote for those who have taken aconitum as a drink. The leaves pounded into small pieces and applied with oil heal burns. Boiled with rain water, wine and black fig leaves they dye the hair. A wine cupful of juice from the leaves helps those bitten by harvest spiders. A decoction of the bark and leaves is a good rinse for toothache. It is milked at harvest time, the roots dug around and cut-in. The next day there will be found some coalesced gum which is good for toothache, dissolves swellings, and purges the bowels. There seem to be some wild mulberries similar to (the fruit) of the bramble but more astringent, the juice is less spoiled and good in warm packs for inflammation, healing ulcerated jaws, and to fill up wounds with flesh. They grow in shady and cold places.

Gerard wrote of Mulberry:

A. Mulberries being gathered before they be ripe, are cold and dry almost in the third degree, and do mightily bind; being dried they are good for the lask and bloody flux, the powder is used in meat, and is drunk with wine and water

B. They stay bleedings, and also the reds; they are good against inflammations or hot swellings of the mouth and jaws, and for other inflammations newly beginning.

C. The ripe and new gathered Mulberries are likewise cold and be full of juice, which hath the taste of wine, and is something drying, and not without a binding quality: and therefore it is also mixed with medicines for the mouth, and such as help the hot swellings of the mouth, and almonds of the throat; for which infirmities it is singular good.

D. Of the juice of the ripe berries is made a confection with sugar, called Diamorum: that is, after the manner of a syrup, which is exceeding good for the ulcers and hot swellings of the tongue, *throat, and almonds, or uvula of the throat, or any other malady arising in those parts.*

E. These Mulberries taken in meat, and also before meat, do very speedily pass through the belly, by reason of the moisture and slipperiness of their substance, and make a passage for other meats, as Galen saith.

F. They are good to quench thirst, they stir up an appetite to meat, they are not hurtful to the stomach, but they nourish the body very little, being taken in the second place, or after meat, for although they be less hurtful than other like fruits, yet are they corrupted and putrefied, unless they speedily descend.

G. The bark of the root is bitter, hot and dry, and hath a scouring faculty: the decotion hereof doth open the stoppings of the liver and spleen, it purgeth the belly, and driveth forth worms.

H. The same bark being steeped in vinegar helpeth the toothache: of the same effect is also the decoction of the leaves and bark, saith Dioscorides, who showeth that about harvest time there issueth out of the root a juice, which the next day after is found to be hard, and that the same is very good against the toothache; that it wasteth away Phyma, and purgeth the belly.

I. Galen saith, that there is in the leaves and first buds of this tree a certain middle faculty, both to bind and scour.

Culpepper wrote:

Mercury rules the tree, therefore are its effects variable as his are. The mulberry is of different parts; the ripe berries, by reason of their sweetness and slippery moisture, opening the body, and the unripe binding it, especially when they are dried, and then they are good to stay fluxes, lasks, and the abundance of women's courses. The bark of the root kills the broad worms in the body. The juice, or the syrup made of the juice of the berries, helps all inflammations or sores in the mouth, or throat, and palate of the mouth when it is fallen down. The juice of the leaves is a remedy against the biting of serpents, and for those that have taken aconite. The leaves beaten with vinegar, are good to lay on any place that is burnt with fire. A decoction made of the bark and leaves is good to wash the mouth and teeth when they ache. If the root be a little slit or cut, and a small hole made in the ground next thereunto, in the Harvest-

time, it will give out a certain juice, which being hardened the next day, is of good use to help the tooth-ache, to dissolve knots, and purge the belly. The leaves of Mulberries are said to stay bleeding at the mouth or nose, or the bleeding of the piles, or of a wound, being bound unto the places. A branch of the tree taken when the moon is at the full, and bound to the wrists of a woman's arm, whose courses come down too much, doth stay them in a short space.

Mrs. Grieves gives us a long history of the cultivation of Mulberry, especially to feed silk worms. Of its medicinal properties, she writes only:

The sole use of Mulberries in modern medicine is for the preparation of a syrup, employed to flavour or colour any other medicine. Mulberry Juice is obtained from the ripe fruit of the Mulberry by expression and is an official drug of the British Pharmacopoeia. It is a dark violet or purple liquid, with a faint odour and a refreshing, acid, saccharine taste. The British Pharmacopceia directs that Syrupus Mori should be prepared by heating 50 fluid drachms of the expressed juice to boiling point, then cooling and filtering. Ninety drachms of sugar is then dissolved in the juice, which is warmed up again. When once more cooled, 6.25 drachms of alcohol is added: the product should then measure about 100 drachms (20 fluid ounces). The dose is 2 to 1 fluid drachm, but it is, as stated, chiefly used as an adjuvant rather than for its slightly laxative and expectorant qualities, though used as a gargle, it will relieve sore throat.

However, she includes the following recipe for Mulberry wines and jam:

Mulberry Wine

On each gallon of ripe Mulberries, pour 1 gallon of boiling water and let them stand for 2 days. Then squeeze all through a hair sieve or bag. Wash out the tub or jar and return the liquor to it, put in the sugar at the rate of 3 lb. to each gallon of the liquor; stir up until quite dissolved, then put the liquor into a cask. Let the cask be raised a little on one side until fermentation ceases, then bung down. If the liquor be clear, it may be bottled in 4 months' time. Into each bottle put 1 clove and a small lump of sugar and the bottles should be kept in a moderate temperature. The wine may be used in a year from time of bottling.

Mulberries are sometimes used in Devonshire for mixing with cider during fermentation, giving a pleasant taste and deep red colour. In Greece, also, the fruit is subjected to fermentation, thereby furnishing an inebriating beverage.

Scott relates in Ivanhoe that the Saxons made a favourite drink, Morat, from the juice of Mulberries with honey, but it is doubtful whether the Morum of the Anglo-Saxon 'Vocabularies' was not the Blackberry, so that the 'Morat' of the Saxons may have been Blackberry Wine.

Mulberry Jam

Unless very ripe Mulberries are used, the jam will have an acid taste. Put 1 lb. of Mulberries in a jar and stand it in a pan of water on the fire till the juice is extracted. Strain them and put the juice into a preserving pan with 3 lb. of sugar. Boil it and remove the scum and put in 3 lb. of very ripe Mulberries and let them stand in the syrup until thoroughly warm, then set the pan back on the fire and boil them very gently for a short time, stirring all the time and taking care not to break the fruit. Then take the pan off and let them stand in the syrup all night. Put the pan on the fire again in the morning and boil again gently till stiff.

King's American Dispensatory, 1898 tells us:

Action, Medical Uses, and Dosage.—Mulberries possess very slightly nutritive qualities; they are refrigerant and laxative, and their juice forms a pleasant and grateful drink for patients suffering under febrile diseases, as it checks the thirst, relieves febrile heat, and when taken freely, gently relaxes the bowels. The juice, formed into a syrup and added to water, answers the same purpose, and forms a pleasant adjunct to gargles in quinsy. If the berries are eaten to excess they are apt to induce diarrhoea. The bark of the tree is reputed purgative and vermifuge, having expelled tapeworm.

Plants for A Future Lists Mulberry as:

The root bark is anthelmintic and cathartic. A tea made from the roots has been used in the treatment of weakness, difficult urination, dysentery, tapeworms and as a panacea. The sap is used in the treatment of ringworm. Another report says that the milky juice obtained from the axis of the leaf is used. The fruits are used to reduce fevers.

Peterson Field Guides Eastern and Central Medicinal Plants tells us:

Red Mulberry: American Indians drank root tea for weakness, difficult urination, dysentery, tapeworms; panacea; externally, sap used for ringworms. Nutritious fruits used for lowering fever. Warning: large doses cause vomiting.

White Mulberry: in China, leaf tea used for headaches, hyperemia (congestion of blood), thirst, coughs; "Liver cleanser". Experimentally, leaf extracts or antibacterial. Young twig tea used for arthralgia, edema. Fruits eaten for blood deficiency, to improve vision in circulation, and for diabetes. Inner bark tea used for lung ailments, asthma, coughs, and edema.

Botany In a Day states:

Medicinally, a bark of the tea is used as a laxative and to expel tapeworms. The Milky juice and the unripe fruit may cause hallucinations, nervousness and upset stomach.

Nyssa, Tupelo

Three varieties of Tupelo have been found useful in herbal medicine: Nyssa aquatica - Water Tupelo Synonym, Nyssa ogeche - Ogeechee Lime, Nyssa sylvatica - Black Tupelo

Three varieties of Tupelo grow in my region: Nyssa aquatica (Water Tupelo), Nyssa biflora (Swamp Tupelo, Swamp Blackgum), Nyssa sylvatica (Blackgum, Black Tupelo, Pepperidge)

Tupelos are new world trees, so little if any record of their use exists in the old British and European herbals. I will have to do more research for Native American use of these trees and update this book when/if I find something useful. Anyone who buys this version may request a free, updated eBook as they become available. For me, the Tupelos are a tree of childhood memory. My great grandfather was a remarkable farmer and bee keeper. He placed his hives near the Tupelos that grew in the swamps. The honey made from those trees was as dark as molasses, slightly biting to the throat and by far the very best I have ever tasted. Tupelo honey is famous in the American South, but I have never found any so dark and rich.

Herbal Remedies of the Lumbee Indians states:

Some Lumbee healers would scrape the bark from the roots of the black gum tree and boil it to make a tea to treat colic, cramps or worms. The inner bark was made into a tea to treat milky urine and diarrhea. Some local healers would also boil the branches of the black gum with Gall of the Earth to obtain a tonic used to treat high blood pressure.

Plants for A Future states:

Medicinal use of Black Tupelo: The bark is emetic, ophthalmic and vermifuge. An infusion has been used as a bath and also given to children with worms. A strong decoction is used to cause vomiting when unable to retain food. A strong ooze from the roots is used as eye drops.

Ostrya, Hophornbeam or Ironwood

There are two species of Ostrya: Ostrya carpinifolia - Hop Hornbeam and Ostrya virginiana – Ironwood. Both are found in my region.

King's American Dispensatory, 1898 tells us:

Action, Medical Uses, and Dosage.—Iron-wood is antiperiodic, tonic, and alterative. It has been used with efficacy in intermittent fevers, neuralgic affections, dyspepsia, scrofula, and all diseases where an antiperiodic tonic is indicated. Dose of the decoction, 1 or 2 fluid ounces, 3 or 4 times a day; of the fluid extract, 1 fluid drachm.

Plants for A Future states:

Medicinal use of Ironwood: The bark is astringent, blood tonic and haemostatic. A decoction of the bark is used to bathe sore muscles. An infusion of the bark can be held in the mouth to relieve the pain of toothache. An infusion of the heartwood has been used in the treatment of lung haemorrhages, coughs and colds, catarrh and kidney problems. It is also used as a herbal steam bath in the treatment of rheumatism.

Botany In a Day states:

A tea of the bark is taken for intermittent fevers and nervousness.

Oxydendrum arboretum, Sourwood

This is the tree that made Appalachian Mountain "Sourwood Honey" famous. It is the opposite of the Tupelo of the swamps. Sourwood honey is champaign colored and remarkably light. The genuine article is hard to find, as much wildflower honey is mixed with light corn syrup to make a counterfeit Sourwood Honey. As the old folks would say, "Sour Wood honey is so good that if you put it on a biscuit, and put that biscuit on your head, your tongue would beat your brains out trying to get to it!" This was the honey from which most of the old Appalachian cough syrups and cold remedies were made, and it was believed to have particularly strong medicinal properties.

King's American Dispensatory, 1898 tells us:

Action, Medical Uses, and Dosage.—Sorrel tree leaves are tonic, refrigerant, and strongly diuretic. Fever patients will find a decoction of the leaves a pleasant, cooling, and diuretic drink. A tincture of the leaves and twigs in whiskey is said to have been a popular remedy in Kentucky for the kidney and bladder ailments of aged men, being employed to increase the renal secretion, and to relieve the unpleasant symptoms attending prostatic enlargement, vesical calculi, and chronic irritation of the neck of the bladder. The remedy was specially recommended in the treatment of dropsies by Dr. J. W. Davis, of Lewisburg, Ky., in 1881 (Ec. Med. Jour., 1881, p. 497). Its strong diuretic powers were generally recognized, and several experimenters reported remarkable success from its employment in anasarca, hydrocele, pleuritic effusions, and hydropericardium. It was asserted to give marked relief in urinary troubles, with frequent desire to urinate, with burning pain at urethral outlet, and the urine passing in drops, mixed with blood. It was subsequently employed in bowel troubles from exposure to cold, as when a determination of blood to the viscera occurred, causing diarrhoea or dysentery. It undoubtedly acts by giving increased tone to relaxed capillaries. Pills of a solid extract, containing 3 to 6 grains may be given every 2 hours; specific oxydendron, 1 to 20 minims every 2 or 3 hours.

Specific Indications and Uses.—Anasarca, ascites, and other forms of dropsy; the urinary difficulties of old men; painful micturition, with scanty renal secretion.

Plans for A Future lists it as Sorrel Tree, indicating its sourness:

Medicinal use of Sorrel Tree: The leaves are cardiac, diuretic, refrigerant and tonic. A tea made from the leaves has been used in the treatment of asthma, diarrhoea, indigestion and to check excessive menstrual bleeding. It is diuretic and is a folk remedy for treating fevers, kidney and bladder ailments. The bark has been chewed in the treatment of mouth ulcers.

Peterson Field Guides Eastern and Central Medicinal Plants tells us:

American Indians chewed bark for mouth ulcers. Leaf tea used for "nerves", asthma, diarrhea, indigestion, and to check excessive menstrual bleeding. Leave tea, a Kentucky folk remedy for kidney and bladder elements diarrhetic, fevers, diarrhea, and dysentery. Flowers yield the famous sourwood honey.

Paulownia tomentosa, Princesstree

Princesstree has been naturalized in my region. It is an interesting tree, traditionally used to make musical instruments and carvings used for gifts and associated with royalty in Asia. In the era before Styrofoam and bubble wrap, the seeds of the Princesstree were used as packing material. When one sees a Princesstree now, it is most likely growing in an area where the seeds fell from a train in the era when they were used for that purpose. The rail lines are mostly gone, but the trees remain.

Plants for A Future states:

A decoction of the leaves is used to wash foul ulcers and is also said to promote the growth of hair and prevent greying. The leaves are also poulticed onto bruises. The leaf juice is used in the treatment of warts. The flowers are used in the treatment of skin ailments. A tincture of the inner bark is used in the treatment of fevers and delirium. It is astringent and vermifuge.

Peterson Field Guides Eastern and Central Medicinal Plants tells us:

In China, a wash of the leaves in capsules was used in daily applications to promote the growth of hair and prevent greying. Leaf tea was used as a foot bath for swollen feet. Inner bark tincture soaked in two parts whiskey, given for fevers and delirium. Leaves or ground bark were fried in vinegar, poulticed and bruises. Flowers were mixed with other herbs to treat liver ailments. In Japan the leaf juice is used to treat warts. Warning: contains potentially toxic compounds.

Persea, Bay Laurel

Five varieties of Bay have been found useful in Herbal Medicine: Persea borbonia - Red Bay, Persea duthiei, Persea edulis, Persea gammieana, Persea villosa

Two Bays are native to my region: Persea borbonia (Redbay) and Persea palustris (Swampbay)

These are coastal trees that are somewhat shrubby. Their foliage is bright and shiny, and their scent is unmistakable. All the Bays are highly aromatic.

Plants for A Future states:

Medicinal use of Red Bay: Red bay was widely employed medicinally by the Seminole Indians who used it to treat a variety of complaints, but especially as an emetic and body cleanser. It is little, if at all, used in modern herbalism. The leaves are abortifacient, analgesic, antirheumatic, appetizer, emetic and febrifuge. An infusion can be used to abort a foetus up to the age of four months. An infusion is also used in treating fevers, headaches, diarrhoea, thirst, constipation, appetite loss and blocked urination. A strong decoction is emetic and was used as a body purification when treating a wide range of complaints. A decoction of the leaves is used externally as a wash on rheumatic joints and painful limbs.

Picea, Spruce

Sixteen varieties of Spruce have been found to be useful in Herbal Medicine: Picea abies - Norway Spruce, Picea asperata - Chinese Spruce, Picea brachytyla - Sargent Spruce, Picea breweriana - Weeping Spruce, Picea engelmannii - Mountain Spruce, Picea glauca - White Spruce, Picea glehnii - Sakhalin Spruce, Picea jezoensis - Yezo Spruce, Picea mariana - Black Spruce, Picea omorika - Serbian Spruce, Picea orientalis - Caucasian Spruce, Picea pungens - Blue Spruce, Picea purpurea - Purple-Coned Spruce, Picea rubens - Red Spruce, Picea sitchensis - Sitka Spruce, Picea smithiana - Morinda Spruce

Only Picea rubens (Red Spruce), is native to my region… which, at least saves me from having to discriminate between Caucasian Spruce, White Spruce, Chinese Spruce and Black Spruce… or saluting a tree as Sargent Spruce…botanical humor! Picea abies, Norway Spruce has been naturalized.

Spruce is particularly good medicine. It is astringent. Topically, it is good for wounds. Spruce stops bleeding and prevents infection.

Both the needles and inner bark are used. The bark is astringent and stimulant. Spruce tightens tissue and stimulates blood flow. This allows blood to carry the congestion/inflammation out. It increases arterial blood to tissues, so they can heal. Spruce is also diuretic.

Herbalist, Michael Moore considered Spruce good for, "Chronic pharyngitis with thick tenacious mucus. Chronic bronchitis with profuse secretions. Heartburn with vomiting, diarrhea, stomach pain. Prolapse of rectal mucosa. Asthenia with poor digestion, vascular weakness, pale mucosa."

Dioscorides included an interesting recipe for Spruce wine in his Materia Medica:

OINOS RETINITES

Rosin from Spruce Firs, Pines — Rosin Wine

Rosin wine is made in many nations. It is abundant in Galatia because the grapes remain unripe because of the cold, and the wine grows sour if it is not mixed with Picea resina [spruce]. The rosin is pounded with the bark, and a quarter pint is mixed to nine gallons of wine; some strain it after it is boiled, taking away the rosin; others leave it alone. Growing old, these become sweet. They all cause headaches and vertigo, and yet are digestive and urinary. They are good for those with dripping mucus and coughs, for the abdominal cavity, dysentery, dropsy, and women's menstrual flows, and it is a syringe for deep ulcers. The black is more binding than the white.

Saint Hildegard von Bingen wrote:

Spruce pitch is very hot. It is healthful in drinking vessels. If maggots eat a person, place spruce pitch over the wound. It will draw the worms to itself, so that it is possible to pull them out and scrape them off. When they have been removed, place spruce pitch on the wound a second time, until the worms are completely gone. After the flesh has been purged of them, anoint the place with olive oil and other good ointments, and it will be healed.

Brother Aloysius wrote of Spruce:

In the spring, the young shoots covered with brown scales, are gathered and made into a tea to cleanse the blood; this tea is also useful for eczema, skin rashes and phlegm in the lungs. Boil 1 cup of dried, finely chopped shoots in 2 cups water; take 1 to 2 cups daily. For seminal discharge, take 3 teaspoons of powder from the finely ground, dried needles with red wine and a fresh egg.

Plants for A Future states:

Medicinal use of Red Spruce: A tea made from the boughs has been used in the treatment of colds and to "break out" measles. The pitch from the trunk has been used as a poultice on rheumatic joints, the chest and the stomach in order to relieve congestion and pain. A decoction of the bark has been used in the treatment of lung complaints and throat problems.

Sacred and Healing Herbal Beers says of Spruce:

Spruce has been traditionally used by indigenous peoples for coughs, colds, and flu as an infusion in sweat baths, and the inner bark has been applied to stubborn skin infections. They have also used it for kidney infections, much like juniper.

Peterson Field Guides Eastern and Central Medicinal Plants tells us:

Black spruce: American Indians poulticed inner bark on inflammations. Inner bark tea a folk medicine for kidney stones, stomach problems, rheumatism. Resin poulticed on sores to promote healing. Needles used to make beer that was drunk for scurvy.

Red spruce: American Indians used tea of boughs for colds and to break out measles. Pitch formally poulticed on rheumatic joints, chest, and stomach to relieve congestion in pain.

Botany In a Day states:

A tea of the shoots is expectorant and diaphoretic, ideal for coughs and bronchitis.

The Physicians' Desk Reference for Herbal Medicine tells us:

Indications and usage spruce needle oil, approved by Commission E: common cold, cough/bronchitis, fevers and colds, inflammation of the mouth and pharynx, neuralgias, rheumatism, tendency to infection. The essential oil is used internally for catarrhal conditions of the respiratory tract. Externally it is used for catarrhal conditions of the respiratory tract, rheumatic and neuralgic pain. Unproven uses: for tension states. Spruce shoots fresh approved by Commission E: common cold, cough bronchitis, fevers and colds, inflammation of the mouth and pharynx, muscular and nerve pain, tendency to infection. The drug is used internally in respiratory tract catarrh and externally for muscle pains and neuralgia. Unproven uses: in folk medicine it is used internally for tuberculosis and externally as a bath additive for patients with neurological illnesses. Contraindications include bronchial asthma and whooping cough. Patients with extensive skin injuries, acute skin diseases, fevers or infectious diseases, cardiac insufficiency, or hypotonia should not use the drug as a bath additive. No health hazards or side effects are known in conjunction with the proper administration of designated therapeutic dosages, although bronchial spasm could be worsened.

Pinus, Pine

Sixty-three varieties of Pine have been found useful in Herbal Medicine!!!!

Pinus albicaulis - White-Bark Pine, Pinus aristata - Bristle-Cone Pine, Pinus armandii - Chinese White Pine, Pinus ayacahuite - Mexican White Pine, Pinus banksiana - Jack Pine, Pinus bungeana - Lace-Bark Pine, Pinus californiarum, Pinus cembra - Swiss Stone Pine, Pinus cembra sibirica - Siberian Pine, Pinus cembroides - Mexican Pine Nut, Pinus cembroides orizabensis - Mexican Pine Nut, Pinus contorta - Beach Pine, Pinus contorta latifolia - Lodgepole Pine, Pinus coulteri - Big-Cone Pine, Pinus culminicola - Cerro Potosi Pinyon, Pinus densiflora - Japanese Red Pine, Pinus discolor, Pinus edulis - Rocky Mountain Pinon, Pinus echinata - Short-Leaf Pine, Pinus flexilis - Limber Pine, Pinus gerardiana - Chilghoza Pine, Pinus halepensis - Aleppo Pine, Pinus henryi Synonym: Pinus tabuliformis henryi, Pinus jeffreyi - Jeffrey Pine, Pinus johannis, Pinus koraiensis - Korean Nut Pine, Pinus lambertiana - Sugar Pine, Pinus leiophylla - Smooth-Leaf Pine, Pinus massoniana - Chinese Red Pine, Pinus monophylla - Single Leaf Pinon, Pinus montezumae - Montezuma Pine, Pinus monticola - Western White Pine, Pinus mugo - Dwarf Mountain Pine, Pinus muricata - Bishop's Pine, Pinus nelsonii, Pinus nigra - Austrian Pine, Pinus nigra laricio - Corsican Pine, Pinus palustris – Pitne, Pinus parviflora - Japanese White Pine, Pinus patula - Mexican Weeping Pine, Pinus pinaster - Maritime Pine, Pinus pinea - Italian Stone Pine, Pinus ponderosa - Ponderosa Pine, Pinus pumila - Dwarf Siberian Pine, Pinus pungens - Prickle Pine, Pinus quadrifolia - Parry Pinon, Pinus radiata - Monterey Pine, Pinus remota - Paper-Shell Pinon, Pinus resinosa - Red Pine, Pinus rigida - Northern Pitch Pine, Pinus roxburghii - Chir Pine, Pinus sabiniana - Digger Pine, Pinus serotina - Pond Pine, Pinus strobiformis - Southwestern White Pine, Pinus strobus - White Pine, Pinus sylvestris - Scot's Pine, Pinus tabuliformis - Chinese Red Pine, Pinus taeda - Loblolly Pine, Pinus teocote - Twisted Leaf Pine, Pinus thunbergii - Japanese Black Pine, Pinus torreyana - Soledad Pine, Pinus veitchii, Pinus virginiana - Scrub Pine, Pinus wallichiana - Himalayan Blue Pine

Only eight Pines are native to my region: Pinus echinata (Shortleaf Pine), Pinus palustris (Longleaf Pine), Pinus pungens (Table Mountain Pine), Pinus rigida (Pitch Pine), Pinus serotina (Pond Pine), Pinus strobus (Eastern White Pine), Pinus taeda (Loblolly Pine), Pinus virginiana (Virginia Pine). Naturalized Pines include: Pinus clausa (Sand Pine), Pinus elliottii var. elliottii (Slash Pine), Pinus pinaster (Maritime Pine), Pinus resinosa (Red Pine), Pinus thunbergiana (Japanese Black Pine)

The state of my birth, North Carolina, is known as "The land of the longleaf pine" although, the loblolly is far more common. It was the Pine that was the backbone of the early economy of the Carolinas. The Pine tar industry was essential for ship building and is why North Carolinians were called "Tar heels". Pines are strongly medicinal and are excellent first aid. The virtues of turpentine, made from Pine are well known and have been in our medicine cabinets for centuries. I recently taught a class, entitled Four Ways Pines Can Save Your Life. My points were:

1) The Pine is among our most edible trees. It has been said that every part of the pine can be eaten... but, that would take a desperate effort.

2) Pine pitch can stop bleeding and disinfect a wound.

3) Pine needle tea or wine can prevent a sore throat from becoming life-threateningly severe, can help break a fever and is good against viruses and other infections.

4) Inhaling the vapors from immature male pollen cone can lower blood pressure and heartrate and help stop an asthma attack.

Dioscorides wrote extensively on the medical uses of Pine, below is a brief selection out of around 100 mentions:

PITUS, PEUKE

SUGGESTED: Pinus rigida, Peuce [Pliny] — Pitch Pine

Pin, Pinus, Pinus pinea, Pinus sativa — Italian Stone Pine

Pitys is a well-known tree. There is another similar tree called peuce which differs in shape. The bark of both of them is astringent. Pounded into small pieces and a poultice then made of it, it is good with sediment [of wine] and manna [exudation of trees] for chafing, dermatitis, superficial ulcers and for burns. Taken with myrica wax ointment it brings boils to a scar in those with tender skin; and pounded into small pieces with blacking from a shoemaker it represses serpentia [snakebite]. It expels the birth and afterbirth out of the uterus taken asinhalations (smoke, fumes); and taken as a drink it stops discharges of the intestines and encourages urine. Their leaves pounded into small pieces and made into a poultice lessen inflammation and keep wounds from being inflamed. Pounded into small pieces and boiled in vinegar they lessen toothache when [the teeth are] washed with the warm liquid. One teaspoon of the leaves (taken as a drink with water, or honey and water) is good for liver disorders. The bark from the cones and the split leaves (taken in a drink) are good for the same purposes. A toeda [a piece of the heart of the tree] cut in small pieces in a decoction boiled with vinegar and held in to a tooth that suffers, lessens toothache. A paste is made from them suitable for preparations for enemas and suppositories. When they are burning a soot is taken, good to make writing ink, and good also to be put in medicines for the eyelids. It is also good for erosions at the corners of the eyes, weeping eyes and bald eyelids.

PITUIDES

SUGGESTED: *Pinus rigida, Peuce* — Pitch Pine

Pinus mughus, Pinus nigra, Pinus maritima — Pineseeds, Pine

Pityides are the fruit of the pines [and of the pinus picea] found in the cones. They are astringent and somewhat warming. They help coughs and disorders of the chest taken either by themselves or with honey.

STROBILOI

SUGGESTED: *Pinus mughus, Pinus nigra,*

Pinus maritima, Pinus pinea, Pinus rigida — Pine Cones

Fir cones cleaned and eaten or taken in a drink with passum [raisin wine] and cucumber seed are diuretic, and dull irritations of the bladder and kidneys. They also lessen rosiones [gnawing corrosion] of the stomach. Taken with juice of purslane they strengthen infirmity of the body, and dull the infection of fluids. Fir cones gathered whole from the trees, pounded while they are fresh, and boiled in passum [raisin wine] are good for old coughs and consumptive wasting if three cups of this liquid is taken every day.

Gerard wrote of the virtues of the Pine:

A. The kernels of these nuts do concoct and moderately heat, being in a mean between cold and hot: it maketh the rough parts smooth; it is a remedy against an old cough, and long infirmities of the chest, being taken by itself or with honey, or else with some other licking thing.

B. It cureth the phthisic, and those that pine and consume away through the rottenness of their lungs: it recovereth strength; it nourisheth and is restorative to the body. It yieldeth a thick and good juice, and nourisheth much, yet is it not altogether easy of digestion, and therefore it is mixed with preserves, or boiled with sugar.

C. The same is good for the stone in the kidneys, and against frettings of the bladder, and scalding of the urine, for it allayeth the sharpness, mitigateth pain, and gently provoketh urine: moreover, it increaseth milk and seed, and therefore it also provoketh fleshly lust.

D. The whole Cone or Apple being boiled with fresh Horehound, saith Galen, and afterwards boiled again with a little honey till the decoction be come to the thickness of honey, maketh an excellent medicine for the cleansing of the chest and lungs.

E. The like thing hath Dioscorides; the whole cones, saith he, which are newly gathered from the trees, broken and boiled in sweet wine are good for an old cough, and consumption of the lungs, if a good draught of that liquor be drunk every day.

F. The scales of the Pine apple, with the bark of the tree, do stop the lask and the bloody flux, they provoke urine; and the decoction of the same hath the like property.

Mrs. Grieves preferred the White pine for medicinal value, as doI: "Medicinal Action and Uses---Expectorant, demulcent, diuretic, a useful remedy in coughs and colds, having a beneficial effect on the bladder and kidneys." I would caution though, that pine can irritate the kidneys with prolonged use or in large amounts.

An Irish Herbal states:

The bark, eaves and cones are of a dry, astringent nature. They stop diarrhea and dysentery and provoke urine. Boiled in vinegar, the leaves alleviate toothache. The kernels of the pine apples are beneficial for the lungs, kidneys, liver and spleen. They loosen phlegm and are good for consumptive cough.

Fr. Kneipp recommended a bath of Pine:

The pine-sprig bath. It is prepared as follow : The sprigs (the fresher the better), small branches, even very resinous pine-cones, all cut in pieces, are thrown into hot water and boiled for half an hour , the rest as above said. This bath, too, is of good effect against diseases of the kidneys and bladder, but not so strong as the bath of oat-straw. Its chief effect is on the skin, which is brought to activity by it, and on the interior vessels which it strengthens.

This fragrant and strengthening bath, is the proper bath for more aged people.

Brother Aloysius wrote of Larch Pine:

A fungus, called larch fungus, grows all over the trunk of old larch trees. The white, loose substance within the fungus, is very useful in curbing excessive perspiration of consumptives if given every evening in a dose of ½ to 1 gram. A dose of 2 to 4 grams has a purgative action.

Resources of the Southern Fields and Forests states:

This tree shoots up into a straight shaft, devoid of branches sometimes for fifty or sixty feet; the heart is very durable, and the wood is employed for almost every purpose. It is, indeed, one of the great gifts of God to man, for it furnishes to every one an abundant material for fuel, fire, warmth and light. The forests of pine are not only useful but beautiful. The characteristic moan of the winds through their branches, their funereal aspect, almost limitless extent, and the health-giving influences which attend their presence, all contribute to make the pine an object of peculiar interest to the people of the Southern States. The terebinthinate odor of the tree, somaelectrical influence of its long, spear-like leaves, a certain modification of " ozone," (an allotropic condition of oxygen, according to Faraday,) are severally esteemed to modify the atmosphere and diminish the effects of malaria. They also create a mechanical barrier to the ingress of malaria, and hence the pine land residences, though condemned for their sterile aspect, have proved a blessing to the Southern planters in affording a comparatively safe refuge from the unhealthy emanations of the neighboring plantations. I need not describe the processes for making Tar. It is a very compound substance, (see Rural Cyc.,) and contains modified resin, oil of turpentine, empyreumatic oil, acetic acid, charcoal and water, and when inspissated by boiling is converted into pitch. It is extensively used in the cordage, caulking and sheathing of ships, to preserve them from the weather. It is of great service in many of the arts and medicinal usages connected with agriculture. I will add what Wilson states of its economical employment, as it may be made of great service on our plantations and in veterinary medicine. It serves well as a paint to coarse kinds of boarding and paling but is improved in its use by the addition of tallow or other coarse fat. It is applied as a covering to cuts on animals, and to parts affected by the fly. It serves, either alone or in combination with some fatty substance, to defend the sore or diseased feet of cattle from being further injured by wet or abrasion ; when spread upon coarse cloth it is a prime covering for broken horns, and makes an excellent application to various kinds of wounds and punctures in cattle. It is given internally to horses as a remedy for cough; also as a detergent and local remedy for scaly and eruptive diseases. Rural Cyc. It is used to cover the lower surface of posts to prevent their rotting, and grain soaked in it is not eaten by birds. Tar water was formerly much used in medicine, but at present wood naphtha and pyroligneous acid, etc., are commonly employed. The buds of the pine or the inside barks steeped in water is a favorite domestic remedy on our plantations for colds and coughs. Bits of fat pine steeped, in gin are also used. A decoction of the inside bark is given daily as a remedy in chronic diarrhea. Pills of resin are often employed as a simple diuretic. Resin also enters into the composition of strengthening plasters. Wilson, in his Rural Cyc, articles "Fuel" and "Charcoal," gives the best mode of preparation, including the quality and yield of several trees. See Salix, in this volume, for manufacture of charcoal. The chief consumption of charcoal is as fuel. It is also employed as a tooth powder and to purify tainted meat. No mode of preparation for the first of these objects is at all necessary, and for the two last it must merely be reduced to a fine powder. It forms a part of all reducing fluxes. It is the basis of most black paints and varnishes. It is used to polish brass and copper, and is an excellent clarifier. It is used in farriery, in combination with linseed meal, as an anti-septic cataplasm for foul and fetid ulcers. Powdered charcoal must be heated to redness in a covered crucible, with an opening in the middle of the cover, and kept in that state till no flame issues out; it must then be withdrawn, allowed to cool, and then put into close vessels. Whenever either wine, vinegar, or other fluid is to be clarified it is simply to be mixed with the liquor; a froth appears at the surface, and after filtration it is pure and colorless. Charcoal is also used as a valuable manure, fully described in Wilson's Eural Cyc. Charcoal and sand placed in the bottom of a barrel or hogshead will purify water passed through it. (See Salix.) It is generally believed that it will prevent contagion, yellow fever, etc., if taken during the prevalence of an epidemic. It is also used as a mild mechanical laxative in dyspepsia with foul stomach. See *medical authors. Its power of absorbing gases and vapors is well known.*

Euell Gibbons tells us:

Dried white pine bark is still a valuable ingredient in cough remedies. It is an official drug in the US Pharmacopoeia, The National Formulary and the US Dispensatory. Its medicinal properties are expectorant and diuretic. It is most often prescribed in the title role of Compound White Pine Syrup, or, as a doctor would write it on your prescription, Syrupus Pini Albae Compositus. This is a real herbal mixture and a good illustration of the fact that modern medicine does not disdain remedies if they are effective. This compound contains, not only white pine bark, but wild cherry, spikenard, poplar buds, bloodroot, sassafras root bark and Amaranth.

Unfortunately, while Gibbons' statement was true when he wrote Stalking The Healthful Herbs in 1966, such is no longer the case. Pharmacists rarely compound medicines these days, as the pharmaceutical industry has become far more powerful and influential. Chemicals have replaced herbs or "crude drugs" as they were called then… and, extremely flawed, even fraudulent, studies prohibit the sale of sassafras.

Plants for A Future States of our native Pines:

Medicinal use of Loblolly Pine, Pitch Pine, Prickle Pine, Pond Pine, Loblolly Pine, Scrub Pine and Short Leaf Pine: The turpentine obtained from the resin of all pine trees is antiseptic, diuretic, rubefacient and vermifuge. It is a valuable remedy used internally in the treatment of kidney and bladder complaints and is used both internally and as a rub and steam bath in the treatment of rheumatic affections. It is also very beneficial to the respiratory system and so is useful in treating diseases of the mucous membranes and respiratory complaints such as coughs, colds, influenza and TB. Externally it is a very beneficial treatment for a variety of skin complaints, wounds, sores, burns, boils etc and is used in the form of liniment plasters, poultices, herbal steam baths and inhalers.

Medicinal use of White Pine: White pine was employed medicinally by several native North American Indian tribes who valued it especially for its antiseptic and vulnerary qualities, using it extensively in the treatment of skin complaints, wounds, burns, boils etc. It is also very beneficial to the respiratory system and so was used in treating coughs, colds, influenza and so on. The turpentine obtained from the resin of all pine trees is antiseptic, diuretic, rubefacient and vermifuge. It is a valuable remedy used internally in the treatment of kidney and bladder complaints and is used both internally and as a rub and steam bath in the treatment of rheumatic affections. It is also very beneficial to the respiratory system and so is useful in treating diseases of the mucous membranes and respiratory complaints such as coughs, colds, influenza and TB. Externally it is a very beneficial treatment for a variety of skin complaints, wounds, sores, burns, boils etc and is used in the form of liniment plasters, poultices, herbal steam baths and inhalers. A poultice of pitch has been used to draw out toxins from boils and reduce the pain. The dried inner bark is demulcent, diuretic and expectorant. An infusion was used as a treatment for colds and it is still used as an ingredient in commercial cough syrups, where it serves to promote the expulsion of phlegm. A poultice made from the pounded inner bark is used to treat cuts, sores and wounds. The wetted inner bark can be used as a poultice on the chest in treating strong colds. The dried inner bark contains 10% tannin, some mucilage, an oleoresin, a glycoside and a volatile oil. A tea made from the young needles is used to treat sore throats. It is a good source of vitamin C and so is effective against scurvy. An infusion of the young twigs has been used in the treatment of kidney disorders and pulmonary complaints. The powdered wood has been used as a dressing on babies chaffed skin, sores and improperly healed navels.

Sacred and Healing Herbal Beers tells us:

Pine needles are strongly antiscorbutic and impart a pleasing taste to tea. They also posses expectorant, diuretic and antiseptic activity as well. The resin is the most strongly expectorant element of the plant, for this purpose and amount about the size of a raisin is chewed and swallowed. Pine helps soften bronchial mucous and move it out of the system through expectoration. In any condition where the lungs are congested without fruitful expectoration, it is useful. As a diuretic and antiseptic, it is useful for urinary tract infections. Pine is strong, and as a result, it is easy to take too much, which can aggravate active kidney and urethral inflammation. The bark is fairly high in tannins and mucilaginous constituents. These, combines with its antibacterial activity make it a highly useful herb for external wound poultices, as it will help stop bleeding, help damaged tissue bind together, soothe inflamed tissues and help prevent infection. These same actions make it useful in stomach ulceration and especially in cough syrups for upper respiratory infections…. In traditional medicinal herbalism, pine bark or resin has been used as a stimulant, laxative, expectorant, diuretic, pectoral, vermifuge, detergent, balsamic and vulnerary. Indigenous practice has used it frequently for colds and flus, sore throats, stubborn wounds, sores or ulcers, inflammations and rheumatism. It was one of the most important herbal medicines for the Menominee Indians of North America.

Peterson Field Guides Eastern and Central Medicinal Plants tells us pine

Shortleaf Pine: American Indians used the inner bark end tea to induce vomiting called tea of buds once used as a worm experiment pitched he used as a laxative for tuberculosis also for kidney elements causing backaches.

Longleaf pine: turpentine derived from sap formally used for colic' chronic diarrhea, worms, to arrest bleeding from tooth sockets. Rubefacient. Folk remedy from abdominal tumors.

White pine: used extensively by American Indians. Pitch poultice to draw out boils abscesses also for rheumatism broken bones cuts bruises sores felons and inflammations. Twig tea usd for kidney an lung ailments; emetic. Bark and or leaf tea used for colds coughs gripe sore throats lung ailments, poultice for headaches backaches, etc. Inner bark formerly used in cough syrups.

Botany In a Day states:

Medicinally, the Pines are quite resinous and aromatic; the tea is useful as an expectorant but can irritate the kidneys. It is reported that the needles of some Pines cause abortion in cattle, so caution is advised here. Externally, the resin has a disinfectant quality, like Pinesol. The bark of some species contains powerful antioxidants.

The Physicians' Desk Reference for Herbal Medicine tells us:

Pine shoots indications in usage, approved by Commission E: blood pressure problems, common cold, cough/bronchitis, fevers and colds, inflammation of the mouth and pharynx, neuralgia's, tendency to infection. Pine shoots are used internally for catarrh, conditions of the upper and lower respiratory tract. Externally it is used for mild muscular pain and neuralgia, coughs, an acute bronchial diseases and topically for nasal congestion hoarseness. Pine oil, approved by Commission E: common cold, coughs/bronchitis, fevers and colds, inflammation of the mouth and pharynx, neuralgias, rheumatism, tendency to infection. The essential oil is used internally and externally for congestive diseases of the upper lower respiratory tract. Externally it is used for rheumatic and neuralgic ailments. Turpentine oil purified, approved by Commission E: cough bronchitis, inflammation the mouth and pharynx, rheumatism. Purified turpentine oil is used internally and externally for chronic diseases of the bronchi with profuse secretions it is used externally for rheumatic and neuralgic ailments. Unproven uses: folk medicine use includes bladder catarrh, gallstones, and phosphorus poisoning.

Platanus occidentalis, American Sycamore or Buttonwood

Plants for A Future states:

The inner bark is astringent, diuretic, emetic and laxative. It has been used as a tea in the treatment of dysentery, coughs, colds, lung ailments, haemorrhages, measles, milky and difficult urination etc and also as a blood tonic. Externally, it has been used as a wash on wounds. An infusion of the bark and roots has been used as a foot soak for treating rheumatism. The bark ooze has been used as a wash on infected sores and an infusion has been given in the treatment of infant rash. An infusion of the bark, mixed with honey locust bark (Gleditsia triacanthos), has been used as a gargle to treat hoarseness and sore throat.

Peterson Field Guides Eastern and Central Medicinal Plants tells us:

American Indians used inner bark tea for dysentery, colds, lung ailments, measles, coughs; Also as a "blood purifier", ,an emetic to induce vomiting, laxative. Bark once suggested for rheumatism and scurvy efficacy unconfirmed.

Pistacia chinensis, Chinese Pistacio

Pistachios are known for their delicious nuts, but they may also have some medicinal value. According to Plants for A Future, "Resin from the related P. lentiscus is analgesic, antitussive, expectorant and sedative. It would be worthwhile examining this species."

Populus - Poplar, Cottonwood or Aspen

Twenty-three varieties of Populus have been found useful in Herbal Medicine; they go by various names: Populus alba - White Poplar, Populus angustifolia - Narrowleaf Cottonwood, Populus 'Balsam Spire', Populus balsamifera - Balsam Poplar, Populus ciliata - Himalayan Poplar, Populus deltoides - Eastern Cottonwood, Populus deltoides monilifera - Plains Cottonwood, Populus deltoides wislizenii - Rio Grande Cottonwood, Populus euphratica, Populus fremontii – Cottonwood, Populus grandidentata - Canadian Aspen, Populus heterophylla - Swamp Cottonwood, Populus maximowiczii – Doronoki, Populus nigra - Black Poplar, Populus pseudosimonii, Populus sieboldii - Japanese Aspen, Populus simonii, Populus tremula - Aspen Poplar, Populus tremuloides - American Aspen, Populus trichocarpa - Western Balsam Poplar, Populus x canadensis - Canadian Poplar, Populus x canescens - Grey Poplar, Populus x jackii - Balm Of Gilead

Four varieties of Populus are native to my region: Populus deltoides (Eastern Cottonwood) , Populus grandidentata (Bigtooth Aspen), Populus heterophylla (Swamp Cottonwood), Populus tremuloides (Quaking Aspen). Naturalized are: Populus alba (White Poplar), Populus ×canadensis [deltoides × nigra] (Hybrid Black Poplar),

Populus ×canescens [alba × tremula] (Gray Poplar), Populus ×jackii [balsamifera × deltoides] (Balm-of-Gilead), Populus nigra (Lombardy Poplar), Populus simonii (Chinese Poplar)

Chief among the virtues of Poplar is its ability to relieve plan and reduce fevers, like the Willows and other plants that contain salycin. The tree was sought out and utilized wherever it grew, and it seems there have always been many names used for Populus.

Gerard wrote:

There be divers trees under the title of Poplar, yet differing yery notably, as shall be declared in the descriptions, whereof one is the white, another the black, and a third sort set down by Pliny, which is the Aspen, named by him Lybica, and by Theophrastus, Kerkis: likewise there is another of America, or of the Indies, which is not to be found in these regions of Europe.

A. The White Poplar hath a cleansing faculty, saith Galen, and a mixed temperature, consisting of a watery warm essence, and also a thin earthy substance.

B. The bark, as Dioscorides writeth, to the weight of an ounce (or as others say, and that more truly, of little more than a dram) is a good remedy for the sciatica or ache in the huckle bones, and for the strangury.

C. That this bark is good for the sciatica, Serenus Sammonicus doth also write:

Sæpius occultus victa coxendice morbus

Perfurit, & gressus diro languore moratur:

Populus alba dabit medicos de cortice potus.

An hidden disease doth oft rage and reign,

The hip overcome and vex with the pain,

It makes with vile aching one tread slow and shrink;

The bark of white Poplar is help had in drink.

D. The same bark is also reported to make a woman barren, if it be drunk with the kidney of a mule, which thing the leaves likewise are thought to perform, being taken after the flowers or reds be ended.

211

E. The warm juice of the leaves being dropped into the ears doth take away the pain thereof.

F. The resin or clammy substance of the black Poplar buds is hot and dry, and of thin parts, attenuating and mollifying: it is also fitly mixed acopis & malagmatis ["into a salve used to ease fatigue or pain, or as a poultice]": the leaves have in a manner the like operation for all these things, yet weaker, and not so effectual, as Galen teacheth.

G. The leaves and young buds of black Poplar do assuage the pain of the gout in the hands or feet, being made into an ointment with May butter.

H. The ointment made of the buds is good against all inflammations, bruses, squats, falls, and such like: this ointment is very well known to the apothecaries.

I. Paulus Ægineta teacheth to make an oil also hereof, called Ægyrinum, or oil of black Poplar

Saint Hildegard von Bingen wrote:

The aspen is hot and designates excess. When an infant lying in its cradle is wounded and suffused with blood between his skin and flesh, so that he is in much pain, take new, fresh aspen leaves. Put them on an unfolded linen cloth and wrap the infant with these leaves in the cloth. Place him for sleeping and cover him with clothing, so that he emits perspiration. The power of the leaves will draw it out and he will get well.

But, if one is virgitchtiget or has a cold stomach, he should take the bark of this tree, when it is green, and wood from the exterior, down to but not including the inner heart. He should cut them into minute bits and cook them in water. The, he should pour this water, with the wood, into a cask and bathe in it. If he does this often, the gitch will leave him, or his stomach will be warm, and each malady will be better.

Also, in May, take the bark of this tree, and wood from the outside, into he heart, and cut it into small bits. Pound this in a mortar, and express the juice. Add this juice to other ointments which you prepare. They will be much better against all diseases that trouble *a person in his head, torso, loins, stomach and other parts, and these unguents will check the bad humors to a greater degree.*

Culpeper wrote of Black and White Poplar:

Saturn hath dominion over both, white poplar, saith Galen, is of a cleansing property. The weight of an ounce in powder, of the bark thereof, being drank, saith Dioscorides, is a remedy for those that are troubled with the sciatica, or the stranguary. The juice of the leaves dropped warm into the ears, eases the pains in them. The young clammy buds or eyes, before they break out into leaves, bruised, and a little honey put to them, is a good medicine for a dull sight. The Black Poplar is held to be more cooling than the White, and therefore the leaves bruised with vinegar and applied, help the gout. The seed drank in vinegar, is held good against the falling-sickness. The water that drops from the hollow places of this tree, takes away warts, pushes, wheals, and other the like breakings- out of the body. The young Black Poplar buds, saith Matthiolus, are much used by women to beautify their hair, bruising them with fresh butter, straining them after they have been kept for some time in the sun. The ointment called Populneon, which is made of this Poplar, is singularly good for all heat and inflammations in any part of the body, and tempers the heat of wounds. It is much used to dry up the milk of women's breasts when they have weaned their children.

The leaves and buds are used to make the unguent populcon; but as the black poplar is hot, the ointment cannot receive itso cooling virtue from those leaves or buds, but from the other ingredients which are put in it. Schroeder says, that women in Germany use the buds to make their hair grow thick and ornamental.

Mrs. Grieves wrote specifically of the "Trembling Poplar: or Quaking Aspen:

Febrifuge and tonic, chiefly used in intermittent fevers. It has been employed as a diuretic in urinary affections, gonorrhoea and gleet. The infusion has been found helpful in debility, chronic diarrhcea, etc. Is a valuable and safe substitute for Peruvian bark.

Peruvian Bark was Chinchona, the main source of quinine. It was widely used for malaria and fevers.

An Irish Herbal states of White Poplar and of Trembling Poplar, called the "Asp Tree":

The juice of the leaves of this tree eases the pains of the ears and hears ulcers and eruptions on the skin. The bark is useful for promoting the discharge of urine and is therefore good against strangury.

Brother Aloysius wrote of Poplar:

The leaf decoction is used externally in the form of a compress for sciatica; internally, ¾ to 1 cup per 2 cups water for difficult urination.

Jolanta Wittib writes of Poplar:

Poplar bud tincture is highly valued in our region. Maybe because poplar is a rare tree here. Trees protect their buds with resin. Bees know that. They have been collecting resin from the buds for thousands of years and have been turning it into propolis - the highly protective, antibacterial, antiviral, antifungal substance with which they protect and disinfect their beehive.

We, humans, most probably have learned that from the bees, but, as we cannot turn it into Propolis with our bodies, like bees do, we make tinctures.

I collect some buds and with the help of high percentage Alcohol I get the resin from them and turn it into tincture. Diluted internally it is used for inflammations, colds, flu; externally for rashes, small wounds, muscle pain. I use it for gurgling when I feel that I might develop a sore throat.

Since I have bees, I have stopped collecting poplar buds. Instead, I take a little bit of Propolis from my bee hives, turn it into tincture and use it in the same way as poplar bud tincture. I like toothpaste with Propolis. It does so much more than just cleaning the teeth.

The Thomsonian System of Medicine states:

POPLAR BARK. Populus Tremuloides.(Dr. Thomson.)

There are several species of the poplar tree that grow common in the country. One kind is called the white poplar, and another the stinking poplar. The barks of both these kinds are good for medicine; but the latter is the best, being the most bitter. It has tags hanging on the limbs, which remain on till it leaves out, which is about a week later than the other kind. It has short brittle twigs, which are extremely bitter to the taste. The inner bark given as a tea is one of the best articles to regulate the bile and restore the digestive powers of anything I have ever used. The bark may be taken from the body of the tree, the limbs or the roots, and the outside shaved off. Preserve the inner bark, which should be dried and carefully preserved for use. To make the bitters No. 4, it should be pounded or ground fine, and mixed with the other articles, or it may be used alone for the same purpose. To make a tea, take a handful of the bark, pounded or cut into small strips, and put into a quart mug, and fill it with boiling water. This, if taken freely, will relax the system, will relieve headache, faintness at the stomach, and many other complaints caused by bad digestion. It is good for obstructions of the urine, and weakness in the loins; and those of a consumptive habit will find great relief in using this tea freely. In chronic diarrhoea, chronic dysentery, cholera infantum, it is a tonic, not an astringent. It is of much use in kidney and bladder trouble. It gradually increases the urine and relieves the aching back. If given with Uva ursi, it will give good results in cystic and renal catarrh and in congestions. It is also indicated in uterine, vaginal and anal weakness, and can be used as a wash or internally. Is good as a wash in skin diseases and sores caused by gonorrhoea or syphilis. The dose of the Tincture is from 30 to 60 minims.

King's American Dispensatory, 1898 tells us:

Action, Medical Uses, and Dosage.—Poplar bark is tonic and febrifuge, and has been used in intermittent fever with advantage. An infusion of it is reputed a valuable remedy in emaciation and debility, after protracted fevers and reproductive disorders of the nervous and hysterical, lumbricoid worms, impaired digestion, chronic diarrhoea, intermittent fevers, etc. As a diuretic, it has been beneficially used in urinary affections, gonorrhoea, gleet, etc. Both populus and populin have a decided affinity for the genito-urinal tract. It is thought to aid the recuperative powers of the kidney when undergoing granular degeneration. In tenesmic vesical irritation and in tenesmus after urination it is decidedly effective. Minute doses—

fraction of a drop—are most beneficial here. It is suggested by Prof. Webster for trial in stubborn uterine congestion and prostatic hypertrophies. The Large aspen, P. grandidentata, is said to be the most active and bitter. Dose of the powdered bark, 1 drachm, 2 or 3 times a day; of a saturated tincture of the fresh bark, from a fraction of a drop to 30 drops; of populin, 1 x trituration, 1 grain every 2 or 4 hours.

Specific Indications and Uses.—Marked debility with impairment of digestion; tenesmic vesical irritation; tenesmus after micturition.

Plants for A Future states:

Medicinal use of White Poplar: The stem bark is anodyne, anti-inflammatory, antiseptic, astringent, diuretic and tonic. The bark contains salicylates, from which the proprietary medicine aspirin is derived. It is used internally in the treatment of rheumatism, arthritis, gout, lower back pains, urinary complaints, digestive and liver disorders, debility, anorexia, also to reduce fevers and relieve the pain of menstrual cramps. Externally, the bark is used to treat chilblains, haemorrhoids, infected wounds and sprains. The bark is harvested from side branches or coppiced trees and dried for later use. The leaves are used in the treatment of caries of teeth and bones. The twigs are depurative.

Medicinal use of Eastern Cottonwood: The bark contains salicin, a glycoside that probably decomposes into salicylic acid (aspirin) in the body. The bark is therefore anodyne, anti-inflammatory and febrifuge. It is used especially in treating rheumatism and fevers, and also to relieve the pain of menstrual cramps. An infusion of the bark has been used in the treatment of whooping cough and tuberculosis. A decoction of the bark has been used to rid the body of intestinal worms. The bark has been eaten as a treatment for colds. A tea made from the inner bark is used in the treatment of scurvy. The inner bark, combined with black haw bark (Crataegus douglasii) and wild plum bark (Prunus spp) has been used as a female tonic. A poultice of the leaves has been used as a treatment for rheumatism, bruises, sores and boils.

Rodale's Illustrated Encyclopedia of Herbs states:

The entire poplar genus contains salicylate precursors, which are related to aspirin and share its properties as an anti-inflammatory, antipyretic and analgesic. The species vary greatly in their medicinal properties; those with highly resinous buds are usually the most effective.

Peterson Field Guides Eastern and Central Medicinal Plants tells us:

Balsam Poplar, balm of Gilead: buds boiled to separate resin then dissolved in alcohol, once used as preservative in ointments. Folk remedy (balm) used for sores; Tincture for toothaches, rheumatism, diarrhea, wounds; Tea used as a wash for inflammation, frostbite, sprains, and muscle strain. Internally, bud tea used for cough, lung ailments expectorant. Inner bark tea used for scurvy, also as an eyewash, "blood tonic". Root tea used as a wash for headaches. Probably contain salicin, explaining its aspirin like qualities.

Cottonwood: inner bark tea used for scurvy, as a female tonic. Tree held sacred by American Indians of the prairies. Bark contains the aspirin-like compound, salicin.

Quaking aspen: American Indians used root bark tea for excessive menstrual bleeding; poultice roots for cuts, wounds. Inner bark tea used for stomach pain, venereal disease, urinary elements, worms, colds, fevers, an as an appetite stimulant. Leaf buds used in a salve for colds, coughs, irritated nostrils. Bark tincture contains salicin, a folk remedy used for fevers, rheumatism, arthritis, colds, worms, urinary infections, and diarrhea. Bark contains aspirin like salicin which is anti-inflammatory, analgesic; Reduces fevers.

Botany In a Day states:

Medicinally, the buds are diaphoretic, expectorant and diuretic. The leaves were used as a poultice. Cotton wood and Aspen leaf buds contain a sticky, aromatic resin that can be collected in the early spring an used in an oil based ointment for burns and skin irritations. It is popularly known as "Balm of Gilead". The buds are soaked in olive oil for a week to extract constituents.

The Physicians Desk Reference for Herbal Medicine tells us:

Poplar buds have antiphlogistic antibacterial and wound healing effects Poplar bark and leaves have antiphlogistic, analgesic, antibacterial and spasmolytic effects. Unproven uses: Poplar bark and leaves are used for pain and rheumatism therapy an in micturition complaints due to prostate hypertrophy. Poplar leaf buds approved by Commission E: hemorrhoids, wounds and burns. Unproven uses: Poplar buds are used for frostbite and sunburn. Contraindications: contraindicated in cases of hypersensitivity to salicylate. No health hazards or side effects are known in conjunction with proper administration of designated therapeutic dosages.

Prunus, Plumb, Cherry, Peach, Apricot, Nectarine, Almond, Damson Sloe, etc.

One hundred and twenty-four varieties of Prunus have been found useful in Herbal Medicine!!!! Prunus alabamensis - Alabama Cherry, Prunus alleghaniensis - Allegheny Plum, Prunus americana - American Plum, Prunus americana lanata, Prunus andersonii - Desert Peach, Prunus angustifolia - Chickasaw Plum, Prunus angustifolia watsonii - Sand Plum, Prunus apetala - Clove Cherry, Prunus arabica, Prunus armeniaca – Apricot, Prunus avium - Wild Cherry, Prunus besseriana - Dwarf Almond, Prunus besseyi - Western Sand Cherry, Prunus bifrons, Prunus bokharensis - Bokhara Plum, Prunus brigantina - Briançon Apricot, Prunus buergeriana, Prunus campanulata - Taiwan Cherry, Prunus canescens - Greyleaf Cherry, Prunus capsica, Prunus caroliniana - American Cherry Laurel, Prunus cerasifera - Cherry Plum, Prunus cerasifera divaricate, Prunus cerasoides - Wild Himalayan Cherry, Prunus cerasus - Sour Cherry, Prunus cerasus austera - Morello Cherry, Prunus cerasus caproniana - Kentish Red Cherry, Prunus cerasus frutescens - Bush Sour Cherry, Prunus cerasus marasca - Maraschino Cherry, Prunus cocomilia, Prunus consociiflora - Chinese Wild Peach, Prunus cornuta - Himalayan Bird Cherry, Prunus cortapico, Prunus davidiana - Chinese Wild Peach, Prunus dawyckensis - Dawyck Cherry, Prunus dielsiana, Prunus domestica - Plum, Prunus dulcis – Almond, Prunus emarginata - Bitter Cherry, Prunus fasciculata - Desert Almond, Prunus fenzliana, Prunus fruticosa - Mongolian Cherry, Prunus glandulosa - Korean Cherry, Prunus gracilis - Sour Plum, Prunus grayana - Japanese Bird

Cherry, Prunus gymnodonta, Prunus hortulana - Hog Plum, Prunus humilis - Bush Cherry, Prunus ilicifolia - Holly-Leaved Cherry, Prunus incana, Prunus incisa - Fuji Cherry, Prunus insititia – Damson, Prunus iranica, Prunus jamasakura – Yamazakura, Prunus japonica - Korean Cherry, Prunus japonica nakai - Japanese Plum, Prunus jenkinsii, Prunus kansuensis, Prunus korshinskyi, Prunus lannesiana - Oshima Cherry, Prunus laurocerasus - Cherry Laurel, Prunus lusitanica - Portugal Laurel, Prunus lyonii - Catalina Island Cherry, Prunus mahaleb - Mahaleb Cherry, Prunus mandschurica - Manchurian Apricot, Prunus maritima - Beach Plum, Prunus maximowiczii - Miyama Cherry, Prunus media, Prunus mexicana - Mexican Plum, Prunus macrocarpa, Prunus mira - Smoothpit Peach, Prunus mume - Japanese Apricot, Prunus munsoniana - Wild Goose Plum, Prunus napaulensis, Prunus nigra - Canadian Plum, Prunus nipponica - Japanese Alpine Cherry, Prunus orthosepala, Prunus padus - Bird Cherry, Prunus pedunculata, Prunus pensylvanica - Pin Cherry, Prunus persica – Peach, Prunus persica nucipersica – Nectarine, Prunus pilosiuscula, Prunus prostrata - Mountain Cherry, Prunus pseudocerasus - Cambridge Cherry, Prunus pumila - Dwarf American Cherry, Prunus pumila susquehanae - Dwarf American Cherry, Prunus rivularis - Creek Plum, Prunus rufa - Himalayan Cherry, Prunus salicifolia - Capulin Cherry, Prunus salicina - Japanese Plum, Prunus sargentii, Prunus serotina - Rum Cherry, Prunus serrula - Birch Bark Cherry, Prunus serrulata – Yamazakura, Prunus sibirica - Siberian Apricot, Prunus simonii - Apricot Plum, Prunus Sogdiana, Prunus spinosa – Sloe, Prunus ssiori - Japanese Bird Cherry, Prunus subcordata - Pacific Plum, Prunus subhirtella - Rosebud Cherry, Prunus takesimensis, Prunus tangutica, Prunus tenella - Dwarf Russian Almond, Prunus tomentosa - Nanking Cherry, Prunus triloba - Flowering Almond Synonym:, Prunus triloba simplex - Flowering Almond, Prunus umbellata - Black Sloe, Prunus undulata, Prunus ursina, Prunus ussuriensis, Prunus virens - Wild Cherry, Prunus virginiana – Chokecherry, Prunus virginiana demissa - Western Chokecherry, Prunus virginiana melanocarpa - Rocky Mountain Chokecherry, Prunus x cistena - Purple-Leaf Sand Cherry, Prunus x dasycarpa - Black Apricot, Prunus x eminens, Prunus x fontanesiana, Prunus x gondouinii - Duke Cherry, Prunus x sultana, Prunus x utahensis, Prunus x yedoensis - Tokyo Cherry

Although it would be wonderful to all that tasty fruit, I can honestly say that it is somewhat of a relief that we only have eight varieties of Prunus native to my region… I can't imagine having to learn to identify them all! Native are: Prunus alleghaniensis var. alleghaniensis (Allegheny Plum), Prunus americana (American Plum), Prunus angustifolia (Chickasaw Plum), Prunus caroliniana (Carolina Laurelcherry), Prunus pensylvanica (Pin Cherry), Prunus serotina var. serotina (Black Cherry), Prunus umbellata (Hog Plum, Flatwoods Plum), Prunus virginiana var. virginiana (Chokecherry). Naturalized are: Prunus avium (Sweet Cherry), Prunus cerasus (Sour Cherry), Prunus glandulosa (Flowering Almond), Prunus mahaleb (Mahaleb Cherry), Prunus munsoniana (Wild Goose Plum), Prunus persica (Peach)

Among the Appalachian folks, wild Cherry bark is the most used of the Prunuses, as a medicinal herb. It is used for coughs, congestion and asthma. But, that is barely scratching the surface of these useful trees. I feel safe in saying that if you have access to any member of this family of trees, you will find an herbal use for it. So, let's dig into the history of the Prunus, as best we can.

Dioscorides wrote of Almond Oil:

Amagdalinum oil or metopium is made as follows. Having picked and dried four quarts of bitter almonds beat them gently with a wooden pestle in a mortar until they are pulped. Pour on them one pint of hot water and let them absorb it for half an hour, from which time beat it strongly again. Then press it on a board, squeeze it out, and take that which sticks to your fingers into a spoon. Afterwards pour a half-pint of water into that which was squeezed out, and allow it to be absorbed, and repeat as before. Four quarts of seeds make one half-pint of oil. It is effective against womb pains,constriction, the womb turning around, and things that darken the same places, as well as headaches, ear problems, resonance, and tinnitus. It helps inflammation of the kidneys, illness meientes [urination], stones [urinary, kidney], asthma and splenitis. Furthermore it removes spots from the face, sunburn, and wrinkles on the skin mixed with honey, the root of lily and Cyprian rosewax. With wine it mends moisture of the pupils of the eye, and removes penetrative ulcers and dandruff.

The root of the bitter almond tree bruised and boiled takes away spots on the face caused by sunburn, as well as the almonds themselves, applied as a poultice. Applied to the forehead or temples with vinegar and rosaceum they drive out the menstrual flow and help headaches. They are good with wine for epinyctides [pustules which appear at night], rotten ulcers, and shingles [herpes], and with honey for dog bites. Almonds if eaten take away pains and soften the bowels, cause sleep and are diuretic. They are good for bloody vomit taken with amyl [starch] and mint. They are good for inflamed kidneys and pneumonia taken as a drink with water or as a linctus [syrup] with resina terminthos. Taken with passum [raisin wine] they help those troubled with painful urination and urinary stones. They help diseased livers, coughs, and inflation of the colon, the amount of a nut of the avellana [hazel] taken in a linctus [syrup] with milk and honey. They keep away drunkenness if five to seven of them are taken before indulging. It kills foxes when they eat it with something else. The gum of the tree is astringent and heats, and is taken in drink as a remedy for bloody vomit. Rubbed on with vinegar it takes away impetigo [skin infection] on the surface of the skin. Taken in a drink with diluted wine it cures old coughs, and it is good taken in a drink with passum [raisin wine] for those troubled with urinary stones. The sweet edible almond has a great deal less strength than the bitter, yet that also reduces symptoms and is diuretic. Green almonds eaten with their shells heal moistness of the stomach.

Of the Cherry or Sour Cherry, he wrote:

Cerasia that are eaten when fresh are good for the intestines, and dried they stop discharges of the bowels. The gum from cerasia heals an old cough taken with diluted wine. It causes a good colour, sharpness of sight and appetite. Taken in a drink with wine it is good for those troubled with kidney stones.

Of Peaches:

The fruit of persica are good for the stomach and for the intestines too if ripe, but the unripe are astringent in the intestines. Dried they are more astringent, and a decoction of them dried and taken stops a stomach and intestines troubled with excessive discharges.

Plum or Prune:

Coccymelia is a known tree whose fruit is edible and bad for the stomach, softening the bowels, especially fruit of those from Syria and those growing in Damascus. Dried, it is good for the stomach and therapeutic for the bowels. A decoction of the leaves (used or prepared in wine and gargled) stops the excessive discharge that falls on the uva [uvula], gingiva [gums] and tonsils. The fruit of wild plums dried when it is ripe does the same. Boiled with sapa [syruped new wine] it becomes better for the stomach and more astringent to the bowels. The gum of the plum tree closes open cuts and sores, and taken as a drink with wine breaks kidney stones. Rubbed on with vinegar it heals lichen [papular skin disease] on children

Cherry Laurel:

Chamaedaphne sends out single-branched rods a foot long — straight, thin and smooth; the leaves of this are similar to the [other] bay but much smoother, thinner and greener. The fruit is round and red, growing near to the leaves. The leaves of this (pounded into small pieces and smeared on) helps headaches and burning of the stomach. They cease griping, taken as a drink with wine. The juice (given to drink with wine) expels the menstrual flow and urine, and applied in a pessary it does the same. Some have called this alexandrina, daphnitis, or hydragogon, the Romans, laureola, some lactago, and the Gauls, ousubim.

Saint Hildegard von Bingen wrote of Almond:

The Almond Tree is very hot and has a bit of moisture in it. Its bark, leaves and sap are not much used in medicine, because all of its power is in the fruit. One whose brain is empty, and whose face has a bad color from a pain in the head, should frequently eat the inmost kernels of this fruit. They fill his brain and give him the correct color. Also, one who ails in his lungs, or whose liver is weak, should often eat of these kernels, either raw or cooked. They give strength to the lungs, since they in no way burden a person. Neither do they make a person dry, but render him strong.

Of Cherry:

Take the inmost kernels of this fruit, when raw, and pound them well. Dissolve bear fat in a small dish, and mix this with it, making an ungent. Use it often to anoint one whose body has bad ulcers, which are very like leprosy, but are not, and he will be cured.

One who has wretching pains in his belly, although not from worms, should often eat the kernels raw, and he will eb better. One who has worms in his belly should place the kernels in vinegar and often eat them on an empty stomach, and the worms will die.

One who has pains in his eyes, so that they are red from the pain and ulcerous, should take warm crumbs of rye bread and put the gum of a cherry tree ont hem. He should tie them with a band, so the gum is placed on the skin of the eyes. If he does this often, it will draw the drips from his eyes and he will be cured.

If some disease or bad humors fall upon one's ears, so that he becomes deaf and his ears ring, he should take the forenamed gum and dissolve it in a small dish over the fire. He should pour it, thus warmed over crumbs of rye bread and place this in the openings of his ears at night. He should also cover his ears and temples with these crumbs smeared with the gum and tie a linen cloth over them. If he does this often, bad humors and ringing will be chased away, and he will be cured.

Medlar:

The medlar is very hot. It signifies sweetness. Its bark and leaves are not much good as medicine, because all of its strength is in its fruit. Nevertheless, a person who suffers from ague should, at the onset of this infirmity, pulverize its root and drink this powder in warm wine, before breakfast, with meals and at night. He should do this frequently and he will eb cured. The fruit of this tree is good and useful for healthy and sick people, however much they eat. It increases their flesh and cleanses their blood.

Peach:

One who is in various illnesses, has any kind of spots on his body should take the inner bark of this tree before it fruit matures. He should pound the bark, express its sap, and add a little vinegar to it, and as much cooked honey as there is of the other two things. He should place this in a new clay jar, and frequently anoint his body where the bad spots are, until they are diminished.

When one's breath stinks badly, he should take the fruits of the peach tree that are ripe. He should pound them, then take a handful of licorice, a bit of pepper and some honey, and cook these things in pure win, and so prepare a spiced wine. He should drink this often, with a meal and at night. It will make his breath fragrant and take rottenness away from his body and chest.

For one with worms in his stomach or belly, the root and leaves of betony should be pulverized. Add to this twice as much pulverized leaves of the peach tree, taken when it has just sent out flowers.

Cook this in a new pot with good, pure wine. Drink it often, before breakfast and at night, and the worms will die.

Take also the raw, inmost kernels of the fruit and, having thrown away the shell, pound them to a milk and squeeze five spoonfuls through a cloth. Then pulverize three pennyweight of galingale, two of licorice, and half a pennyweight of spurge, and add this to the peach-kernel milk. Prepare a small cake of whole wheat flour and garden spurge, and dry it gently in the sun or a warm oven. Then mix this cake with a half pennyweight of the forenamed milk. Before sunrise, take spoonfuls of this – equal to the weight of two and a half pennies – after heating it on a fire. Then put yourself to bed for a short while. This checks the gicht and carries congestion away from your chest, and mucus away from your stomach. As a pleasant potion, it gently purges you. If you need to, take it twice a month, and on the day you take it, refrain from strong food, rye bread, peas and lentils. Eat soft foods and drink wine.

One who has pains in his chest, so that his throat is a bit constricted, either because some bad thing is growing on it or there is some bad vapor in it, with no ulcer or tumor, should take a paste of wheat flour and dissolve it in the gum of the peach tree. He should often place this, warm, over his throat for a little while, and he will eb better. If, however, there is pain in his throat from an ulcer or tumor, he should not place this on it, because it would be painful. If a person has glands on his neck that are contracted or more distinct than usual, and if there is no ulcer or tumor, he should place the same prepared paste on them. If the neck were ulcerated or tumescent, this paste would make it worse.

One who has pain in his head should take the wheat paste, dissolve it in the gum of the peach tree, and place it, warm, on the top of his head for some time, and he will be better.

For one whose eyes water, press gum from the peach tree, or from the shell of a walnut, and warm it a bit on a hot tile. Then place it around the eyes, until they grow warm. Do this once a day, every four days, lest in doing it too often the eyes are harmed. The gum of the peach tree has in it the first strength of the wood and draws to itself natural moisture.

Plum:

If some worms are eating the flesh of a person, take the upper bark of that tree, down to the sap, and its leaves and pulverize them.

Dry them in the sun or in a pot by the fire. Put this powder in the place where the worms are eating the person. When the worms begin to move from there, so that the person feels it, take vinegar mixed with a bit of honey and pour it where the worms are, and they will die. When they have fallen from the wound, d *ead, dip a linen cloth in wine and place it over the wounds. It will draw out the rotten matter, and the person will become well.*

Also, make ashes from the bark of the leaves of this tree. From these ashes make lye, and if your head is either pockmarked or withered, wash it often with this lye. Your head will be cured and it will be beautiful, will produce much beautiful hair.

If someone through magic or by evil words is rendered insane, take the earth which is around the roots of this tree and warm it vigorously in the fire, until it burns a little bit. When it has burned a bit by the fire, place rue and a little less pennyroyal on it. Let it absorb their sap and odor. If you do nor have pennyroyal, place fresh fenugreek on it. If it is winter, place on it the seeds of these herbs, moderately warmed. After the person has eaten, place this, with the herbs, on his head, naked stomach, and naked sides, and tie it with a cloth. Put him in bed and cover him with clothing so that he might sweat a bit with that earth. Do this for three or five days, and he will be better. For when the ancient serpent hears magic and evil words, he takes them up and sets traps for the one for whom they were said, unless God stops him

Take the gum of this tree and, if someone's lips swell up, or if he reports gicht springing up in them, heat this gum moderately and at night when he goes to bed tie it, with a cloth, on his lips where it hurts. Do this often and the pain will cease. One whose fingers and hands are always moving from the tremor of the gicht should tie this same gum, warmed, over his whole hand and the tremor will cease.

Whoever has a dry cough should take the inmost kernels of this fruit and, throwing away their covering, place them in wine. They should soak in the wine until they have swelled a bit. Then, he should eat them often and prepare a drink with good wine. He should consume this by sipping, and he will quickly be cured. Every id of plum tree has these powers in their bark and leaves, and the same nature in their fruit, except the trees which are larger and bring forth larger fruits with greater strength.

Gerard wrote of Almond:

A. Sweet almonds when they be dry be moderately hot; but the bitter ones are hot and dry in the second degree. There is in both of them a certain fat and oily substance, which is drawn out by pressing.

B. Sweet almonds being new gathered are pleasant to the taste, they yield some kind of nourishment, but the same gross and earthy, and grosser than those that be dry, and not as yet withered. These do likewise slowly descend, especially being eaten without their skins; for even as the husks or branny parts of corn do serve to drive down the gross excrements of the belly, so do likewise the skins or husks of the almonds: therefore those that be blanched do so slowly descend, as that they do withal bind the belly; whereupon they are given with good success to those that have the lask or the bloody flux.

C. There is drawn out of sweet almonds, with liquor added, a white juice like milk, which over and besides that it nourisheth, and is good for those that are troubled with the lask and bloody flux, it is profitable for those that have the pleurisy and spit up filthy matter, as Alexander Trallianus witnesseth: for there is likewise in the almonds an opening and concocting quality, with a certain cleansing faculty, by which they are medicinable to the chest and lungs, or lights, and serve for the raising up of phlegm and rotten humours.

D. Almonds taken before meat do stop the belly, and nourish but little; notwithstanding many excellent meats and medicines are therewith made for sundry griefs, yea very delicate and wholesome meats, as almond butter, cream of almonds, marchpane, and such like, which dry and stay the belly more than the extracted juice or milk; and they are also as good for the chest and lungs.

E. They do serve also to make the physical barley water, and barley cream, which are given in hot fevers, as also for other sick and feeble persons, for their further refreshing and nourishments.

F. The oil which is newly pressed out of the sweet almonds is a mitigator of pain and all manner of aches. It is given to those that have the pleurisy, being first let blood; but especially to those that are troubled with the stone of the kidneys; it slackens the passages of the urine, and maketh them glib or slippery, and more ready to suffer the stone to have free passage: it maketh the belly soluble, and therefore it is likewise used for the colic.

G. It is good for women that are newly delivered; for it quickly removeth the throes which remain after their delivery.

H. The oil of almonds makes smooth the hands and face of delicate persons, and cleanseth the skin from all spots, pimples, and lentils.

I. Bitter Almonds do make thin and open, they remove stoppings out of the liver and spleen, therefore they be good against pain in the sides: they make the body soluble, provoke urine, bring down the menses, help the strangury, and cleanse forth of the chest and lungs clammy humours: if they be mixed with some kind of lohoch or medicine to lick on: with starch they stay the spitting of blood.

L. And it is reported that five or six being taken fasting do keep a man from being drunk.

M. These also cleanse and take away spots and blemishes in the face, and in other parts of the body; they mundify and make clean foul eating ulcers.

N. With honey they are laid upon the biting of mad dogs; being applied to the temples with vinegar or oil of roses, they take away the headache, as Dioscorides writeth.

O. They are also good against the cough and shortness of wind.

P. They are likewise good for those that spit blood, if they be taken with the fine flour of Amylum.

Q. There is also pressed out of these an oil which provoketh urine, but especially if a few scorpions be drowned, and steeped therein.

R. With oil it it singular good for those that have the stone, and cannot easily make water: but with extremity of pain, if the share and place between the cods and fundament be anointed therewith.

S. Dioscorides saith, that the gum doth heat and bind, which qualities notwithstanding are not perceived in it.

T. It helpeth them that spit blood, not by a binding faculty, but through the clamminess of his substance, and that is by closing up of the passages and pores, and so may it also cure old coughs, and mitigate extreme pains that proceed of the stone, and especially *take away the sharpness of urine, if it be drunk with bastard, or with any other sweet potion, as with the decoction of Liquorice, or of raisins of the sun. The same doth likewise kill tetters in the outward parts of the body (as Dioscorides addeth) if it be dissolved in vinegar.*

Of Cherry:

A. The best and principal cherries be those that are somewhat sour: those little sweet ones which be wild and soonest ripe be the worst: they contain bad juice, they very soon putrefy, and do engender ill blood, by reason whereof they do not only breed worms in the belly, but troublesome agues, and often pestilent fevers: and therefore in well governed commonwealths it is carefully provided, that they should not be sold in the markets in the plague time.

B. Spanish cherries are like to these in faculties, but they do not so soon putrefy: they be likewise cold, and the juice they make is not good.

C. The Flanders or Kentish cherries that are thorough ripe, have a better juice, but watery, cold and moist: they quench thirst, they are good for an hot stomach, and profitable for those that have the ague: they easily descend and make the body soluble: they nourish nothing at all.

D. The late ripe cherries which the Frenchmen keep dried against winter, and are by them called Morelle, and we after the same name call them Morell cherries, are dry, and do somewhat bind; these being dried are pleasant to the taste, and wholesome for the stomach, like as prunes be, and do stop the belly.

E. Generally all the kinds of cherries are cold and moist of temperature, although some more cold and moist than others: the which being eaten before meat do soften the belly very gently, they are unwholesome either unto moist and rheumatic bodies, or for unhealthy and cold stomachs.

F. The common black cherries do strengthen the stomach, and are wholesomer than the red cherries, the which being dried do stop the lask.

G. The distilled water of cherries is good for those that are troubled with heat and inflammations in their stomachs, and prevaileth against the falling sickness given mixed with wine.

H. Many excellent Tarts and other pleasant meats are made with cherries, sugar, and other delicate spices, whereof to write were to small purpose.

I. The gum of the Cherry tree taken with wine and water, is reported to help the stone; it may do good by making the passages slippery, and by tempering & allaying the sharpness of the humours; and in this manner it is a remedy also for an old cough. Dioscorides addeth, that it maketh one well coloured, cleareth the sight, and causeth a good appetite to meat.

Peach:

A. Peaches be cold and moist, and that in the second degree, they have a juice and also a substance, that doth easily putrefy, which yieldeth no nourishment, but bringeth hurt, especially if they be eaten after other meats; for then they cause the other meats to putrefy. But they are less hurtful if they be taken first; for by reason that they are moist and slippery, they easily and quickly descend; and by making the belly slippery, they cause other meats to slip down the sooner.

B. The kernels of the peaches be hot and dry, they open and cleanse; they are good for the stopB pings of the liver and spleen.

C. Peaches before they be ripe do stop the lask, but being ripe they loose the belly, and engender naughty humour, for they are soon corrupted in the stomach.

D. The leaves of the Peach tree do open the stopping of the liver, and do gently loosen the belly: and being applied plasterwise unto the navel of young children, they kill the worms, and drive them forth.

E. The same leaves boiled in milk, do kill the worms in children very speedily.

F. The same being dried, and cast upon green wounds, cure them.

G. The flowers of the Peach tree infused in warm water for the space of ten or twelve hours, and strained, and more flowers put to the said liquor to infuse after the same manner, and so iterated six or eight times, and strained again, then as much sugar as it will require added to the same liquor and boiled unto the consistence or thickness of a syrup, and two spoonfuls hereof taken, doth so singularly well purge the belly, that there is neither Rhubarb, Agaric, nor any other purger comparable unto it; for this purgeth down waterish humours mightily, and yet without grief or trouble, either to the stomach, or lower parts of the body.

H. The kernel within the peach stone stamped small, and boiled with vinegar until it be brought to the form of an ointment, is good to restore and bring again the hair of such as be troubled with the alopecia.

I. There is drawn forth of the kernels of peaches with Pennyroyal water, a juice like unto milk; which is good for those that have the apoplexy: if the same be oftentimes held in the mouth it draweth forth water and recovereth the speech.

K. The gum is of a mean temperature, but the substance thereof is tough and clammy, by reason whereof it dulleth the sharpness of thin humours: it serveth in a lohoch or licking medicine for those that be troubled with the cough, and have rotten lungs, and stoppeth the spitting and raising up of blood, and also stayeth other fluxes.

Plum:

A. Plums that be ripe and new gathered from the tree, what sort soever they are of; do moisten and cool, and yield unto the body very little nourishment, and the same nothing good at all: for as Plums do very quickly rot, so is also the juice of them apt to putrefy in the body, and likewise to cause the meat to putrefy which is taken with them: only they are good for those that would keep their bodies soluble and cool; for by their moisture and slipperiness they do mollify the belly.

B. Dried plums, commonly called prunes, are wholesomer, and more pleasant to the stomach, they yield more nourishment, and better, and such as cannot easily putrefy. It is reported, saith Galen in his book Of the Faculties of Nourishments, that the best do grow in Damascus a city of Syria; and next to those, they that grow in Spain: but these do nothing at all bind, yet divers of the damask damson prunes very much; for damask damson prunes are more astringent, but they of Spain be sweeter. Dioscorides saith, that damask prunes dried do stay the belly; but Galen affirmth, in his books of the faculties of simple medicines, that they do manifestly loose the belly yet lesser than they that be brought out of Spain; being boiled with mead or honeyed water, which hath a good quantity of honey in it, they loose the belly very much (as the same author saith) although a man take them alone by themselves, and much more if the mead be supped after them. We most commend those of Hungary being long and sweet; yet more those of Moravia the chief and principal city in times past of the Province of the Marcomans: for these after they be dried, that the watery humour may be consumed away, be most pleasant to the taste, and do easily without any trouble so mollify the belly, as that in that respect they go beyond Cassia and Manna, as Thomas Iordanus affirmeth.

C. The leaves of the Plum tree are good against the swelling of the uvula, the throat, gums, & kernels under the throat and jaws; they stop the rheum and falling down of humours, if the decoction thereof be made in wine, and gargled in the mouth and throat.

D. The gum which cometh out of the Plum tree doth glue and fasten together, as Dioscorides saith.

E. Being drunk in wine it wasteth away the stone, and healeth lichens in infants and young children; if it be laid on with vinegar, it worketh the same effects that the gum of the Peach and Cherry tree doth.

F. The wild plums do stay and bind the belly, and so do the unripe plums of what sort soever, whiles they are sharp and sour, for then are they astringent.

G. The juice of sloes doth stop the belly, the lask and bloody flux, the inordinate course of women's terms, and all other issues of blood in man or woman, and may very well be used instead of Acatia, which is a thorny tree growing in Egypt, very hard to be gotten, and of a dear price, and therefore the better for wantons; albeit our plums of this country are equal unto it in virtues.

Culpepper wrote of Cherry:

It is a tree of Venus. Cherries, as they are of different tastes, so they are of different qualities. The sweet pass through the stomach and the belly more speedily, but are of little nourishment; the tart or sour are more pleasing to an hot stomach, procure appetite to meat, and help to cut tough phlegm and gross humours; but when these are dried, they are more binding to the belly than when they are fresh, being cooling in hot diseases, and welcome to the stomach, and provoke urine. The gum of the cherry-tree, dissolved in wine, is good for a cold, cough, and hoarseness of the throat;

231

mendeth the colour in the face, sharpeneth the eyesight, provoketh appetite, and helpeth to break and expel the stone; the black cherries bruised with the sotnes, and dissolved, the water thereof is much used to break the stone, and to expel gravel and wind.

Of Peach:

Lady Venus owns this tree, and by it opposes the ill effects of Mars, and indeed for children and young people, nothing is better to purge choler and the jaundice, than the leaves or flowers of this tree being made into a syrup or conserve. Let such as delight to please their lust regard the fruit; but such as have lost their health, and their children's, let them regard what I say, they may safely give two spoonfuls of the syrup at a time; it is as gentle as Venus herself. The leaves of peaches bruised and laid on the belly, kill worms, and so they do also being boiled in ale and drank, and open the belly likewise; and, being dried, is a far safer medicine to discuss humours. The powder of them strewed upon fresh bleeding wounds stays their bleeding, and closes them up. The flowers steeped all night in a little wine standing warm, strained forth in the morning, and drank fasting, doth gently open the belly, and move it downward. A syrup made of them, as the syrup of roses is made, works more forcibly than that of roses, for it provokes vomiting, and spends waterish and hydropic humours by the continuance thereof. The flowers made into a conserve, work the same effect. The liquor that dropped from the tree, being wounded, is given in the decoction of Coltsfoot, to those that are troubled with a cough or shortness of breath, by adding thereunto some sweet wine, and putting some saffron also therein. It is good for those that are hoarse, or have lost their voice; helps all defects of the lungs, and those that vomit and spit blood. Two drams hereof given in the juice of lemons, or of radish, is good for them that are troubled with the stone, the kernels of the stones do wonderfully ease the pains and wringings of the belly through wind or sharp humours, and help to make an excellent medicine for the stone upon all occasions, in this manner: I take fifty kernels of peach-stones, and one hundred of the kernels of cherry-stones, a handful of elder flowers fresh or dried, and three pints of Muscadel; set them in a close pot into a bed of horse-dung for ten days, after which distil in a glass with a gentle fire , and keep it for your use. You may drink upon occasion three or four ounces at a time. The milk or cream of these kernels being drawn forth with some Vervain water and applied to the forehead and temples, doth much help to procure rest and sleep to sick persons wanting it. The oil drawn from the kernels, the temples being therewith anointed, doth the like. The said oil put into clysters, eases the pains of the wind cholic: and anointed on the lower part of the belly, doth the like, and dropped into the ears, eases pains in them; the juice of the leaves doth the like. Being also anointed on the forehead and temples, it helps the megrim, and all other pains in the head. If the kernels be bruised and boiled in vinegar, until they become thick, and applied to the head, it marvellously procures the hair to grow again upon bald places, or where it is too thin.

Plum:

All plums are under Venus, and are, like women, some better, and some worse. As there is great diversity of kinds, so there is in the operation of Plums, for some that are sweet moistens the stomach, and make the belly soluble; those that are sour quench thirst more, and bind the belly; the moist and waterish do sooner corrupt in the stomach, but the firm do nourish more, and offend less. The dried fruit sold by the grocers under the names of Damask Prunes, do somewhat loosen the belly, and being stewed, are often used, both in health and sickness, to relish the mouth and stomach, to procure appetite, and a little to open the body, allay choler, and cool the stomach. Plum-tree leaves boiled in wine, are good to wash and gargle the mouth and throat, to dry the flux of rheum coming to the palate, gums, or almonds of the ear. The gum of the tree is good to break the stone. The gum or leaves boiled in vinegar, and applied, kills tetters and ringworms. Matthiolus saith, The oil preserved out of the kernels of the stones, as oil of almonds is made, is good against the inflamed piles, the tumours or swellings of ulcers, hoarseness of the voice, roughness of the tongue and throat, and likewise the pains in the ears. And that five ounces of the said oil taken with one ounce of muskadel, drives forth the stone, and helps the cholic.

Mrs. Grieves wrote of Almonds:

Fresh Sweet Almonds possess demulcent and nutrient properties, but as the outer brown skin sometimes causes irritation of the alimentary canal, they are blanched by removal of this skin when used for food. Though pleasant to the taste, their nutritive value is diminished unless well masticated, as they are difficult of digestion, and may in some cases induce nettlerash and feverishness. They have a special dietetic value, for besides containing about 20 per cent of proteids, they contain practically no starch, and are therefore often made into flour for cakes and biscuits for patients suffering from diabetes.

Sweet Almonds are used medicinally, the official preparations of the British Pharmacopoeia being Mistura Amygdalae, Pulvis Amygdalae Compositus and Almond Oil.

On expression they yield nearly half their weight in a bland fixed oil, which is employed medicinally for allaying acrid juices, softening and relaxing solids, and in bronchial diseases, in tickling coughs, hoarseness, costiveness, nephritic pains, etc.

When Almonds are pounded in water, the oil unites with the fluid, forming a milky juice - Almond Milk - a cooling, pleasant drink, which is prescribed as a diluent in acute diseases, and as a substitute for animal milk: an ounce of Almonds is sufficient for a quart of water, to which gum arabic is in most cases a useful addition. The pure oil mixed with a thick mucilage of gum arabic, forms a more permanent emulsion; one part of gum with an equal quantity of water being enough for four parts of oil. Almond emulsions possess in a certain degree the emollient qualities of the oil, and have this advantage over the pure oil, that they may be given in acute or inflammatory disorders without danger of the ill effects which the oil might sometimes produce by turning rancid. Sweet Almonds alone are employed in making emulsions, as the Bitter Almond imparts its peculiar taste when treated in this way.

Blanched and beaten into an emulsion with barley-water, Sweet Almonds are of great use in the stone, gravel, strangury and other disorders of the kidneys, bladder and biliary ducts.

By their oily character, Sweet Almonds sometimes give immediate relief in heartburn. For this, it is recommended to peel and eat six or eight Almonds.

Of Cherry:

Astringent tonic, pectoral, sedative. It has been used in the treatment of bronchitis of various types. Is valuable in catarrh, consumption nervous cough, whooping-cough, and dyspepsia.

Laurel Cherry:

Sedative, narcotic. The leaves possess qualities similar to those of hydrocyanic acid, and the water distilled from them is used for the same purpose as that medicine. Of value in coughs, whooping-cough, asthma, and in dyspepsia and indigestion.

Peach:

The fruit is wholesome and seldom disagrees if eaten ripe, though the skin is indigestible. The quantity of sugar is only small.

All Peaches have in the kernel a flavour resembling that of noyau, which depends on the presence of prussic or hydrocyanic acid. Not only the kernels, but also the young branches and flowers, after maceration in water, yield a volatile oil, which is chemically identical with that of bitter almonds, and is the cause of this flavour. Infused in white brandy, sweetened with barley sugar, Peach leaves have been said to make a fine cordial, similar to noyau, and the flowers when distilled furnish a white liquor, which communicates a flavour resembling the kernels of the fruit.

The leaves, bark, flowers and kernels have medicinal virtue. Both the leaves and bark are still employed for their curative powers. They have demulcent, sedative, diuretic and expectorant action. An infusion of 1/2 OZ. of the bark or 1 OZ. of the dried leaves to a pint of boiling water has been found almost a specific for irritation and congestion of the gastric surfaces. It is also used in whooping cough, ordinary coughs and chronic bronchitis, the dose being from a teaspoonful to a wineglassful as required.

The fresh leaves were stated by the older herbalists to possess the power of expelling worms, if applied outwardly to the body as a poultice. An infusion of the dried leaves was also recommended for the same purpose.

In Italy, at the present day, there is a popular belief that if fresh Peach leaves are applied to warts and then buried, the warts will fall off by the time the buried leaves have decayed.

A syrup and infusion of Peach flowers was formerly a preparation recognized by apothecaries, and praised by Gerard as a mildly acting efficient purgative. The syrup was considered good for children and those in weak health, and to be good against jaundice.

A tincture made from the flowers has been said to allay the pain of colic caused by gravel.

Prune:

Dried prunes are mildly laxative and are frequently employed in decoction. They form a pleasant and nourishing diet for invalids when stewed; they enter into the composition of Confection of Senna. A medicinal tincture is prepared from the fresh flower-buds of the Blackthorn. Some 20 per cent of oil is obtainable by crushing the Plum kernel - this is clear, yellow in colour and has an agreeable almond flavour and smell. It is used for alimentary purposes. The residue after pressing is used in the manufacture of a brandy, which is largely consumed in Hungary.

An Irish Herbal states of Almond:

Bitter almonds are used against all diseases of the lungs , liver and spleen and is therefore good against shortness of breath, coughs, inflammation and exulceration of the lungs. It should be taken in a sweet wine, and is also an excellent cure against the headache when it is applied to the forehead with the oil of roses and vinegar. It is said that if a man takes five or six almonds, before breaking his fast, that he will not become drunk that day.

Take 2 ounces of the oil of sweet almonds, the same quantity of fresh butter, sugar candy and clarified honey, a quarter of grated nutmeg, which mixed together and taken off a licorice stick, is an exceeding good cure for the cough.

Of Cherry:

Red Cherry. This tree bears red cherries which are of a cooling, moist nature. They purge and comfort the stomach, assuage thirst and ease the condition of the stone, gravel and epilepsy.

Black Cherry. These cherries are good for all uneasiness of the head and nerves, such as epilepsy, convulsions and paralysis. They also provoke urination and break up the stone, and in general, the distilled water of these cherries is of great use in mediceine.

Medlar:

Medlars have a cold, dry, astringent nature. When hard and green, they are very useful in stopping diarrhea. If the crushed stones of medlar are drunk in a solution, the break up the stones in the bladder.

Peach:

The leaves open the liver and spleen and aid digestion. If applied to the navels of young children, they expel worms, and if crushed and applied to wounds, they cure and heal them. The kernels are beneficial for the liver and chest, and if they are finely crushed and boiled in vinegar until they dissolve and become like a pap, they wonderfully restore the hair. The flowers are purgative and open obstructions.

Fr. Kneipp wrote of Almond Oil:

The sweet almond-oil deserves one of the first places among the oils in the apotheca. It operates on various infirmities and complaints , interior as well as exterior ones, in a softening, cooling and dissolving manner. It dissolves phlegm in the wind-pipe, or in the stomach, and in the latter case it restores appetite and digestion. In inflammations, especially in the drea-ded inflammation of the lungs, it cools. Such patients ought to take one tea- spoonful of almond oil, three or four times a day. When applied externally, this oil is of especial service to those who suffer from various diseases. The almond oil is to my knowledge the best anodyne and dissolving remedy for such complaints as humming in the ears, sharp pains in the ears, cramps in the ears, obdurate ear-wax. Pour six or eight drops into the suffering ear and stop it with cotton-wool. If your hearing is becoming difficult through cold, draught, or rheumatism, pour seven or eight drops into one ear, and on the next day pour the same quantity into the other ear each time stopping the ear with cotton- wool. After a few days you may wash the interior of the ear with hike -warm water, and you will see the result. It would be better to let a competent man syringe the ear with an ear-syringe. Tumours with great heat (inflammation) should be rubbed softly with almond-oil ; it will ease the piercing pain and cool the burning heat. The so-called, often so painful "chinks" of country people, wounds originating from sitting, lying or riding, etc., no matter on what part of the body, they may be exceedingly well treated by a soft, rubbing with sweet almond-oil.

Brother Aloysius wrote of Almond

Almond milk is particularly used for intestinal inflammation, bladder complaints, gravel, dry cough hoarseness and fever.

… the oil dissolves hardened ear wax, as well.

Of Peach:

The leaves are used medicinally. The infusion should contain ¼ to 1/3 cup per 2 cups water and is recommended for constipation; it has a mild purgative action. One should never take more than the prescribed dose; more would be dangerous and even fatal.

Resources of the Southern Fields and Forests states:

Wild Cherry: This is, undoubtedly, one of the most valuable of our indigenous plants. The bark unites with a tonic power the property of calming irritation and diminishing nervous excitability, adapted to cases where the digestive powers are impaired, and with general and local irritation existing at the same time." It is peculiarly suited to the hectic fever attending scrofula and consumption, owing to the reduction of excitability which it induces, it is supposed, by the hydrocyanic acid contained in it. Eberle states that the cold infusion had the effect of reducing his pulse from seventy-five to fifty strokes in the minute. In a case of hypertrophy with increased action of the heart, I tried the infusion of this plant, taken in large quantities, according to Dr. Eberle's plan, but without very satisfactory results. It was persisted in for three weeks; the patient, a gentleman aged twenty-five, of nervous temperament, drinking several ounces of it three times a day. The force of the circulation was at first diminished; but the abatement was not progressive; the individual was not made any worse by it. Tincture of digitalis had been likewise used with no beneficial effects. Dr. Wood speaks of the employment of the wild cherry in the general debility following inflammatory fever. It is valuable, also, in dyspepsia, attended with neuralgic symptoms. Mer. and de L. Diet, de M. Med. v, 159 ; Bull des Sci. Med. xi, 303. The bark is indicated whenever a tonic is necessary, from impairment of the constitution by syphilis, dyspepsia, pulmonary or lumbar abscess, etc. I am informed by a correspondent that he finds equal parts of this bark, rhubarb, and the gum exuding from the peach tree, (Amygdalus communis,') which like- wise affords Prussic acid, when combined with brandy and white sugar, an excellent remedy in dysentery and diarrhoea; one ounce of each is added to one pint of brandy, with a sufficient quantity of white sugar, a tablespoonful of which is taken every half hour. The sensible, as well as the medicinal properties of this plant, are impaired by boiling; cold water extracts its virtues best. The inner bark is officinal. The bark of all parts of the tree is used, but that from the root is most active. The bark is stronger, if collected from the root in autumn, and it deteriorates by keeping. It is tonic, sedative, expectorant. The officinal infusion is thus made: Bark bruised, half an ounce to one pint of cold water; macerate for twenty-four hours. Dose, two or three fluid ounces three or four times a day. To make the officinal syrup: Take of wild cherry}' bark, in coarse powder, five ounces; sugar, refined, two pounds; water sufficient to moisten the bark thoroughly. Let it stand for twenty-four hours in a close vessel; then transfer it to a percolator, and pour cold water upon it gradually until a pint of filtered liquor is obtained. To this add the sugar, in a bottle, and agitate occasionally until it is dissolved. Dose one-half fluid ounce. By Proctor's analysis, it contains starch, resin, tannin, gallic acid, fatty matter, lignin, salts of lime potassa and iron, and a volatile oil associated with hydrocyanic acid. This proved fatal to a cat in less than five minutes. See Journal Phil. Coll. Pharm. vi, 8 ; Am. Journal Pharm. x, 197. The leaves, also, are sedative and anti-spasmodic; used in coughs, angina pectoris, etc. The dose of the powdered root is from twenty grains to one drachm. The infusion is the most convenient form. A syrup is also made; beside several secret preparations. The method of making the "Cherry cordial" by the Southern matrons in the lower country of South Carolina, is as follows:

Fill the vessel with cherries, (not washed, if gathered clean,) and cover with whiskey. After several weeks pour off all the clear liquor and press the cherries through a sieve. Put into the juice thus pressed out five pints of brown sugar, and boil with syrup enough to sweeten the whole. Pour five pints of water on the thick part; boil and strain to make the syrup with the sugar. " Blackberry cordial " is made in the same way; or it can be stewed, strained, sweetened and whiskey added. In the above, the sugar is to be boiled in the water which is obtained from the thick part as directed. Plum cordial is thus made in S. C: Fill the vessel with plums after sticking each one. Pour whiskey enough to cover them. After six weeks preserve the plums in half their weight of. sugar. Put all together and shake the jug well. The common wild plum is used. The gum which exudes from the red cherry, the plum and peach, is used in place of *gum arable in increasing the brilliancy of starch and in sealing envelopes. The wood of this tree is highly valuable, being compact, fine grained and brilliant, and not liable to warp when perfectly seasoned. When chosen near the ramifications of the trunk, it rivals mahogany in the beauty of its curls. Farmer's Encyc.*

The Thomsonian System of Medicine states of Peach and Cherry

PEACH MEATS. (Dr. Thomson.)

The meats that are in the peach stones have long been used as medicine, and need but little to be said about them, except that they are of great value to strengthen the stomach and bowels, and restore the digestion; for which purpose I have made much use of them, and always to good advantage. Made into a cordial, with other articles, in the manner as directed under No. 5, it forms one of the best remedies I know of to recover the natural tone of the stomach after long sickness. A tea may be made of the leaves and bark of the peach tree and answers almost the same purpose as the peach meats. CAUTION. Do not allow the infusion to stand over eight hours, as by fermentation prussic acid will be formed and cause poisoning. It should be made fresh every time it is used. The tincture, syrup or fluid extract can be kept any length of time. The dose of the Tincture is from 30 to 60 minims.

CHERRY STONES. (Dr. Thomson.)

The meats of the Wild Cherry stones are very good, and may be used instead of the peach meats, when they cannot be had. Get the stones as clean as possible, and when well dried, pound them in a mortar, and separate the meats from the stones, which is done with little trouble ; take the same quantity as is directed of the peach meats, and it will answer equally as well. A tea made of the cherries, pounded with the stones, and steeped in hot water, sweetened with loaf sugar, to which is added a little brandy, is good to restore the digestive powers and create an appetite. Bitter almonds may be used as a substitute for the peach meats or cherry stones, when they cannot be had.

King's American Dispensatory, 1898 tells us of wild Cherry:

Action, Medical Uses, and Dosage.—Wild cherry bark has a tonic and stimulating influence on the digestive apparatus, and a simultaneous sedative action on the nervous system and circulation. It is, therefore, valuable in all those cases where it is desirable to give tone and strength to the system, without, at the same time, causing too great an action of the heart and blood vessels, as, during convalescence from pleurisy, pneumonia, acute hepatitis, and other inflammatory and febrile diseases. Its chief property is its power of relieving irritation of the mucous surfaces, making it an admirable remedy in many gastro-intestinal, pulmonic, and urinary troubles. Like lycopus, it lessens vascular excitement, though it does not control hemorrhages like that agent. It is best adapted to chronic troubles. It is also useful in hectic fever, cough, colliquative diarrhoea, some forms of irritative dyspepsia, whooping-cough, irritability of the nervous system, etc., and has been found an excellent palliative in phthisis, the syrup being employed to moderate the cough, lessen the fever, and sustain the patient's strength. It has likewise been of service in scrofula and other diseases attended with much debility and hectic fever. Wild cherry is an excellent sedative in cardiac palpitation, not due to structural wrongs. It is particularly useful in this disorder when there is nervous fever, tuberculosis, or the debility consequent upon irritative dyspepsia, anemia, chlorosis, or nervous diseases. Externally, it has been found useful, in decoction, as a wash to ill-conditioned ulcers and acute ophthalmia. Dose of the powdered bark, 1 or 2 drachms; of the infusion, 1 ounce of bark to 1 pint of cold water, and allowed to stand a few hours, from 1 to 4 fluid ounces, 4 or 5 times a day, and which is the best mode of using it; syrup of wild cherry, 1 fluid drachm. This agent may be used as a vehicle for Fowler's solution and other medicines. Specific prunus, 1 to 20 drops.

Specific Indications and Uses.—Rapid, weak circulation; continual irritative cough, with profuse muco-purulent expectoration; cardiac palpitation, from debility; dyspnoea; pyrexia; loss of appetite; and cardiac pain

Plants for A Future states:

Medicinal use of Almond: As well as being a tasty addition to the diet, almonds are also beneficial to the overall health of the body, being used especially in the treatment of kidney stones, gallstones

and constipation. Externally, the oil is applied to dry skins and is also often used as a carrier oil in aromatherapy. The seed is demulcent, emollient, laxative, nutritive and pectoral. When used medicinally, the fixed oil from the seed is normally employed. The seed contains "laetrile", a substance that has also been called vitamin B17. This has been claimed to have a positive effect in the treatment of cancer, but there does not at present seem to be much evidence to support this. The pure substance is almost harmless, but on hydrolysis it yields hydrocyanic acid, a very rapidly acting poison - it should thus be treated with caution. In small amounts this exceedingly poisonous compound stimulates respiration, improves digestion and gives a sense of well-being. The leaves are used in the treatment of diabetes. The plant contains the antitumour compound taxifolin.

Medicinal uses of Apricot: Apricot fruits are nutritious, cleansing and mildly laxative. The flowers are tonic, promoting fecundity in women. The bark is astringent. The inner bark and/or the root are used for treating poisoning caused by eating bitter almond and apricot seeds (which contain hydrogen cyanide). Another report says that a decoction of the outer bark is used to neutralize the effects of hydrogen cyanide. The decoction is also used to soothe inflamed and irritated skin conditions. The seed is analgesic, anthelmintic, antiasthmatic, antispasmodic, antitussive, demulcent, emollient, expectorant, pectoral, sedative and vulnerary. It is used in the treatment of asthma, coughs, acute or chronic bronchitis and constipation. The seed contains "laetrile", a substance that has also been called vitamin B17. This has been claimed to have a positive effect in the treatment of cancer, but there does not at present seem to be much evidence to support this. The pure substance is almost harmless, but on hydrolysis it yields hydrocyanic acid, a very rapidly acting poison - it should thus be treated with caution. In small amounts this exceedingly poisonous compound stimulates respiration, improves digestion and gives a sense of well-being.

Medicinal use of Wild Cherry: The fruit stalks are astringent, diuretic and tonic. A decoction is used in the treatment of cystitis, oedema, bronchial complaints, looseness of the bowels and anaemia. An aromatic resin can be obtained by making small incisions in the trunk. This has been used as an inhalant in the treatment of persistent coughs. Although no specific mention has been seen for this species, all members of the genus contain amygdalin and prunasin, substances which break down in water to form hydrocyanic acid (cyanide or prussic acid). In small amounts this exceedingly poisonous compound stimulates respiration, improves digestion and gives a sense of well-being.

Medicinal use of Damson: The bark of the root and branches is febrifuge and considerably styptic. An infusion of the flowers has been used as a mild purgative for children. Although no specific mention has been seen for this species, all members of the genus contain amygdalin and prunasin, substances which break down in water to form hydrocyanic acid (cyanide or prussic acid). In small amounts this exceedingly poisonous compound stimulates respiration, improves digestion and gives a sense of well-being.

Medicinal use of Peach: Antihalitosis. The leaves are astringent, demulcent, diuretic, expectorant, febrifuge, laxative, parasiticide and mildly sedative. They are used internally in the treatment of gastritis, whooping cough, coughs and bronchitis. They also help to relieve vomiting and morning sickness during pregnancy, though the dose must be carefully monitored because of their diuretic action. The dried and powdered leaves have sometimes been used to help heal sores and wounds. The leaves are harvested in June and July then dried for later use. The flowers are diuretic, sedative and vermifuge. They are used internally in the treatment of constipation and oedema. A gum from the stems is alterative, astringent, demulcent and sedative. The seed is antiasthmatic, antitussive, emollient, haemolytic, laxative and sedative. It is used internally in the treatment of constipation in the elderly, coughs, asthma and menstrual disorders. The bark is demulcent, diuretic, expectorant and sedative. It is used internally in the treatment of gastritis, whooping cough, coughs and bronchitis. The root bark is used in the treatment of dropsy and jaundice. The bark is harvested from young trees in the spring and is dried for later use. The seed contains "laetrile", a substance that has also been called vitamin B17. This has been claimed to have a positive effect in the treatment of cancer, but there does not at present seem to be much evidence to support this. The pure substance is almost harmless, but on hydrolysis it yields hydrocyanic acid, a very rapidly acting poison - it should thus be treated with caution. In small amounts this exceedingly poisonous compound stimulates respiration, improves digestion and gives a sense of well-being.

Medicinal use of Nectarine: Antihalitosis. The leaves are astringent, demulcent, diuretic, expectorant, febrifuge, laxative, parasiticide and mildly sedative. They are used internally in the treatment of gastritis, whooping cough, coughs and bronchitis. They also help to relieve vomiting and morning sickness during pregnancy, though the dose must be carefully monitored because of their diuretic action. The dried and powdered leaves have sometimes been used to help heal sores and wounds. The leaves are harvested in June and July then dried for later use. The flowers are diuretic, sedative and vermifuge. They are used internally in the treatment of constipation and oedema. A gum from the stems is alterative, astringent, demulcent and sedative. The seed is antiasthmatic, antitussive, emollient, haemolytic, laxative and sedative. It is used internally in the treatment of constipation in the elderly, coughs, asthma and menstrual disorders. The bark is demulcent, diuretic, expectorant and sedative. It is used internally in the treatment of gastritis, whooping cough, coughs and bronchitis. The root bark is used in the treatment of dropsy and jaundice. The bark is harvested from young trees in the spring and is dried for later use. The seed contains "laetrile", a substance that has also been called vitamin B17. This has been claimed to have a positive effect in the treatment of cancer, but there does not at present seem to be much evidence to support this. The pure substance is almost harmless, but on hydrolysis it yields hydrocyanic acid, a very rapidly acting poison - it should thus be treated with caution. In small amounts this exceedingly poisonous compound stimulates respiration, improves digestion and gives a sense of well-being.

Medicinal use of Sloe: The flowers, bark, leaves and fruits are aperient, astringent, depurative, diaphoretic, diuretic, febrifuge, laxative and stomachic. An infusion of the flowers is used in the treatment of diarrhoea (especially for children), bladder and kidney disorders, stomach weakness et. Although no specific mention has been seen for this species, all members of the genus contain amygdalin and prunasin, substances which break down in water to form hydrocyanic acid (cyanide or prussic acid). In small amounts this exceedingly poisonous compound stimulates respiration, improves digestion and gives a sense of well-being.

Peterson Field Guides Eastern and Central Medicinal Plants tells us:

Black or wild Cherry: aromatic inner bark traditionally used in tea or syrup for coughs, "blood tonic", fevers, colds, sore throats, diarrhea, long ailments, bronchitis, pneumonia, inflammatory fever diseases, and dyspepsia. Useful for general debility with persistent cough, poor circulation, lack of appetite; Mild sedative, expectorant. Fruits used as poor man's cherry substitute. Warning: bark, leaves and seeds contain a cyanide like glycoside, prunasin, which converts when digested to the highly toxic hydrocyanic acid. Toxins are most abundant in bark harvested in the fall.

Chokecherry: non-aromatic bark similar to that of black cherry. Externally used for wounds. Dried powdered berries once used to stimulate appetite, treat diarrhea, bloody discharge of bowels. Warning: as with black cherry, seeds, bark, and leaves may cause cyanide poisoning.

The Physicians' Desk Reference for Herbal Medicines 3rd edition states of almond:

Sweet almonds are used topically in skin care and liniments. No health hazards or side effects are known in conjunction with proper administration of design therapeutic topical doses of sweet almond. Bitter almonds were used in the past as a remedy for coughs vomiting and nausea in the form of bitter water almond water. Bitter almonds to be used only under the supervision of an expert qualified in the appropriate use of this substance. 10 bitter almonds are said to be fatal for a child, 64 an adult a fatal dosage would presumably be reached at a lower level, given advantageous conditions, E.G. Higher cyanide levels in the almonds, intensive chewing.

Of Cherry:

Wild cherry bark is an astringent, antitussive and sedative. Unproven uses: wild cherry bark is used for coughs, bronchitis and whooping cough. It is also used in the treatment of nervous digestive disorders and diarrhea. No health hazards or side effects are known in conjunction with proper administration of designated therapeutic dosages. Cyanide poisonings from the drug are unlikely, due to both its low cyanogenic glycoside content and the lack of inclination to digest it.

Ptelea, Hoptree

Three varieties of Ptelea have been found useful in Herbal Medicine: Ptelea baldwinii, Ptelea trifoliata - Hop Tree, Ptelea trifoliata mollis - Hop Tree

Of these tree type members of the Rue family, only one is native to my region, Ptelea trifoliata (Hoptree)

It is said that the fruit of this tree may be used in place of Hops in the bittering and preservation of beer, hence the name. Hop Tree was known to the ancient Greek herbalists. Dioscorides wrote:

The leaves, branches and bark of ptelea are all astringent. The leaves, pounded into small pieces with vinegar and so applied, are good for leprosy and heal wounds; but especially the bark, if it is wrapped around like a bandage, for it is flexible like a girdle. A measure of the thicker bark (taken in a drink with wine or cold water) expels phlegm. A decoction of the leaves or bark of the roots, applied with hot cloths, consolidates by drawing a callum [hard skin] over the fracture of a bone sooner. The moisture which is found in the bladders [undeveloped fruit] at their first sprouting clears the face when rubbed on it. The same moisture, dried, is formed into little creatures like gnats. The newly emerged leaves are used for sauce like vegetables.

Resources of the Southern Fields and Forests states:

HOP TREE, (Ptelea trifoliata, L.) Fla. and northward. Chap. N. C. A small genus of shrubs peculiar to America and India. This species is said by Schoepf, Mat. Med. Am., to be anthelmintic, a string infusion of the leaves and young shoots being used. The fruit is aromatic and bitter, and is stated to be a good substitute for hops.

King's American Dispensatory, 1898 tells us:

Action, Medical Uses, and Dosage.—Ptelea is tonic, and surpassed in this line only by hydrastis. Used after intermittent fevers, remittent fevers, and all cases of debility where tonics are indicated. Said also to be anthelmintic. Equal parts of ptelea and Euonymus atropurpureus, have been found very useful in pulmonary affections. A tincture of ptelea, made in whiskey, is reputed to have cured several cases of asthma, and is said to cause, in many instances where it has been used, a troublesome external erysipelatous inflammation, either general or local, but which, if the use of the tincture be persisted in, finally disappears, and the patient becomes, at the same time, permanently cured of the disease for which he was treated. This would certainly indicate other valuable properties in this plant, than those with which we are acquainted, which deserve a further and thorough investigation. Prof. I. G. Jones stated that this bark is a pure, unirritating tonic, having rather a soothing influence when applied to irritated mucous membranes. He has employed it advantageously in convalescence after fevers, and in debility connected with gastro-enteric irritation. It promotes the appetite, enables the stomach to endure suitable nourishment, favors the early reestablishment of digestion, and will be tolerated by the stomach when other tonics are rejected. He employed it in cold infusion, of which ½ fluid ounce may be given every 2, 3, or 4 hours, according to circumstances. It is also said to cure intermittent fever, and is considered by some to be equal to quinine. It may be used in powder, tincture, or extract. Dose of the powder, 10 to 30 grains, 3 or 4 times a day; of the tincture, 1 or 2 fluid drachms; of the extract, 5 to 10 grains; specific ptelea, 1 to 20 drops.

Specific Indications and Uses.—Asthmatic breathing; chronic diseases, with sense of constriction in the chest, and short breathing.

According to Plants for A Future:

Medicinal use of Hop Tree: The root-bark is anthelmintic, antibacterial, antiperiodic, stomachic and tonic. It has been mixed with other medicines in order to give added potency. It has a soothing influence on the mucous membranes and promotes the appetite, being tolerated when other tonics cannot be retained. It is also taken in the treatment of intermittent fevers such as malaria, heartburn, roundworms, pinworms and poor digestion. Externally it is applied to wounds. The roots are harvested in the autumn, the bark peeled off and dried for later use. The roots are a tonic, used in the treatment of asthmatic breathing, fevers, poor appetite etc. The leaves are said to be useful in the treatment of wounds and also in the destruction of intestinal worms.

Peterson Field Guides Eastern and Central Medicinal Plants tells us:

American Indians added root to strengthen other medicine. Historically used by physicians as a tonic (surpassed only by golden seal) for asthmatic breathing, fevers, poor appetite, gastroenteritis, irritated mucous membranes. A tea of the young leaves and shoots was once considered useful as a warm experiment. The bitter slightly aromatic fruits were once thought to be a useful substitute to hops in the manufacturer beer.

Pyrus, Pear

Two Pear trees have been naturalized in my region, Pyrus calleryana (Callery Pear, Bradford Pear) and Pyrus communis (Common Pear)

Dioscorides wrote of Pear:

There are many kinds of pears and they are all astringent and therefore fit to put into repellent poultices. A decoction of the dried ones (or if they are taken raw) stops discharges of the intestines, but if they are eaten they hurt those who eat them while fasting.

Achras is a kind of wild pear which takes long to ripen. It is more astringent than the pear, as a result it is good for the same purposes. The leaves of it are also astringent. Ash from the wood effectively helps those suffocated from eating mushrooms [antidote]. There are some who say that if anyone boils wild pears together with mushrooms they become harmless.

Saint Hildegard von Bingen wrote:

The pear tree is more cold than hot and is powerful and strong. It is to the apple tree as the liver is to the lungs. For, just as the liver, it is stronger and more useful, and indeed more harmful, than the apple....

The fruit of the tree is powerful heavy and harsh. If someone eats too much when it is raw, it gives his head a migraine and makes vapor in his chest. The lungs draw in the pear sap, which hardens like lead slag and tartar around the liver and the lungs, creating great infirmities in those organs. Just as a person is sometimes filled with the odor of wine, so also his breath mixes with the sap of the pear and takes its sharpness. Whence, after eating the raw pear, he will have difficulty drawing breath. Many infirmities come into the chest from this, since pears grow from dew at the close o day when dew's power is weak. Unless they are cooked, pears create noxious humours in people, since they grow when the dew is flagging.

Anyone who wishes to eat pears should place them in water or roast them on a fire. Boiled pears are better than those roasted, since the warm water gradually cooks out the harmful sap which is in them. Fire is too quick and in roasting not all the moisture is expressed from them. Cooked pears sometimes oppress the one who eats them, since they seek out any rotten matter in him and diminish it, breaking it up,. Nevertheless, they give him good digestion since they remove the rotten matter. The fruits are easily digested and do not bring in rotten matter with them. Take pears, cut them, and throw out their cores. Cook them vigorously in water. Then take hog's fennel and a little less galingale, licorice (less than galingale) and savory (less than licorice). If you do not have hog's fennel, take fennel root and reduce it to a powder. Mix it with the other powders and put them in a bit of warm honey. Add the prepared pears, mix this well, and place it in a small container. Every day eat one small spoonful before breakfast; eat two spoonfuls with a meal; eat three spoonfuls at night, in bed. This electuary is very good, and more precious than gold, since it carries away migraine and diminishes vapor which raw pear creates in a person's chest. It consumes all bad humours in a person, and so cleanses the person, just as a vessel is washed of its impurities.

Gerard had similar concerns about uncooked pears, centuries after Saint Hildegard:

A. Leaving the divers and sundry surnames of pears, let us come to the faculties which the physicians ought to know; which also vary according to the differences of their uses: for some pears are sweet, divers fat and unctuous, others sour, and most are harsh, especially the wild pears, and some consist of divers mixtures of tastes, and some having no taste at all, but as it were a waterish taste.

B. All pears are cold, and all have a binding quality and an earthy substance: but the choke pears and those that are harsh be more earthy, and the sweet ones less: which substance is so full of superfluous moisture in some, as that they cannot be eaten raw. All manner of pears do bind and stop the belly, especially the choke and harsh ones, which are good to be eaten of those that have the lask and the bloody flux.

C. The harsh and austere pears may with good success be laid upon hot swellings in the beginning, as may be the leaves of the tree, which do both bind and cool.

D. Wine made of the juice of pears called in English, perry, is soluble, purgeth those that are not accustomed to drink thereof, especially when it is new; notwithstanding it is as wholesome a drink being taken in small quantity as wine; it comforteth and warmeth the stomach, and causeth good digestion.

Culpepper wrote of Pear:

The tree belongs to Venus, and so doth the apple-tree. For their physical use they are best discerned by their taste. All the sweet and luscious sorts, whether manured or wild, do help to move the belly downwards, more or less. Those that are hard and sour, do, on the contrary, bind the belly as much, and the leaves do so also. Those that are moist do in some sort cool, but harsh or wild sorts much more, and are very good in repelling medicines; and if the wild sort be boiled with mushrooms, it makes them less dangerous. The said Pears boiled with a little honey, help much the oppressed stomach, as all sorts of them do, some more, some less: but the harsher sorts do more cool and bind, serving well to be bound to green wounds, to cool and stay the blood, and heal up the green wound without farther trouble, or inflammation, as Galen saith he hath found by experience. The wild Pears do sooner close up the lips of green wounds than others.

Schola Selerni advises to drink much wine after Pears, or else (say they) they are as bad as poison; nay, and they curse the tree for it too; but if a poor man find his stomach oppressed by eating Pears, it is but working hard, and it will do as well as drinking wine.

An Irish Herbal States:

Pears stop the diarrhea, and can also be applied to fresh, green wounds which they heal.

Quercus, Oak

Sixty-nine varieties of Oak can been found useful in Herbal Medicine: Quercus acuta - Japanese Evergreen Oak, Quercus acutissima - Sawthorn Oak, Quercus agrifolia – Encina, Quercus alba - White Oak, Quercus aliena - Oriental White Oak, Quercus aucheri - Boz-Pirnal Oak, Quercus bicolor - Swamp White Oak, Quercus cerris - Turkey Oak, Quercus coccifera - Kermes Oak, Quercus coccinea - Scarlet Oak, Quercus dentata - Japanese Emperor Oak, Quercus douglasii - Blue Oak, Quercus dumosa revoluta - California Scrub Oak, Quercus ellipsoidalis - Northern Pin Oak, Quercus emoryi - Black Oak, Quercus engelmannii - Evergreen Oak, Quercus falcata - Southern Red Oak, Quercus floribunda, Quercus frainetto - Hungarian Oak, Quercus fruticose, Quercus gambelii - Shin Oak, Quercus garryana - Oregon White Oak, Quercus glauca, Quercus hispanica, Quercus chrysolepis - Live Oak, Quercus ilex - Holly Oak, Quercus ilex ballota - Holm Oak, Quercus imbricaria - Shingle Oak, Quercus infectoria - Aleppo Oak, Quercus ithaburensis macrolepis - Valonia Oak, Quercus kelloggii - Californian Black Oak, Quercus laevis - American Turkey Oak, Quercus lamellosa - Bull Oak, Quercus leucotrichophora, Quercus libani - Lebanon Oak, Quercus lineata, Quercus lobata - Californian White Oak, Quercus lyrata - Overcup Oak, Quercus macrocarpa - Burr Oak, Quercus marilandica - Blackjack Oak, Quercus michauxii - Swamp Chestnut Oak, Quercus mongolica, Quercus mongolica grosseserrata, Quercus muehlenbergii - Yellow Chestnut Oak, Quercus myrsinaefolia, Quercus nigra - Water Oak, Quercus oblongifolia - Mexican Blue Oak, Quercus palustris - Pin Oak, Quercus petraea - Sessile Oak, Quercus phellos - Willow Oak, Quercus phillyreoides, Quercus prinoides - Dwarf Chinkapin Oak, Quercus prinus - Rock Chestnut Oak, Quercus pubescens - Downy Oak, Quercus pungens - Sandpaper Oak, Quercus robur - Pedunculate Oak, Quercus rubra - Red Oak, Quercus semecarpifolia, Quercus serrata, Quercus shumardii - Shumard Oak, Quercus stellata - Post Oak, Quercus suber - Cork Oak, Quercus suber occidentalis - Cork Oak, Quercus undulata - Wavyleaf Oak, Quercus variabilis - Chinese Cork Oak, Quercus velutina - Black Oak, Quercus virginiana - Live Oak, Quercus wislizenii - Live Oak, Quercus x bebbiana

A great many oaks are native to my region and are one of the main reasons that North Carolina was called "The Cradle of Forestry In America". Only the Magnolia rivals the Live Oak as emblematic of the American South, the famous "Angel Oak" being a magnificent example. Native to my region are: Quercus alba (White Oak), Quercus austrina (Bluff Oak), Quercus bicolor (Swamp White Oak), Quercus coccinea (Scarlet Oak), Quercus falcata (Southern Red Oak, Spanish Oak), Quercus geminata (Sand Live Oak), Quercus georgiana (Georgia Oak), Quercus hemisphaerica (Sand Laurel Oak, Darlington Oak), Quercus imbricaria (Shingle Oak), Quercus incana (Bluejack Oak), Quercus laevis (Turkey Oak), Quercus laurifolia (Laurel Oak), Quercus lyrata (Overcup Oak), Quercus margaretta (Sand Post Oak), Quercus marilandica var. marilandica (Blackjack Oak), Quercus michauxii (Swamp Chestnut Oak), Quercus montana (Chestnut Oak), Quercus muehlenbergii (Chinkapin Oak), Quercus nigra (Water Oak), Quercus pagoda (Cherrybark Oak), Quercus palustris (Pin Oak), Quercus phellos (Willow Oak), Quercus prinoides (Dwarf Chinkapin Oak), Quercus rubra var. ambigua (Northern Red Oak), Quercus rubra var. rubra (Northern Red Oak), Quercus shumardii (Shumard Oak), Quercus stellata (Post Oak), Quercus velutina (Black Oak), Quercus virginiana (Live Oak). Two oaks have been naturalized here, Quercus acutissima (Sawtooth Oak) and Quercus variabilis (Chinese Cork Oak)

Dioscorides wrote of Oak:

Each part of the oak is astringent, but the film which lies between the bark and the stock (similar to that under the cup of the acorn) is most therapeutic for the bowels. A decoction of this is given for coeliac [intestinal complaints], dysentery, and to blood-spitters, and pounded into small pieces it is put into suppositories for women troubled with excessive discharges of the womb.

Acorns ...are also diuretic. Eaten as meat they cause headaches and are wind-inducing, but also help poisonous bites. A decoction of them and their bark (taken as a drink with cows' milk) helps poisoning. The unripe ones pounded into small pieces and applied as a poultice relieve inflammation. With salted swines' grease they are good for malignant calluses and injurious ulcers. Those of the ilex [holly oak — Quercus ilex] have greater strength than those of the oak.

Cecides [oak gall] is a fruit of the oak, of which some is called omphacitis. It is little, knobby, heavy and without a hole. Some is smooth and light and has a hole in it, but the omphacitis ought to be chosen as it is the most effective. Either of them is strongly astringent. Pounded into small pieces they stop abnormal growths of the flesh, and stop discharges of the gums and the middle ear, as well as ulcers of the mouth. That which is in the middle of them put into the cavities of teeth eases the pain. Laid on hot coals until they are set on fire and quenched with wine, vinegar, or brine made with vinegar they are able to staunch blood. A decoction of them is good in hip baths for a prolapsed uterus and for discharges. They make the hair black steeped in vinegar or water. They are good for coeliac [intestinal complaints] and dysentery pounded into small pieces and rubbed on, or taken as a drink with wine or water, and also mixed with sauce, or first boiled whole in water (with which you must boil something else too, of things that are good for people). Generally where there is need of an astringent, or to stop or dry, you ought to make use of them.

Gerard wrote of Oak:

A. The leaves, bark, acorn cups, and the acorns themselves, do mightily bind and dry in the third degree, being somewhat cold withal.

B. The best of them, saith Galen, is the thin skin which is under the bark of the tree, and that next, which lieth nearest to the pulp, or inner substance of the acorn; all these stay the whites, the reds, spitting of blood and lasks: the decoction of these is given, or the powder of them dried, for the purposes aforesaid.

C. Acorns if they be eaten are hardly concocted, they yield no nourishment to man's body, but that which is gross, raw, and cold.

D. Swine are fatted herewith, and by feeding hereon have their flesh hard and sound.

E. The acorns provoke urine, and are good against all venom and poison, but they are not of such a stopping and binding faculty as the leaves and barke.

F. The Oak apples are good against all fluxes of blood and lasks, in what manner soever they be taken, but the best way is to boil them in red wine, and being so prepared, they are good also against the excessive moisture and swelling of the jaws and almonds or kernels of the throat.

G. The decoction of Oak apples stayeth women's diseases, and causeth the mother that is fallen down to return again to the natural place, if they do sit over the said decoction being very hot.

H. The same steeped in strong white wine vinegar, with a little powder of brimstone, and the root of Ireos mingled together, and set in the sun by the space of a month, maketh the hair black, consumeth proud and superfluous flesh, taketh away sun-burning, freckles, spots, the morphew, with all deformities of the face, being washed therewith.

I. The Oak Apples being broken in sunder about the time of their withering, do foreshew the sequel of the year, as the expert Kentish husbandmen have observed by the living things found in them: as if they find an ant, they foretell plenty of grain to ensue: if a white worm like a gentle or maggot, then they prognosticate murrain of beats and cattle; if a spider, then (say they) we shall have a pestilence or some such like sickness to follow amongst men: these things the learned also have observed and noted; for Matthiolus writing upon Dioscorides saith, that before they have an hole through them, they contain in them either a fly, a spider, or a worm: if a fly, then war insueth, if a creeping worm, then scarcity of victuals, if a running spider, then followeth great sickness or mortality.

Culpepper wrote:

It is so well known (the timber thereof being the glory and safety of this nation by sea) that it needs no description. Jupiter owns the tree. The leaves and bark of the Oak, and the acorn cups, do bind and dry very much. The inner bark of the tree, and the thin skin that covers the acorn, are most used to stay the spitting of blood, and the bloody-flux. The decoction of that bark, and the powder of the cups, do stay vomitings, spitting of blood, bleeding at the mouth, or other fluxes of blood, in men or women; lasks also, and the nocturnal involuntary flux of men. The acorn in powder taken in wine, provokes urine, and resists the poison of venomous creatures. The decoction of acorns and the bark made in milk and taken, resists the force of poisonous herbs and medicines, as also the virulency of cantharides, when one by eating them hath his bladder exulcerated, and voids bloody urine. Hippocrates saith, he used the fumes of Oak leaves to women that were troubled with the strangling of the mother; and Galen applied them, being bruised, to cure green wounds. The distilled water of the Oaken bud, before they break out into leaves is good to be used either inwardly or outwardly, to assuage inflammations, and to stop all manner of fluxes in man or woman. The same is singularly good in pestilential and hot burning fevers; for it resists the force of the infection, and allays the heat. It cools the heat of the liver, breaking the stone in the kidneys, and stays women's courses. The decoction of the leaves works the same effects. The water that is found in the hollow places of old Oaks, is very effectual against any foul or spreading scabs. The distilled water (or concoction, which is better) of the leaves, is one of the best remedies that I know of for the whites in women.

Mrs. Grieve included interesting historical bacgkround in her writings on Oak:

The Oak is noted for the slowness of its growth, as well as for the large size to which it attains. In eighty years the trunk is said not to exceed 20 inches in diameter, but old trees reach a great girth. The famous Fairlop Oak in Hainault Forest measured 36 feet in girth, the spreading boughs extending above 300 feet in circumference. The Newland Oak in Gloucestershire measures 46 feet 4 inches at 1 foot from the ground, and is one of the largest and oldest in the kingdom, these measurements being exceeded, however, by those of the Courthorpe Oak in Yorkshire, which Hooker reports as attaining the extraordinary girth of 70 feet. King Arthur's Round Table was made from a single slice of oak, cut from an enormous bole, and is still shown at Winchester.

Humboldt refers to an oak in the Département de la Charente-Inférieure measuring nearly 90 feet in circumference near the base; near Breslau an oak fell in 1857 measuring 66 feet in circumference at the base. These large trees are for the most part decayed and hollow in the interior, and their age has been estimated at from one to two thousand years.

The famous Oak of Mamre, Abram's Oak, was illustrated formerly in the Transactions of the Linnean Society, by Dr. Hooker. It is a fine specimen of the species Q. Coccifera, the prickly evergreen or Kermes Oak, a native of the countries bordering on the Mediterranean; the insect (coccus) from which it derives its name yielding the dye known as 'Turkey red.' Abram's Oak is 22 feet in circumference; it is popularly supposed to represent the spot where the tree grew under which Abraham pitched his tent. There is a superstition that any person who cuts or maims this oak will lose his firstborn son.

The oak of Libbeiya in the Lebanon measures 37 feet in girth, and its branches cover an area whose circumference measured over 90 yards. The Arab name is Sindian.

The Greeks held the Oak sacred, the Romans dedicated it to Jupiter, and the Druids venerated it.

In England the name Gospel Oak is still retained in many counties, relating to the time when Psalms and Gospel truths were uttered beneath their shade. They were notable objects as resting-places in the 'beating of the parish bounds,' a practice supposed to have been derived from the feast to the god Terminus.

The following is a quotation from Withers:

'That every man might keep his own possessions,

Our fathers used, in reverent processions,

With zealous prayers, and with praiseful cheere,

To walk their parish limits once a year;

And well-known marks (which sacrilegious hands

Now cut or breake) so bordered out their lands,

That every one distinctly knew his owne,

And brawles now rife were then unknowne.'

The ceremony was performed by the clergyman and his parishioners going the boundaries of the parish and choosing the most remarkable sites (oak-trees being specially selected) to read passages from the Gospels, and ask blessings for the people.

'Dearest, bury me

Under that holy oke, or Gospel Tree;

Where, though thou see'st not, thou may'st think upon

Me, when you yearly go'st Procession.'

-----HERRICK

Many of these Gospel trees are still alive five in different parts of England.

An old proverb relating to the oak is still a form of speculation on the weather in many country districts.

'If the Oak's before the Ash,

Then you'll only get a splash;

If the Ash before the Oak,

Then you may expect a soak.'

The technical name of the Oak is said to be derived from the Celtic quer (fine) and cuez (tree).

A curious custom in connexion with wearing an oak-leaf (or preferably an oak-apple) on May 29, still exists in some villages in South Wilts. Each one has the right to collect fallen branches in a certain large wood in the district. To claim this privilege each villager has to bring them home shouting 'Grovely, Grovely, and all Grovely!' (this being the name of the large wood).

After the Oak has passed its century, it increases by less than an inch a year, but the wood matured in this leisurely fashion is practically indestructible. Edward the Confessor's shrine in Westminster Abbey is of oak that has outlasted the changes of 800 years. Logs have been dug from peat bogs, in good preservation and fit for rough building purposes, that were submerged a thousand years ago. In the Severn, breakwaters are still used as casual landing-places, where piles of oak are said to have been driven by the Romans.

Medicinal Action and Uses---The astringent effects of the Oak were well known to the Ancients, by whom different parts of the tree were used, but it is the bark which is now employed in medicine. Its action is slightly tonic, strongly astringent and antiseptic. It has a strong astringent bitter taste, and its qualities are extracted both by water and spirit. The odour is slightly aromatic.

Like other astringents, it has been recommended in agues and haemorrhages, and is a good substitute for Quinine in intermittent fever, especially when given with Chamomile flowers.

It is useful in chronic diarrhoea and dysentery, either alone or in conjunction with aromatics. A decoction is made from 1 OZ. of bark in a quart of water, boiled down to a pint and taken in wineglassful doses. Externally, this decoction has been advantageously employed as a gargle in chronic sore throat with relaxed uvula, and also as a fomentation. It is also serviceable as an injection for leucorrhoea, and applied locally to bleeding gums and piles.

An Irish Herbal states:

All parts of oak have a binding nature, and are therefor useful against diarrhea, dysentery, hemorrhages and flows of all kinds. The bark can be used in gargles for dropped uvula.

Fr. Kneipp wrote of Oak Bark:

Bark of oak.

Are we then to use even the bark of oak as a medicine? Certainly, be it fresh from the tree, or dried. Young bark of oak, boil- ed for about half an hour, gives a sanative decoction.

A small towel is dipped into it and tied as a bandage round the neck; such bandages give great help to people afflicted with thick throats, and even with a wen on the' throat, if it has not yet grown too large and firm, this decoction operates as a most effective and harmless remedy. Complaints of the glands are removed just as thoroughly by these bandages.

Whoever is troubled with prolapses of the rectum, may often take sitting baths with a decoction of oak-bark, and also from time to time an enema of a diluted decoction. The troublesome and often dangerous fistules on the rectum are dissolved and healed by the decoction.

Also hard tumours, if they are not inflamed, may be treated and dissolved in the same way.

Tea made of oak -bark operates like resin in a strengthening way on the inner vessels.

Brother Aloysius wrote of Oak:

The acorns, together with the bark and the leaves, are used medicinally. The acorns are gathered in autumn, burned and ground into a powder; when steeped in boiling water to make acorn coffee, they are highly recommended for scrofula and many indispositions which stem from it, such as diarrhea and abdominal swelling, anemia and leukorrhea. Use one sugarspoon powdered acorn in a cup of water.

The bark can be removed from two or three year old branches. It has no smell, but a very astringent taste, and is used externally in the form of compresses, baths, washes, syringes, gargles etc. For a gargle, take 2 to 4 teaspoons bark per 2 cups water; for compresses 2/3 to 1 cup of leaves or bark per 2 cups water. Internally, 1 to 2 teaspoons of powdered bark should be taken in syrup, honey, etc, to control heavy menstrual bleeding, blood spitting and blood in the stools. The bark is also used externally, in the form of a compress for lupus, soft, rotten ulcers, sores, etc.

An excellent remedy for leukorrhea is to boil a handful of oak bark for 15 minutes in 4 cups water, strain and syringe with this quantity every evening.

Frink 1 cup of oak bark teak daily for blood-spitting, heavy bleeding, painful bleeding, urinary incontinence, chronic dysentery and excessive mucus.

Jolanta Wittib writes of Oak:

Oak bark is my strongest anti-inflammatory, antiseptic home medicine. I always have oak bark at home, but, thank God, I very seldom need it. I collect oak bark in the same way as I collect willow bark and keep it dried in a jar. I would use oak bark decoction externally for washing the wounds which do not heal properly, or for very strong perspiration of the feet, although, after what I have read in this book, I might never "heal" sweaty feet. As sweat bodies detoxify themselves, so why hem this process?

I might use oak bark decoction for a very severe diarrhea, but, so far, I have not done that, as I have never had one. Well, it is very important to know the reason for diarrhea, especially when it is severe, thus consulting a doctor is always useful.

I use oak leaves in my recipe for fermented cucumbers. I add a leaf per jar before I finally close it for storing so that cucumbers keep firm, crispy and crunchy.

People still remember times when they used roasted acorns for food. I will definitely try out one of the old recipes. I am sure that there is enormous power in the seeds of such a powerful tree.

Herbal Remedies of the Lumbee Indians tells us of Red Oak:

A handful of red oak bark was boiled until the water became deep red. This wash was used by Lumbee healers to rub on the skin affected by poison oak. The Lumbee also used the red oak in an external was to bathe or aid the treatment of chills and fevers. A tea made from the red oak was used by many Lumbee healers to aid the system, especially after long fevers. The bark was also used as an astringent, a tonic and as an antiseptic. The tea was also drank to serve as an emetic, and to treat indigestion, chronic dysentery, asthma and debility of the system. The bark was used externally and applied to sore, chapped skin.

Resources of the Southern Fields and Forests states:

Black Oak: The bark, a powerful and valuable astringent, is also possessed of purgative properties, in which respect it has an advantage not met with in the Q. falcata. They have both been efficacious in leucorrhoea, amenorrhoea, chronic hysteria, diarrhoea, rheumatism, pulmonary consumption, tabes mesenterica, cynanche tonsillaris and asthma. Oak-balls produced by these are also powerful astringents, and are employed in many cases requiring such remedies—as in diarrhoea, dysentery and hemorrhage; also, in mild cases of intermittent fever. The dose of the powder is forty grains. The powder of this, or of the bark, mixed with hog's lard, is a very simple and effectual remedy in painful hemorrhoids and a decoction is serviceable as a fomentation for prolapsus uteri and ani, and for defluctions from those parts. According to Dr. Cullen, it is applicable in relaxations or impaired conditions of the mucous membranes, on account of its tonic, constringing effect, and as a gargle in inflammation of the fauces, prolapsus uvulae, etc. Mr. Lizars has used it with " wonderful success " in the cure of reducible hernia. It is applied topically in mortification, and to ill-conditioned ulcers. Marasmic and scrofulous children are bathed with great advantage in a bath made of the bark. Although this species acts slightly on the bowels, it contains more tannin and gallic acid than the Q. alba and Q. falcata; hence it is better suited to cases requiring an external astringent.

White Oak: The bark is officinal, and is generally used in similar cases with the above, with the exceptions before mentioned. By some it is preferred to the others on account of its not acting on the bowels. The decoction is sometimes employed as an injection in leucorrhoea and gonorrhoea. The bark contains tannin, gallic acid, and bitter extractive, the former predominating. The bark is officinal, the young bark being preferable. The whiter bark, and the delicate and finely lobed leaves, with the general neat appearance of the tree, serve to distinguish this from the other varieties of the oak, than which it is more acceptable to the stomach. All, however, are valuable for external application. It is astringent and somewhat tonic. Powder: dose, from one-half drachm to one drachm. Extract: dose, half that of the powder. Decoction: bark bruised, one ounce; water, three half-pints ; boil to one pint. Dose, one wineglassful. Surg. McLauglin and others of Lynchburg, re- port through the Surgeon-General's office C. S. A. a favorable notice of the decoctions and syrups of the Quercus alba and Hubiis villosus in chronic diarrhoea, stating that the tinctures of R. V. and of Ooniiis Florida make an excellent astringent tonic.

King's American Dispensatory, 1898 tells us:

Action, Medical Uses, and Dosage.—Oak bark is slightly tonic, powerfully astringent, and antiseptic. It is useful, internally in chronic diarrhoea, chronic mucous discharges, passive hemorrhages, and wherever an internal astringent is required. In colliquative sweats, the decoction is usually combined with lime-water. It is, however, more generally used in decoction, as an external agent, which forms an excellent gargle for relaxed uvula and sore throat, a good stimulating astringent lotion for ulcers with spongy granulations, and an astringent injection for leucorrhoea, prolapsus ani, hemorrhoids, etc. The ground bark, made into a *poultice, has proved useful in gangrenous or mortified conditions. In sickly, debilitated children, and in severe diarrhoeas, especially when the result of fevers, the decoction, given internally, and used as a bath to the body and limbs, 2 or 3 times a day, will be found very efficient. When given for diarrhoea or dysentery, it should be combined with aromatics, and sometimes with castor oil. A bath is often advantageous in some cutaneous diseases. The green bark of elder and white oak bruised together, or in strong decoction, forms a very useful and valuable application to abrasions. Dose of the decoction, 1 to 2 fluid ounces; of the extract, from 5 to 20 grains. A coffee made from roasted acorns, has been highly recommended in the treatment of scrofula.*

Specific Indications and Uses.—Relaxation of mucous membranes, with unhealthy discharge; ulcerations, with spongy granulations.

Plants for A Future lists the medical uses of the oaks similarly, but states of White Oak:

White oak was often used medicinally by several native North American Indian tribes, who valued it especially for its antiseptic and astringent properties and used it in the treatment of many complaints. It is little, if at all, used in modern herbalism. The inner bark contains 6 - 11% tannin, it has powerful antiseptic and astringent properties and is also expectorant and tonic. The bark is boiled and the liquid drunk in the treatment of bleeding piles and diarrhoea, intermittent fevers, coughs and colds, consumption, asthma, lost voice etc. The bark has been chewed as a treatment for mouth sores. Externally, it is used as a wash for skin eruptions, burns, rashes, bruises, ulcers etc and as a vaginal douche. It has also been used as a wash for muscular pains. The bark is best collected in the spring. Any galls produced on the tree are strongly astringent and can be used in the treatment of haemorrhages, chronic diarrhoea, dysentery etc.

Peterson Field Guides Eastern and Central Medicinal Plants tells us of white oak:

Astringent inner bark tea once used for chronic diarrhea, dysentery, chronic mucus discharge, bleeding, anal prolapse, piles; As a gargle for sore throats and a wash for skin eruptions, Poison Ivy rash, burns, hemostatic. Folk cancer remedy. Contains tannins. Experimentally, tannic acid is antiviral, antiseptic, anti-tumor and carcinogenic. Warning: tannic acid is potentially toxic

Botany In a Day states:

Medicinally, the oaks are astringent throughout, due to the tanning. The bark also contains quercin, a compound similar to salicin (like aspirin). The astringency is used internally for gum inflammations, sore throat and diarrhea. Externally it is used for first and second degree burns. The tannin binds to proteins and amino acids, sealing off the burns from weeping and from bacterial infections. The leaves can be chewed into a mash and use for an astringent poultice. Oak galls also have a high tannin content, as much as 60 to 70% in the galls.

The Physicians" Desk Reference for Herbal Medicine tells us:

Indications and usage approved by Commission E: cough-bronchitis, diarrhea, inflammation of the mouth and pharynx, inflammation of the skin. Oak is used internally for nonspecific diarrhea. In smaller doses is used to the stomach tonic. The drug is used externally for inflammatory skin diseases and inflammation of the mouth and throat. Unproven uses: in folk medicine, oak is used for inflammation of the genital and anal area, suppurating eczema, hyperhidrosis, interigo, an as an adjutant treatment of chilblains. Oak is also used in folk medicine internally for hemorrhagic stool, non-menstrual uterine bleeding, hemoptysis, and chronic inflammation of the gastrointestinal tract. External uses include hemorrhoid bleeding, varicose veins, uterine bleeding, vaginal discharge, rashes, chronic itching, scaly and suppurating eczema, and eye inflammations.

Oak gall: the astringent quality of the drug can be explained by the tannins it contains. The dry extract, exhibits analgetic, hypoglycemic, and sedative-hypnotic efficacy. Unproven uses external use includes treatment of inflammation of the skin and frostbite and as an adjuvant in the treatment of infectious skin conditions. Oak gall is used externally for chilblains and gingivitis, for which efficacy appears plausible but is not yet been sufficiently documented.

Rhododendron

Although Rhododendrons have varying levels of toxicity, eighteen varieties have been found useful in Herbal Medicine: Rhododendron anthopogon, Rhododendron arboretum, Rhododendron aureum – Rosebay, Rhododendron campanulatum, Rhododendron ferrugineum – Alpenrose, Rhododendron griersonianum, Rhododendron indicum - Rhododendron,, Rhododendron japonicum, Rhododendron kaempferi, Rhododendron lapponicum - Lapland Rosebay, Rhododendron lutescens, Rhododendron luteum - Honeysuckle Azalea, Rhododendron maximum - Rosebay Rhododendron, Rhododendron molle - Chinese Azalea, Rhododendron mucronulatum, Rhododendron 'PJM', Rhododendron ponticum – Rhododendron, Rhododendron x praecox

The beautiful flowers of the Rhododendron draw nearly as many visitors to my region of Appalachia as do the colors of the fall hardwood leaves. We have two native Rhododendron, Rhododendron catawbiense (Catawba Rhododendron) and Rhododendron maximum (Rosebay Rhododendron, Great Laurel)

Resources of the Southern Fields and Forests states:

MOUNTAIN LAUREL; WILD ROSEBAY, (Rhododendron maximum, L.) Grows among the mountains. Fl. July. Lind. Nat. Syst. Bot. 221. " It is well known to be possessed of poisonous properties." Mer. and de L. Diet, de M. Med. vi, 75 Employed with success in chronic rheumatism, gout, and glandular enlargements. The petioles act as a sternutatory. Coxe, Am. Disp. 526 ; Big. Am. Med. Bot. iii, 103. It is a resinous astringent, the leaves containing tannin ; but its supposed poisonous, narcotic power is doubted by some, as Bigelow swallowed an entire leaf, and no bad effects resulted. B. S. Barton, however, in his Collections, i, 18, says it is certainly poisonous. The brown powder attached to the foot-stalks possesses considerable power as an errhine. The purple variety, one of the most beautiful, grows in South Carolina.

King's American Dispensatory, 1898 tells us:

Action, Medical Uses, and Dosage.—Yellow rhododendron contains a stimulant, narcotic principle; for it increases the heat of

the body, excites thirst, and produces diaphoresis, or an increased discharge of the other secretions or excretions, and which are generally followed by a decrease of action of the arterial system. With some persons it causes emeto-catharsis, inebriation, and delirium. The Siberians use a decoction of it in chronic rheumatism and gout. They put about 2 drachms of the dried shrub in an earthen pot, with about 10 ounces of boiling water, keeping it near a boiling heat for a night, and this they take in the morning. Beside its other effects, it is said to produce a sensation of prickling or creeping in the painful parts; but in a few hours the pain and disagreeable symptoms are relieved, and 2 or 3 doses generally complete the cure. The use of liquids is not allowed during its operation, as this is apt to induce vomiting (Ed.—Coxe). It is a valuable remedy, used in Russia, Germany, and sometimes in France and England, but scarcely at all in this country. That it possesses a decided control over the circulation, acting like the special sedatives, slowing the quickened pulse by giving increased heart power and removing capillary obstruction, seems well established. Myalgic pains, whether rheumatic or not, but especially of the facial and ocular region, appear to be the special indication for its use. It has been employed in acute testicular, and ovarian affections, as well as in chronic orchitis and hydrocele. The dose should be minute, from a fraction of a drop to a drop of a saturated tincture. Probably our native species would be fully as effective.

Specific Indications and Uses.—Myalgic pain, particularly of the face; "face-ache"; pain in the ocular muscles.

Plants for a Future states:

Medicinal use of Rosebay Rhododendron: The poulticed leaves are used to relieve arthritic pain, headaches etc. A decoction of the leaves is occasionally employed internally in domestic practice in the treatment of rheumatism. The leaves are taken internally in controlled dosage for the treatment of heart ailments. Caution is advised, see the notes on toxicity.

Known hazards of Rhododendron maximum: The leaves are poisonous. Ingestion can cause convulsions and coma. The pollen of many if not all species of rhododendrons is also probably toxic, being said to cause intoxication when eaten in large quantities.

Rhus, Sumac

Twenty-five varieties of Rhus are commonly discussed in Herbal Medicine… some as the cause of terrible rashes that must be cured using other herbs, and some as useful herbs or edible berries: Rhus ambigua, Rhus aromatica - Lemon Sumach, Rhus copallina – Dwarf, Rhus coriaria - Elm-Leaved, Rhus diversiloba - Western Poison Oak, Rhus glabra – Smooth, Rhus chinensis - Chinese Gall, Rhus integrifolia - Lemonade Berry, Rhus microphylla – Desert, hus ovata - Sugar Bush, Rhus potaninii, Rhus punjabensis, Rhus punjabensis sinica, Rhus radicans - Poison Ivy, Rhus sempervirens, Rhus succedanea - Wax Tree, Rhus sylvestris, Rhus toxicodendron - Eastern Poison Oak, Rhus trichocarpa, Rhus trilobata - Skunk Bush, Rhus typhina - Stag's Horn Sumach, Rhus verniciflua - Lacquer Tree, Poison Sumach, Rhus wallichii, Rhus x pulvinata

The Sumac family may be seen as one in which some are helpful and pleasant, while near relatives should be avoided like poison! Fortunately, the tree or bush type Sumacs that grow in my region are among the nicer members of the family (although, we certainly have a ton of poison ivy and poison oak): Rhus copallinum var. copallinum (Winged Sumac, Shining Sumac), Rhus copallinum var. latifolia (Eastern Winged Sumac), Rhus copallinum var. leucantha (Southern Winged Sumac), Rhus glabra (Smooth Sumac), Rhus typhina (Staghorn Sumac)

Sumac berries are a popular spice in some countries. Dioscorides mentioned this in his Materia Medica:

Rhus (which is sprinkled among sauces and also called erythrum) is the fruit of rhus coriaria, which is called this because tanners use it for thickening their hides. It is a little tree which grows on rocks — two feet high, the leaves somewhat long and red, jagged all around. The fruit is like little bunches of grapes — thick, the size of that of terminthos, and somewhat broad. That which encloses the fruit is very useful. The leaves are astringent and good for the same purposes as acacia. A decoction dyes the hair black, and is a suppository for dysentery. It is a liquid medicine, hip bath, and an instillation for discharges of the ears. The leaves applied as a poultice with vinegar or honey stop pterygium [membrane on the eye] and gangrene. The juice of the dried leaves boiled with water to the consistency of honey are as useful for as many things as lycium. The fruit does the same things (being food) in mixing it with meat for coeliac [intestinal complaints] and dysentery. Applied as a plaster with water it prevents inflammation of fractures, desquamation or skin peeling, and blueness of wounds. It cleans rough tongues with honey. It prevents the excessive discharges called whites [leucorrhoea — a mucosal vaginal discharge] and cures haemorrhoids, applied with oak coals pounded into small pieces. The boiled liquid of this fruit gathers a cream that is better for these purposes than the fruit itself. It also leaves a gum which is put into the cavities of teeth to take away their pain.

Gerard wrote of Currior Sumac and Myrtle Sumac in the Rhus family:

A. The leaves of Sumach boiled in wine and drunken, do stop the lask, the inordinate course of women's sicknesses, and all other inordinate issues of blood.

B. The seed of Sumach eaten in sauces with meat, stoppeth all manner of fluxes of the belly, the bloody flux, and all other issues, especially the white issues of women.

C. The decotion of the leaves maketh hairs black, and is put into stools to fume upward into the bodies of those that have the dysentery, and is to be given them also to drink.

D. The leaves made into an ointment or plaster with honey and vinegar, stayeth the spreading nature of gangrenes and pterygia.

E. The dry leaves sodden in water until the decoction be as thick as honey, yield forth a certain oiliness, which performeth all the effects of Licium.

F. The seed is no less effectual to be strewed in powder upon their meats which are Cœliaci or Dysenterici.[Suffereing from colic or dysentery]

G. The seeds pounded, mixed with honey and the powder of oaken coals, healeth the hæmorrhoids.

H. There isseth out of the shrub a gum, which being put into the hollowness of the teeth, taketh away the pain, as Dioscorides writeth.

I am not sure which Rhus Culpepper referred to as "Sumach":

The seeds dried, reduced to powder, and taken in small doses, stop purges and hæmorrhages; the young shoots have also great efficacy in strengthening the stomach and bowels; they are best given in a strong infusion. The bark of the roots has the sam virtues, but in an inferior degree.

Mrs. Grieves used the name "Sumachs" for both the Smooth (Rhus glabra) and Sweet (Rhus aromatica) Sumac, but gave medicinal uses for only the Smooth Sumac:

The bark is tonic, astringent, and antiseptic; the berries refrigerant and diuretic.

A strong decoction, or diluted fluid extract, affords an agreeable gargle in angina, especially when combined with potassium chlorate. Where tannin drugs are useful, as in diarrhoea, the fluid extract is an excellent astringent.

The bark, in decoction or syrup, has been found useful in gonorrhoea, leucorrhoea, diarrhoea, dysentery, hectic fever, scrofula and profuse perspiration from debility. Combined with the barks of slippery elm and white pine and taken freely, the decoction is said to have been greatly beneficial in syphilis. As an injection for prolapsus uteri and ani, and for leucorrhoea, and as a wash in many skin complaints, the decoction is valuable. For scald-head it can be simmered in lard, or the powdered root-bark can be applied as a poultice to old ulcers, forming a good antiseptic.

A decoction of the inner bark of the root is helpful for the sore-mouth resulting from mercurial salivation, and also for internal use in mercurial diseases. A free use of the bark will produce catharsis.

The berries may be used in infusion in diabetes, strangury bowel complaints, and febrile diseases; also as a gargle in quinsy and ulcerations of the mouth and throat, and as a wash for ringworm, tetters, offensive ulcers, etc.

The astringent excrescences, when powdered and mixed with lard or linseed oil, are useful in haemorrhoids.

The mucilagic exudation, if the bark be punctured in hot weather, has been used advantageously in gleet and several urinary difficulties.

The Thomsonian System of Medicine states:

SUMACH. Rhus Glabra. (Dr. Thomson.)

This appears to be a new article in medicine, entirely unknown to the medical faculty, as no mention is made of it by any author. The first of my knowledge that it was good for canker was when at Onion River, in 1807, attending the dysentery. Being in want of something to clear the stomach and bowels in that complaint, found that the bark, leaves or berries answered the purpose extremely well, and have made much use of it ever since. It is well known, and is found in all parts of the country; some of it grows from eight to twelve feet high, and has large spreading branches ; the berries grow in large bunches, and when ripe are a deep red color, of a pleasant sour taste ; and are used by the country people to dye with. The leaves and young sprouts are made use of in tanning morocco leather. For medicine, the bark should be peeled when full of sap, the leaves when full grown, and the berries when ripe; they should be carefully dried, and when used as part of No. 3 should be pounded, and may be used altogether, or either separate. A tea made of either or altogether is very good, and may be given with safety in almost all complaints, or put into the injection. It will scour the stomach and bowels, and is good for strangury, as it promotes urine and relieves difficulties in the kidneys by removing obstructions and strengthening those parts. I have been in the habit of late years of making use of this article with bayberry bark and lily root, or hemlock bark, equal parts, for No. 3, and it has, always answered a good purpose. The leaves are the least astringent, but are valuable in dysentery and hemorrhages of lungs or uterus. The bark is more stimulating, astringing and toning, and is valuable for leucorrhoea, inflammation of the bladder, and for rectal troubles, chronic diarrhoea and rectal hemorrhages. The berries are a pleasant acid astringent. Fill a vessel full of berries, cover with boiling water and steep a half-hour. Then strain and sweeten to suit taste. This is a good beverage to allay irritation of the bladder and in the treatment of diabetes and for the relief of bloody urine.

King's American Dispensatory, 1898 tells us of several plants:

Rhus Aromatica.—Fragrant Sumach.

Action, Medical Uses, and Dosage.—This exceedingly valuable medicine was introduced by J. T. McClanahan, M. D., Booneville, Mo. (Ec. Med. Jour., 1879, p. 317). At first, the use of this remedy *was confined to the treatment of diabetes, and other excessive discharges from the kidneys and the bladder, as well as to cases of incipient albuminuria. More recently, in addition to the above-named diseases, it has been largely employed with advantage in urethral irritations, uterine leucorrhoea, cholera infantum, diarrhoea, dysentery, chronic laryngitis, chronic bronchitis, and especially in the enuresis of children and of aged persons.*

While it is of undoubted value in many hemorrhagic states, particularly in chronic hematuria, a malarial form of which is quite common in the southern states, its chief value is in enuresis, with marked atony and chronic irritability of the urinary passages, whether in young or old subjects. The favorite remedies for "bed-wetting" are Rhus aromatica, belladonna, and thuja. Sometimes this affection yields to Rhus aromatica alone; sometimes a combination, as indicated, must be used. Fragrant sumach is indicated in all cases of over-activity of the kidneys, but is always contraindicated when there is active inflammation. A patient suffering, for several years, from catarrh of the bladder and hypertrophy of the prostate, with excruciating pain during micturition, necessitating the continued use of a soft catheter, the introduction of which invariably proved painful, was relieved by fragrant sumach. After exhausting the employment of all recognized remedies for the patient's condition, together with the use of the water at the Hot Springs of Arkansas, etc., without the least benefit, as a dernier ressort, the patient was placed upon teaspoonful doses, 3 or 4 times daily, of the fluid extract of Rhus aromatica. In 3 weeks' time the symptoms were all removed, and the prostate so far reduced that the use of the soft catheter became unnecessary. The patient was 65 years old and subsequently voided urine as freely and as painlessly as a boy of 18 years (J. King).

Inflammatory symptoms being absent, it may be employed in passive uterine hemorrhage, hemorrhage of the bowels, as in chronic bloody-flux (not in acute dysentery), chronic painful vesical catarrh, and in phthisis, to control hemorrhage when small in amount, and to restrain the accompanying diarrhoea and night-sweats. In bronchitis, with profuse, blood-streaked expectoration, it may be given with confidence. A good form of administration is as follows: R Specific fragrant sumach, ℥ss; glycerin, ℥ijss. Mix. Sig. Dose, from ½ to 1 teaspoonful every 3 or 4 hours. This remedy is reputed useful in purpura hemorrhagica. The forms of administration now preferred are specific fragrant sumach and the fluid extract, of which the dose of either varies from 5 to 60 minims, repeated every 3 or 4 hours. It may be taken in water, in glycerin and water, and in solution of pure gelatin, or in syrup, when these vehicles are not contraindicated.

Specific Indications and Uses.—Not the remedy for active conditions. As given by its introducer, Dr. McClanahan, the specific indications are: "Stools profuse, skin cool and sallow, pulse small and feeble, loss of flesh, abdomen flabby, tongue pale, trembling and moist, trembling in lower limbs; general sense of lassitude and languor. Dose for infants, 10 to 20 drops in a half-glass of water, teaspoonful as often as necessary; for children, perhaps 5 drops of the first dilution" (Ec. Med. Jour., 1879, p. 317). To these may be added large, painless diarrhoeal discharges; nocturnal enuresis, from weakness of spincter vesicae; prostatic enlargement; and malarial haeematuria.

Rhus Glabra (U. S. P.)—Rhus Glabra.

Action, Medical Uses, and Dosage.—Sumach bark is tonic, astringent, antiseptic, and decidedly alterative; the berries are refrigerant and diuretic. In decoction or syrup, the bark of the root has been found valuable in gonorrhoea, leucorrhoea, diarrhoea, dysentery, hectic fever, scrofula, and in profuse perspiration from debility. Combined with the barks of slippery elm and white pine, in decoction, and taken freely, it is said to have proved highly beneficial in syphilitic ulcerations. Externally, the bark of the root in powder, applied as a poultice to old ulcers, forms an excellent antiseptic. A decoction may also be used in injection for prolapsus uteri and ani, and leucorrhoea, and as a wash in many cutaneous diseases; simmered in lard it is valuable in scald head. A decoction of the inner bark of the root is serviceable in the sore mouth resulting from mercurial salivation, and was formerly much used internally in mercurial diseases. A saturated tincture is useful in ulcerative stomatitis, and for spongy gums attending purpura hemorrhagica and scorbutus. Diarrhoea and dysentery, with intestinal ulceration, seem to be well controlled by it. Dose of the tincture, from 5 to 20 drops. The berries may be used in infusion in diabetes, strangury, bowel complaints, febrile diseases (as a pleasant acidulous drink where acids are indicated), etc., as a gargle in quinsy and ulcerations of the mouth and throat; and as a wash for ringworm, tetter, offensive ulcers, etc. Excrescences are frequently formed on the leaves of this plant, and which are very astringent; when powdered and mixed, with lard or linseed oil, they are said to prove useful in hemorrhoids. In hot weather, if the bark be punctured, a gummy substance flows out, which has been used with advantage in gonorrhoea and gleet, and several urinary affections. Dose of the decoction of sumach bark, or infusion of the berries, from 1 to 4 fluid ounces. A free use of the bark will produce catharsis.

Specific Indications and Uses.—Relaxation of mucous tissues, with unhealthy discharges; mercurial ulcerations; aphthous stomatitis; spongy gums; ulcerative sore throat, with fetid discharges; flabbiness and ulceration of tissues.

Related Species.—There are several species of Rhus, as the Rhus typhina, Staghorn or Velvet sumach; and the Rhus copallina, Mountain or Dwarf sumach, which possess similar virtues, and which must be carefully distinguished from those which possess poisonous properties. The non-poisonous species have their fruit clothed with acid crimson hairs, and their panicles are compound, dense, and terminal; the poisonous varieties have axillary panicles and smooth fruit.

According to Plants for A Future:

Medicinal use of Dwarf Sumach (Rhus copallina): a decoction of the root has been used in the treatment of dysentery. An infusion of the roots has been used in the treatment of VD. A poultice of the root has been applied to sores and skin eruptions. A tea made from the bark has been drunk to stimulate milk flow in nursing mothers. A decoction of the bark has been used as a wash for blisters and sunburn blisters. An infusion of the leaves has been used to cleanse and purify skin eruptions. The berries were chewed in the treatment of bed-wetting and mouth sores. Some caution is advised in the use of the leaves and stems of this plant, see the notes above on toxicity.

Known hazards of Rhus copallina: There are some suggestions that the sap of this species can cause a skin rash in susceptible people, but this has not been substantiated.

Medicinal use of Smooth Sumach (Rhus Glabra): Smooth sumach was employed medicinally by various native North American Indian tribes who used it to treat a variety of complaints. It is occasionally used in modern herbalism where it is valued for its astringent and antiseptic qualities. Some caution should be employed in the use of this species since it can possibly cause skin irritations. It is best only used under the supervision of a qualified practitioner. A tea made from the bark or root bark is alterative, antiseptic, astringent, galactogogue, haemostatic, rubefacient and tonic. It is used in the treatment of diarrhoea, fevers, general debility, sore mouths, rectal bleeding, uterine prolapse etc. It is used as a gargle to treat sore throats and applied externally to treat excessive vaginal discharge, burns and skin eruptions. The powdered bark can be applied as a poultice to old ulcers, it is a good antiseptic. A tea made from the roots is appetizer, astringent, diuretic and emetic. An infusion is used in the treatment of colds, sore throats, painful urination, retention of urine and dysentery. The root is harvested in the autumn and dried for later use. An infusion of the green or dried branches has been used in the treatment of TB. A decoction of the branches, with the seed heads, has been used to treat itchy scalps and as a bathing water for frost-bitten limbs. The milky latex from the plant has been used as a salve on sores. A tea made from the leaves was used in the treatment of asthma, diarrhoea and stomatitis. A poultice of the leaves has been used to treat skin rashes. The leaves have been chewed to treat sore gums and they have been rubbed on the lips to treat sore lips. The berries are diuretic, emetic, emmenagogue, purgative and refrigerant. They are used in the treatment of late-onset diabetes, stranguary bowel complaints, febrile diseases, dysmenorrhoea etc. They have been chewed as a remedy for bed-wetting. The blossoms have been chewed as a treatment for sore mouths. A decoction of the blossoms has been used as a mouthwash for teething children. An infusion of the blossoms has been used as an eye wash for sore eyes.

Known hazards of Rhus glabra: There are some suggestions that the sap of this species can cause a skin rash in susceptible people, but this has not been substantiated.

Medicinal use of Stag's Horn Sumach (Rhus typhina): Stag's horn sumach was often employed medicinally by several native North American Indian tribes who valued it especially for its astringent qualities. It is little used in modern herbalism. Some caution is advised in the use of the leaves and stems of this plant, see the notes above on toxicity. The bark is antiseptic, astringent, galactogogue and tonic. An infusion is used in the treatment of diarrhoea, fevers, piles, general debility, uterine prolapse etc. An *infusion is also said to greatly increase the milk flow of a nursing mother - small pieces of the wood were also eaten for this purpose. The inner bark is said to be a valuable remedy for piles. The roots are astringent, blood purifier, diuretic and emetic. An infusion of the roots, combined with purple coneflower (Echinacea purpurea) has been used in the treatment of venereal disease. A poultice of the roots has been used to treat boils. The leaves are astringent. They have been used in the treatment of asthma, diarrhoea and stomatosis. An infusion of the fruits has been used as a tonic to improve the appetite and as a treatment for diarrhoea. The berries are astringent and blood purifier. They were chewed as a remedy for bed-wetting. A tea made from the berries has been used to treat sore throats. The flowers are astringent and stomachic. An infusion has been used to treat stomach pains. The sap has been applied externally as a treatment of warts. Some caution is advised here since the sap can cause a rash on many people.*

Known hazards of Rhus typhina: There are some suggestions that the sap of this species can cause a skin rash in susceptible people, but this has not been substantiated.

Robinia, Locust

Six varieties of Locust have been found useful in Herbal Medicine: Robinia fertilis - Bristly Locust, Robinia flava, Robinia luxurians, Robinia neomexicana, Robinia pseudoacacia - Black Locust, Robinia viscosa - Clammy Locust

Only Robinia pseudoacacia (Black Locust) is native to my region. Black locust is a very important tree in the Appalachian Mountains. Not only is it valued for timber and firewood, but fence posts made from Locust resist rot. Many homesteads would not have been possible without the Locust tree. One of the key characteristics of this tree is that, when cut, it will grow back – new shoots will come from the stump. Wise people coppice this tree, cutting it off at a certain height, so that firewood may be harvested from it repeatedly.

Resources of the Southern Fields and Forests states:

YELLOW LOCUST TREE; LOCUST; FALSE ACACIA, (Rohinia pseudacacia, L.) Grows in the mountains of N. and S. Carolina; vicinity of Charleston; collected in lower St. John's Berkeley, near Ward's plantation; Newbern. Fl. May. Dem. Elem. de Bot. The flowers are aromatic and emollient. An anti-spasmodic syrup is prepared from them; and Gendrin states that when given to infants, it produces sleep, vomiting, and sometimes slight convulsive movements; he relates a case where it was swallowed by boys, in whom acro-narcotic effects were induced. Mer. and de L. Diet, de M. Med. vi, 101 ; Desfont, Traite des Arbres, ii, 304; Ann. d'Hort. ix, 168; Ann. Clin, de Mont, xxiv, 68. Dr. Wood, in the 12th Ed. U. S. Disp., states that the bark of the root is said to be tonic, and in large doses, emetic and purgative, and he reports from the Ann. de Therap. 1860, p. 64, three cases of poisoning, in children, from eating the root; they all recovered; the symptoms were like those produced by an overdose of Belladonna. One of them who happened to be laboring under intermittent fever at the time, had no return of the paroxysm. He adds, "these facts render caution advisable in the use of the root, yet are also well calculated to stimulateinquiry." Mills states that "the best bows of the Indians were made of this tree."

King's American Dispensatory, 1898 tells us:

Chemical Composition.—From the root of this plant Hlasiwetz (1852) isolated asparagin. The flowers, according to Zwenger and Dronke (1861; see Husemann and Hilger, Pflanzenstoffe, p. 1046), contain a yellow, crystallizable glucosid, robinin ($C_{25}H_{20}O_{16}$), which, upon hydrolysis, is split into quercetin and a non-fermentable sugar. The bark of the locust tree, when chewed, produced violent emeto-catharsis (Amer. Jour. Pharm., 1887, p. 153; F. B. Power and Jacob Cambier, Pharm. Rundschau, 1890, pp. 29-38). The latter authors, searching for the poisonous principle, found it in an albuminous body (phytalbumose, 1.66 per cent), which is tasteless, soluble in water, insoluble in alcohol, and coagulated by heat, with complete loss of its toxic properties; for this reason some declare a decoction of the bark is inert. It is precipitated by tannic acid and by solution of potassium bismuth iodide. It is allied to ricin, the poisonous, albuminous constituent of the castor-oil seed. (For further reactions, see the original paper.) The authors, in addition, found an inert albumin (globulin, characterized by being insoluble in concentrated salt solution);

small quantities of the poisonous alkaloid, choline (of the class known as ptomaïnes), fatty matter, inert resin, cane sugar (4.57 per cent, referred to air-dry bark), starch, gum, some tannin, coloring matter, and probably asparagin. The poisonous principle, in the form of an albuminous body, was likewise obtained by R. Kobert (Jahresb. der Pharm., 1891, p. 146).

Action, Medical Uses, and Dosage.—A decoction of the bark of the root is tonic in small doses, but emetic and purgative in large ones. An ounce of the bark boiled in 3 gills of water, operates as a cathartic in doses of ½ ounce, given morning and evening. The bark is supposed to possess some acro-narcotic properties, as the juice of it has been known to produce coma and slight convulsions. An overdose has produced symptoms very similar to those resulting from an improper dose of belladonna, and at the same time cured a case of fever and ague. The flowers possess antispasmodic properties, and form an excellent and agreeable syrup. The leaves, in doses of 30 grains, every 20 minutes, operate mildly and efficiently as an emetic. The drug should be tested for its effects upon gastro-intestinal and nervous affections.

Plants for A Future states:

Medicinal use of Black Locust: Febrifuge. The flowers are antispasmodic, aromatic, diuretic, emollient and laxative. They are cooked and eaten for the treatment of eye ailments. The flower is said to contain the antitumor compound benzoaldehyde. The inner bark and the root bark are emetic, purgative and tonic. The root bark has been chewed to induce vomiting, or held in the mouth to allay toothache, though it is rarely if ever prescribed as a therapeutic agent in Britain. The fruit is narcotic. This probably refers to the seedpod. The leaves are cholagogue and emetic. The leaf juice inhibits viruses.

Peterson Field Guides Eastern and Central Medicinal Plants states:

American Indians chewed root bark to induce vomiting; held bark in mouth to allay tooth aches. A folk tonic, purgative, emetic. Flower tea used in rheumatism. In China the root bark is also considered purgative an emetic and the flowers are considered diuretic. Flowers contain a glycoside, robinin, which is experimentally diuretic. Warning: all parts are toxic dash even honey derived from the flowers is said to be toxic. The strong odor of the flowers has been reported to cause nausea and headaches in some persons.

Sabal Palmetto, Palmetto

Four varieties of Sabal have been found useful in Herbal Medicine: Sabal etonia - Scrub Palmetto, Sabal mexicana - Mexican Palmetto Synonym: Sabal texana, Sabal minor - Bush Palmetto Synonym: Sabal adansonii, Sabal palmetto - Cabbage Palmetto

Only one Sabal is native to my region, and that is the Cabbage Palmetto. This is the state tree of South Carolina, but also grows in coastal areas of North Carolina. It has historically been used as food, and for weaving baskets and hats, but I have found very little information on its medicinal use.

Plants for A Future states:

Medicinal use of Cabbage Palmetto: The berries or seeds have been used in the treatment of grass sickness, low fever, headaches and weight loss.

Salix, Willow or Osier

Sixty-two varieties of Salix have been found useful in Herbal Medicine: Salix acutifolia - Sharp-Leaf Willow, Salix aegyptiaca, Salix alaxensis - Feltleaf Wiillow, Salix alba - White WillowSalix alb, a caerulea - Cricket Bat Willow, Salix alba vitellina - Golden Willow, Salix 'Americana', Salix amygdaloides - Peach Leaved Willow, Salix appendiculata, Salix arenaria, Salix atrocinerea - Rusty Sallow, Salix aurita - Eared Sallow, Salix babylonica - Weeping Willow, Salix bakko, Salix bebbiana - Beak Willow, Salix 'Bowles hybrid', Salix brachycarpa, Salix caprea - Goat Willow, Salix cinerea - Grey Willow, Salix commutate, Salix daphnoides - Violet Willow, Salix decipiens, Salix eriocephala - Missouri Willow, Salix exigua - Coyote Willow, Salix fluviatilis - River Willow, Salix 'Forbiana', Salix fragilis - Crack Willow, Salix gilgiana, Salix gooddingii - Goodding's Willow, Salix gracilistyla - Rosegold Pussy Willow, Salix hastata - Halberd-Leaved Willow, Salix hookeriana - Dune Willow, Salix chaenomeloides, Salix japonica, Salix koriyanagi, Salix lanata - Woolly Willow, Salix lasiandra - Yellow Willow, Salix lasiolepis - Pacific Willow, Salix lucida - Shining Willow, Salix matsudana, Salix miyabeana, Salix nigra - Black Willow, Salix nipponica, Salix pentandra - Bay Willow, Salix petiolaris - Slender Willow, Salix piperi - Dune Willow, Salix pulchra - Tealeaf Willow, Salix purpurea - Purple Osier, Salix purpurea lambertiana - Purple Osier, Salix repens - Creeping Willow, Salix scouleriana - Scouler's Willow, Salix schwerinii, Salix sitchensis - Sitka Willow, Salix sungkianica, Salix taxifolia - Yew-Leaf Willow, Salix triandra - Almond-Leaved Willow, Salix viminalis – Osier, Salix wallichiana, Salix x mollisima hippophaeifolia, Salix x mollisima undulata, Salix x rubra, Salix x smithiana

Fortunately, I need not get into the specific virtues of all sixty-two trees, as only one variety of Salix is native to my region, the Black Willow (Salix Nigra). Naturalized are: Salix alba (White Willow), Salix atrocinerea (Grey Willow, Common Sallow, Rusty Sallow, Olive-leaf Willow), Salix babylonica (Weeping Willow), Salix caprea (Goat Willow), Salix cinerea (Grey Willow), Salix pentandra (Laurel Willow, Bay Willow)

The Willows are widely used in Herbal Medicine. Their chief value is salic acid. Willows, and a few other plants, are nature's aspirin. They reduce pain and inflammation, thin the blood and lower fevers.

Dioscorides referred to Willow as Itea:

Itea is a tree known to all whose fruit, leaves, bark and juice are astringent. The leaves pounded into small pieces and taken in a drink with a little pepper and wine help those troubled with iliaca passio [painful intestinal obstruction]. Taken by themselves with water they cause inconception [birth control]. The fruit (taken in a drink) is good for those who spit blood, and the bark does the same. Burnt and steeped in vinegar it takes away calluses and corns, rubbed on them. The juice from the leaves and bark warmed with rosaceum in a cup of malum punicum [pomegranate] helps sores in the ears, and a decoction of them is an excellent warm pack for gout. It also cleans away scurf [eczema]. A juice is taken from it at the time of its flowering, the bark being cut, for it is found coalesced within. It has the ability to clean away things that darken the pupils.

Oddly, Saint Hildegard von Bingen did not approve of Willow. She wrote:

The willow is cold, and it designates vices, since it seems to be beautiful. It is not useful for people, except in serving external uses, and is not good for medicine. Its fruit and juice is bitter and not good for human use. If one wishes to eat it, it stirs up and augments melancholy in him, makes him bitter inside, and diminishes his health and happiness.

Gerard wrote of eight varieties of Willow, listing their virtues as:

A. The leaves and bark of Withy or Willows do stay the spitting of blood, and all other fluxes of blood whatsoever in man or woman, if the said leaves and bark be boiled in wine and drunk.

B. The green boughs with the leaves may very well be brought into chambers and set about the beds of those that be sick of fevers, for they do mightily cool the heat of the air, which thing is a wonderful refreshing to the sick patients.

C. The bark hath like virtues: Dioscorides writeth, that this being burnt to ashes, and steeped in vinegar, takes away corns and other like risings in the feet and toes: divers, saith Galen, do slit the bark whilst the Withy is in flowering, and gather a certain juice, with which they use to take away things that hinder the sight, and this is when they are constrained to use a cleansing medicine of thin and subtle parts.

Culpepper wrote of Willow:

The Moon owns it. Both the leaves, bark, and the seed, are used to stanch bleeding of wounds, and at mouth and nose, spitting of blood, and other fluxes of blood in man or woman, and to stay vomiting, and provocation thereunto, if the decoction of them in wine be drank. It helps also to stay thin, hot, sharp, salt distillations from the head upon the lungs, causing a consumption. The leaves bruised with some pepper, and drank in wine, helps much the wind cholic. The leaves bruised and boiled in wine, and drank, stays the heat of lust in man or woman, and quite extinguishes it, if it be long used. The seed also is of the same effect. Water that is gathered from the Willow, when it flowers, the bark being slit, and a vessel fitting to receive it, is very good for redness and dimness of sight, or films that grow over the eyes, and stay the rheums that fall into them; to provoke urine, being stopped, if it be drank; to clear the face and skin from spots and discolourings. Galen says, the flowers have an admirable faculty in drying up humours, being a medicine without any sharpness or corrosion; you may boil them in white wine, and drink as much as you will, so you drink not yourself drunk. The bark works the same effect, if used in the same manner, and the tree hath always a bark upon it, though not always flowers; the burnt ashes of the bark being mixed with vinegar, takes away warts, corns, and superfluous flesh, being applied to the place. The decoction of the leaves or bark in wine, takes away scurff and dandrif by washing the place with it. It is a fine cool tree, the boughs of which are very convenient to be placed in the chamber of one sick of a fever.

In the fifty-third volume of the Philosophical Transactions, page 195, we have an account given by Mr. Stone, of the great efficacy of the bark of this tree, in the cure of intermitting fevers. He gathered the bark in summer, when it was full of sap, and having dried it by a gentle heat, gave a drachm of it in powder every four hours between the fits.

While the Peruvian bark remained at its usual moderate price, it was hardly worth while to seek for a substitute, but since the consumption of that article is become nearly as equal to the supply of it, from South America, we must expect to find it dearer, and very much adulterated every year, and consequently the white Willow bark is likely to become an object worthy the attention of the faculty; and should its success, upon a more enlarged scale of practice, prove equal to Mr. Stone's experiments, the world will be much indebted to that gentleman for his communication.

Mrs. Grieves wrote of both Black and White Willow:

Willow, Black American

Botanical: Salyx nigra

Medicinal Action and Uses---An aphrodisiac sedative, tonic. The bark has been prescribed in gonorrhoea and to relieve ovarian pain; a liquid extract is prepared and used in mixture with other sedatives. Largely used in the treatment of nocturnal emissions.

Willow, White

Botanical: *Salix alba*

Medicinal Action and Uses---Tonic, antiperiodic and astringent. It has been used in dyspepsia connected with debility of the digestive organs. In convalescence from acute diseases, in worms, in chronic diarrhoea and dysentery, its tonic and astringent combination renders it very useful

.

An Irish Herbal states:

A decoction of the leaves, bark, seed and flower in wine, taken internally, stops vomiting, spitting of blood, excessive menstrual flow and all other flows of the blood. The ashes of the bark, mixed with vinegar, causes warts to fall off and soothes hard skin. The sap that flows from the bark is good for inflammations of the eye.

Brother Aloysius wrote of White Willow:

Before the flowering period in April, the bark of two to three year old branches should be gathered and left to dry. The decoction of this very bitter astringent can be fruitfully used for the treatment of fever. It is, indeed, one of the best febrifuge remedies, especially for intermittent fever. It is also highly recommended for blood-spitting , and is a very potent tonic. Boil 3 to 4 tablespoons in 2 cups water until reduced by half; add a little sugar or honey, as it has a rather bitter taste. Take 1 tablespoon every 2 hours; 1 tablespoon ever hour in case of fever. It is a most efficacious remedy for heavy bleeding, also for chronic diarrhea, leukorrhea, excessive mucus, stomach cramps, nervous complaints, spleen and liver disorders, foul or mucus stomach.

Powder from the dried bark of willow can also be used for the same complaints; take 2 to 2 ½ tablespoons as necessary, per day, with a little honey or syrup, in wine. When taken in wine, ½ to ¾ cup should be steeped in 1 quart of wine for 14 days. Dosage, 1 tablespoon 3 times a day. Boil 3 handfuls of willow leaves in ½ cups wine until reduced by two thirds. This is a beneficial remedy for blood-spitting, heavy menstruation and leukorrhea. Dosage: a liqueur glassful, three times a day. A tincture of willow bark can also be prepared by letting 3 parts powdered willow bark steep for 10 days in 10 parts alcohol; it should then be filtered. The dose is 5 drops in a spoon of water one to four times a day.

Fr. Johannes Künzle wrote of Willow:

Old people whose legs are weak, because of old age or because of an illness could strengthen their legs in frequent foot baths in boiled willow bark. The basket weavers sell bark cheaply

Jolanta Wittib writes of Willow:

Willow bark together with Meadowsweet is part of Bayer Aspirin. As I am always careful to have enough willow bark and Meadowsweet at home, I use only my homemade "Aspirin".

In spring, just before the buds start opening I cut a few two or three year old twigs from a willow. The twigs are thinner than the thickness of a finger. I peel the bark, cut it into 1 cm pieces, dry it well and store it in tightly closed dark jars or in a dark place.

Whenever I have fever, flu, pains in joints or muscles or a headache, I make a decoction/infusion: I soak 1 spoon of powdered willow bark in 1 Liter of cold water for half an hour, then heat it on a very low heat for another 20-30 minutes, but do not bring it to a boil. I add a spoon of dried meadowsweet and I might add some lemon verbena or lemon balm or lavender for a better taste and a better sleep. I let the infusion soak for 10 minutes, strain it, pour into thermos and drink half a cup or a cup every three, four hours. I know, I have to wait for the soothing effect of the remedy, as it has to pass through the "chemical factory" of my body before the healing substances of the plants start to work, but then the healing powers start working.

A quicker version is making an infusion: pour 500 ml of very hot, but not boiling water onto 1 teaspoon of powdered willow bark and 1 teaspoon of powdered meadow sweet, leave 15 minutes to draw and drink many times a day.

Well, this is my way of getting rid of infections with fever without ruining my stomach.

Resources of the Southern Fields and Forests states:

SALICACEAE. {The Willow Tribe.)

Bark generally astringent, tonic and stomachic.

BLACK OE SWAMP WILLOW, {Salix nigra, L.) Grows along streams; Eichland ; vicinity of Charleston ; collected in St. John's; Newbern. Fl. May. Bell's Pract. Diet. 403; U. S. Disp. 622. See work of younger Michaux, Ball, and Gar. Mat. Med. 337; Mer. and de L. Diet, de M. Med. vi, 185; Griffith, Med. Bot. 583 ; Schcepf, Mat. Med. 43; Ell. Bot. Med. Notes, ii, 671. The willow is supposed to furnish us with one of the best substitutes for Peruvian bark ; the S. alba, which may be included among the many varieties found in the Southern States, and which are not yet accurately distinguished, seems to be held in high estimation. But this species, also, is considered valuable; the bark possessing some power as a purgative, anti-intermittent and vermifuge. It also furnishes the principle called salicin, which, from the results of late experiments, is found to be much less valuable than quinia, but is a good bitter tonic. See Journal Phil. Coll. Pharm. for the mode of preparation. The bark of the root and branches is officinal It is tonic and somewhat astringent. The decoction made with one ounce of bark to one pint of boiling water, of which the dose is two fluid ounces, should be boiled ten minutes, and strained while hot. Dose of salicin from two to eight grains and increased. It might well attract attention as a substitute for quinine. The large stems of this tree are light and durable, and are used for the timbers of boats. There are several other species in the Southern States. The willow—osier willow, (see article in Farmer and Planter, Sept., 1861,) is cultivated extensively in Germany, France and Belgium for making baskets, hats, screens, etc., etc. After most careful experiment it has been found that the best species to introduce into the Southern States for the purpose, are the Salix forbeyana, Salix purpurea, purple willow and Salix triandra, long-leaved willow. Forbes' willow is very productive and hardy, one of the most valuable species for common work, where unpeeled rods are used. It does not whiten well.

King's American Dispensatory, 1898 tells us:

Action, Medical Uses, and Dosage.—Willow bark is tonic, antiperiodic, and an astringent bitter. It has been given in intermittents, dyspepsia, connected with debility of the digestive organs, passive hemorrhages, chronic mucous discharges, in convalescence from acute diseases, and in worms. Although occasionally substituted for the cinchona bark, it is inferior in activity. In chronic diarrhoea and dysentery, the tonic and astringent combination of the willow renders it very eligible. It may be given in substance, in doses of 1 drachm of the powder, repeated as indicated; or of the decoction, 1 or 2 fluid ounces, 4 or 5 times a day. The decoction has also proved efficient as a local application to foul and indolent ulcers.

Plants for A Future states:

Medicinal use of Black Willow: The bark is anodyne, anti-inflammatory, antiperiodic, antiseptic, astringent, diaphoretic, diuretic, febrifuge, hypnotic, sedative, tonic. It has been used in the treatment of gonorrhoea, ovarian pains and nocturnal emissions. The bark of this species is used interchangeably with S. alba. It is taken internally in the treatment of rheumatism, arthritis, gout, inflammatory stages of auto-immune diseases, diarrhoea, dysentery, feverish illnesses, neuralgia and headache. The bark can be used as a poultice on cuts, wounds, sprains, bruises, swellings etc. The bark is removed during the summer and dried for later use. The leaves are used internally in the treatment of minor feverish illnesses and colic. The leaves can be harvested throughout the growing season and are used fresh or dried. The fresh bark contains salicin, which probably decomposes into salicylic acid (closely related to aspirin) in the human body. This is used as an anodyne and febrifuge and as an ingredient of spring tonics.

Rodale's Illustrated Encyclopedia of Herbs states:

Willow bark is used by herbalists as an anodyne, antipyretic, astringent, detergent, tonic, antiperiodic and antiseptic. It is useful for headache, neuralgia, hay fever, fever, pain and inflammation of joints (like aspirin).

In Weiner's Herbal, herbalist Michael Weiner recommended a decoction of 1 teaspoon of white willow bark slowly boiled in 1 ½ pints of water in a covered container for 30 minutes. After slowly cooling, it should be drunk a mouthful or tablespoonful at a time, "As needed to promote sweating in chills and fever."

Peterson Field Guides Eastern and Central Medicinal Plants tells us:

White Willow: the bark of this Willow and other willows with very bitter and astringent bark has traditionally been used for diarrhea, fevers, pain, arthritis, rheumatism; poultice or wash used for corns, cuts, cancers, ulcers, Poison Ivy rash, etc. Salicylic acid, derived from salicin found in the bark, is a precursor to the most widely used semi synthetic drug, acetyl salicylic acid aspirin, which reduces pain, inflammation, and fever. Aspirin reduce reduces risk of heart disease in males; Experimentally, delays cataract formation.

Botany In a Day states:

Willow is a commonly known wilderness medicine due to its aspirin like qualities. It is used for headaches, fevers, hay fever, neuralgia, and inflammation of the joints. Some of the salicylic acid is excreted in urine, making it useful as an analgesic to the urethra and bladder.

The Physicians' Desk Reference for Herbal Medicine tells us:

The efficacy of the drug is due mainly to the proportion of salicin present. After splitting of the acyl residue, the salicin glycosides converted to salicin, the precursor of salicylic acid. Salicylic acid is antipyretic, antiphlogistic come in analgesic. White Willow bark is the phototherapeutic precursor to salicylic acid aspirin. The salicin component is responsible for the anti-inflammatory an antipyretic affects the tannin content has astringent property on mucous membranes. Indications and usage approved by Commission E: rheumatism and pain. Salicin is useful in diseases accompanied by fever, rheumatic elements, headache and pain caused by inflammation. Unproven uses: folk medicine uses include toothache, gout, gastrointestinal disorders, diarrhea and wound healing. Contra indications: Willow bark is contraindicated in patients that have a hypersensitivity to salicylate. Salicylate should not be used in children with flu like symptoms due to the association of salicylates with Reye's syndrome. Patients with active gastric or duodenal ulcer, hemophilia, asthma, or diabetes should avoid willow bark preparations. Salicylate should be avoided during pregnancy. Salicylate's have been associated with rashes and breast-fed infants; Use is not recommended. General: no health hazards are known in conjunction with the proper administration of designated therapeutic dosages. Stomach complaints could occur as a side effect due to the tanning content.

Sambucus, Elder

The Elderberries and their relatives are not native to my region but can be cultivated.

Dioscorides wrote of two members of this family, calling them Akte and Chamaiakte:

AKTE - Sambucus], Sambcus nigra, Elder Tree, Arn Tree, Boon Tree

Acte has two types; one is like a tree with reed-like branches — round, hollow, whitish and a good length. The three or four leaves are set at distancesaround the stem, like the carya, more jagged, and with a strong smell. On the top are branches or stalks on which are round tufts with white flowers, and a fruit like terminthos of a somewhat purplish black, growing in clusters, full of juice, smacking of wine. It is also called arbor ursi, orsativa; the Romans call itsambucus, the Gauls, scobie, and the Dacians, seba.

CHAMAIAKTE - Ebulus, Sambucus ebulus, Dwarf Elder, Ground Elder, Danewort

BERRIES POISONOUS

The other kind is called chamaiacte. This has a creeping rhizome and is smaller and more herb-like, with a foursquare stalk that has many joints. The leaves are spread out at distances around every joint, like the almond tree, cut-in all around, and longer, with a strong scent, and having a tuft on the top like that above, and with a similar flower and fruit. The long root lies underneath, the thickness of a finger. This has the same properties and uses as that above — drying, expelling water, yet bad for the stomach. The leaves (boiled as vegetables) purge phlegm and bile, and the stalks (boiled as a vegetable) do the same. The roots (boiled with wine and given with meat) are good for dropsy. A decoction (taken as a drink) helps those bitten by vipers. Boiled with water for bathing it softens the womb and opens the vagina, and sets to rights any disorders around it. A decoction of the fruit (taken as a drink with wine) does the same things, and rubbed on it darkens the hair. The new tender leaves (smeared on with polenta) lessen inflammation, and smeared on, they are good for burns and dog bites. Smeared on with bull or goat grease they heal hollow ulcers, and help gout. It is also called heliosacte, sylvestris sambucus, or euboica; the Romans call it ebulus, the Gauls, ducone, and the Dacians, olma.

Saint Hildegard von Bingen wrote of Elder:

... one who has jaundice should enter a sauna bath and place the leaves of the tree on hot rocks. He should pour water over them, and then place a twig in pure wine, so that it takes its flavor. While in the bath, he should drink this in moderation. After he comes out of the bath, he should lie in bed, so that he sweats. He should do this often and he will be better.

Gerard wrote of "Common Elder":

A. Galen attributeth the like faculty to Elder that he doth to Danewort, and saith that it is of a drying quality, gluing, and moderately digesting: and it hath not only these faculties, but others also; for the bark, leaves, first buds, flowers, and fruit of Elder, do not only dry, but also heat, and have withal a purging quality, but not without trouble and hurt to the stomach.

B. The leaves and tender crops of common Elder taken in some broth or pottage open the belly, purging both thick phlegm and choleric humours: the middle bark is of the same nature, but stronger, and purgeth the said humours more violently.

C. The seeds contained within the berries dried are good for such as have the dropsy, and such as are too fat, and would fain be leaner, if they be taken in a morning to the quantity of a dram with wine for a certain space.

D. The leaves of Elder boiled in water until they be very soft, and when they are almost boiled enough a little oil of sweet Almonds added thereto, or a little Linseed oil; then taken forth and laid upon a red cloth, or a piece of scarlet, and applied to the haemorrhoids or piles as hot as can be suffered, and so let to remain upon the part affected, until it be somewhat cold, having the like in a readiness, applying one after another upon the diseased part, by the space of an hour or more, and in the end some bound to the place, and the patient put warm a-bed; it hath not as yet failed at the first dressing to cure the said disease; but if the patient be dressed twice it must needs do good if the first fail.

E. The green leaves pounded with deer's suet or bull's tallow are good to be laid to hot swellings and tumors, and doth assuage the pain of the gout.

F. The inner and green bark doth more forcibly purge: it draweth forth choler and watery humours; for which cause it is good for those that have the dropsy, being stamped, and the liquor pressed out and drunk with wine or whey.

G. Of like operation are also the fresh flowers mixed with some kind of meat, as fried with eggs, they likewise trouble the belly and move to the stool: being dried they lose as well their purging quality as their moisture, and retain the digesting and attenuating quality.

H. The vinegar in which the dried flowers are steeped are wholesome for the stomach: being used with meat it stirreth up an appetite, it cutteth and attenuateth or maketh thin gross and raw humours.

I. The faculty of the seed is somewhat gentler than that of the other parts: it also moveth the belly, and draweth forth watery humours, being beaten to powder, and given to a dram weight: being new gathered, steeped in vinegar, and afterwards dried, it is taken, and that effectually, in the like weight of the dried lees of wine, and with a few Anise seeds, for so it worketh without any manner of trouble, and helpeth those that have the dropsy. But it must be given for certain days together in a little wine, to those that have need thereof.

K. The jelly of the Elder, otherwise called Jew's ear, hath a binding and drying quality: the infusion thereof, in which it hath been steeped a few hours, taketh away inflammations of the mouth, and almonds of the throat in the beginning, if the mouth and throat be washed therewith, and doth in like manner help the uvula.

L. Dioscorides saith, that the tender and green leaves of the Elder tree, with barley meal parched, do remove hot swellings, and are good for those that are burnt or scalded, and for such as be bitten with a mad dog, and that they glue and heal up hollow ulcers.

M. The pith of the young boughs is without quality: This being dried, and somewhat pressed or quashed together, is good to lay upon the narrow orifices or holes of fistulas and issues, if it be put therein.

Of Dwarf Elder, he wrote:

A. The roots of Wallwort boiled in wine and drunken are good against the dropsy, for they purge downwards watery humours.

B. The leaves do consume and waste away hard swellings if they be applied poultice-wise, or in a fomentation or bath.

C. Dioscorides saith, that the roots of Wallwort do soften and open the matrix, and also correct the infirmities thereof, if they be boiled for a bath to sit in; and dissolve the swellings and pains of the belly.

D. The juice of the root of Danewort doth make the hair black.

E. The young and tender leaf quencheth hot inflammations, being applied with barley meal: it is with good success laid upon burnings, scaldings, and upon the bitings of mad dogs; and with bull's tallow or goat's suet it is a remedy for the gout.

F. The seed of Wallwort drunk in the quantity of a dram is the most excellent purger of watery humours in the world, and therefore most singular against the dropsy.

G. If one scruple of the seed be bruised and taken with syrup of Roses and a little sack, it cureth the dropsy, and easeth the gout, mightily purging downwards waterish humours, being once taken in the week.

Culpepper said of both Elder and Dwarf Elder:

Both the elder and dwarf tree are under the dominion of Venus. The first shoots of the common elder boiled like asparagus, and the young leaves and stalks boiled in fat broth, doth mightily carry forth phlegm and choler. The middle or inward bark boiled in water, and given in drink, worketh much more violently; and the berries, either green or dry expel the same humour, and are often given with good success to help the dropsy; the bark of the root boiled in wine, or the juice thereof drank, worketh the same effects, but more powerfully than either the leaves or fruit. The juice of the root taken, doth mightily procure vomitings, and purgeth the watery humours of the dropsy. The decoction of the root taken, cureth the biting of an adder, and biting of mad dogs. It mollifieth the hardness of the mother, if women sit thereon, and openeth their veins, and bringeth down their courses: The berries boiled in wine performeth the same effect; and the hair of the head washed therewith is made black. The juice of the green leaves applied to the hot inflammations of the eyes assuageth them; the juice of the leaves snuffed up into the nostrils, purgeth the tunicles of the brain; the juice of the berries boiled with honey, and dropped into the ears, helpeth the pains of them; the decoction of the berries in wine being drank provoketh urine: the distilled water, of the flowers is of much use to clean the skin from sun-burning, freckles, morphew, or the like; and taketh away the head-ach, coming of a cold cause, the head being bathed therewith. The leaves or flowers distilled in the month of May, and the legs often washed with the said distilled water, it taketh away the ulcers and sores of them. The eyes washed therewith, it taketh away the redness and bloodshot; and the hands washed morning and evening therewith, helpeth the palsy, and shaking of them.

The dwarf elder is more powerful than the common elder in opening and purging choler, phlegm, and water; in helping the gout, piles, and women's diseases, coloureth the hair black, helpeth the inflammations of the eyes, and pains in the ears, the biting of serpents, or mad dogs, burnings and scaldings, the wind cholic, cholic and stone, the difficulty of urine, the cure of old sores and fistulous ulcers. Either leaves or bark of elder, stripped upwards as you gather it, causeth vomiting. Also Dr. Butler, in a manuscript of his, commends dwarfelder to the sky for dropsies, viz to drink it, being boiled in white wine; to drink the decoction I mean, not the elder.

Mrs. Grieves made a point of differentiating the true Elders from those so called in the Acer family:

Medicinal Action and Uses---Expectorant, diuretic, diaphoretic, purgative.

The Dwarf Elder has more drastic therapeutic action than the Common Elder, and it is only the leaves, or very occasionally the berries, that are used medicinally. The leaves are probably more used in herbal practice than those of Sambucus nigra, and are ingredients in medicines for inflammation of both kidney and liver. The drug is said to be very efficacious in dropsy. Dwarf Elder Tea, which has been considered one of the best remedies for dropsy, is prepared from the dried roots, cut up fine or ground to powder; the drug was much used by Kneipp.

The root, which is white and fleshy, has a nauseous, bitter taste and a decoction from it is a drastic purgative. Culpepper states that the decoction cures the bites of mad dogs and adders. The root-juice has been employed to dye hair black.

The leaves, bruised and laid on boils and scalds, have a healing effect, and boiled in wine and made into a poultice were employed in France to resolve swellings and relieve contusions.

A rob made from the berries is actively purgative.

An oil extracted from the seeds has been used as an application to painful joints.

Mice and moles are said not to come near the leaves, and in Silesia there is a belief that it prevents some of the diseases of swine, being strewn in sties.

In the United States, the name of Dwarf Elder is given to an entirely different plant, viz. Aralia hispida (N.O. Araliaceae). In Homoeopathy, it is the American Dwarf Elder which is employed. There it is also called Bristly Sarsaparilla and Wild Elder. It is found growing in rocky places in North America.

The homoeopaths use a tincture from the fresh, root and a fluid extract is also prepared from it. It has sudorific, diuretic and alterative properties and is regarded as very valuable in dropsy, gravel and in suppression of urine. It is particularly recommended as a diuretic in dropsy, being more acceptable to the stomach than other remedies of the same class.

The 'Prickly Elder' of America is a closely related species, A. spinosa, also known as False Prickly Ash (the real Prickly Ash being Xanthoxylum Americanum), which contains a glucoside named Aralin. A decoction of the plant is used for the same purposes as Sarsaparilla.

The 'Poison Elder' of America is again no Elder, but a Sumach, its other name being Swamp Sumach, botanically Rhus verni (Linn.). It is a handsome shrub or small tree, 10 to 15 feet high, growing in swamps from Canada to California, with very small greenish flowers and small greenish-white berries and is extremely poisonous. It was confounded by the older botanists with R. vernicifera (D.C.) of Japan, the Japanese lacquer tree, which has similar poisonous properties. Its synonym is R. venenata (D.C.) See SUMACH.

There is a tree called the 'Box Elder,' mentioned by W. J. Bean in his Trees and Shrubs hardy in the British Isles; this is not a true Elder, however, but one of the American maples that yield sugar.

There are about half a dozen species of Elder hardy in Great Britain. The Common Elder (S. nigra), of which there are many varieties in cultivation, several of which are very ornamental, has leaves often very finely divided and jagged and variegated both with golden and silver blotches, a specially ornamental form being the 'golden cut-leaf Elder,' and another with yellow berries; the American Elder (S. canadensis) (the flowers of which, together with those of S. nigra are official in the United States Pharmacopoeia) has berries smaller and deep purple rather than black, the leaves broader and the flowers more fragrant than our Common Elder, it never attains tree size, but is a shrub of from 6 to 10 feet in height; the Blue Elder (S. glauca), the intensely blue berries of which are used as a food, when cooked, in California; the Red-berried Elder (S. racemosa), a pretty species, native of Central and Southern Europe, cultivated in shrubberies, which flowers in March and towards the end of summer is highly ornamental, with large oval clusters of bright scarlet berries, is so attractive to birds that their beauty is rarely seen, except when cultivated close to a house; the Red-berried American Elder (S. rubens and S. melanocarpa).

An Irish Herbal states:

Elder. The leaves, tender tops and inner bark purge bilious conditions. A small amount of seed pounded and taken in wine will disperse all accumulation of water fluid. The green leaves are good against all sorts of inflammations, while the flowers expel wind from the stomach. The berries can be used in gargles for sore mouths and throats.

Dwarf Elder. It is very beneficial in causing watery evacuations.

Fr. Kneipp wrote with particular enthusiasm of both Elder and Dwarf Elder:

Common Elder.

In the good old times the elder-bush stood nearest to the house, but now it is in many ways displaced and rooted up. It ought to stand near every house as pait of the household, as it were; or if cast aside it should be brought back to its post of honour, for every part of the elder-tree, leaves, blossoms, berries, bark and roots are all efficacious remedies. In spring time, vigorous nature strives to throw off matters that have gathered together in the body during winter. Who does not know these states, the so-called "spring diseases", such as eruptions, diarrhoea, colic, and such like?

Whoever wishes to purify juices and blood by a spring course of medicine, and to get rid of injurious matters in the easiest and most natural way, let hirn take six or eight leaves of the elder-tree, cut them up small, like one cuts tobacco, and let the tea boil for about ten minutes.

Then take daily during the whole course, one cup of this tea, fasting, an hour before breakfast. This most simple blood -purifying tea cleanses the machine of the human body in an excellent manner, and with poor people it takes the place of the pills and Alpine herbs, and such like which now-a-days are found in fine medicine chests, and which have often very strange effects

This course may also be undertaken at any other time of the year. Even the withered leaves make a good purifying tea.

Who has not eaten cakes made with elder flowers, the Suabian so-called "little cakes"? Many people bake them just at the time when the tree is shining in iis white spring-adornments, and they say these flower-cakes are a protection against fever. I know a place which is often visited with the ague, and there in spring you will see these elder-flower or fever-cakes on every table.

I have never examined this minutely and critically; let those people remain in their faith, for such fare is good and wholesome

Elder-flowers also purify, and it, would be good if in every home-dispensary a box of dried flowers were kept.

Winter is long, and cases can occur in which such a dissolving and sudorific little remedy may prove of excellent service. Harm can never be done by it.

From organisms in which dropsy has commenced, elder-root prepared as tea, drives out the water so powerfully, that it is scarcely excelled by any other medicament.

The berries which in autumn are often boiled and eaten as porridge or marmalade, were highly esteemed by our forefathers as a blood-purifying remedy. My departed mother undertook such an elder-flower course every year for a fortnight to three weeks. This was the chief reason why our ancestors forty or fifty years ago, had at least two elder-trees planted before their houses. As the higher classes now-a-days travel, and often to distant lands, to make use of the expensive grape cure, so our parents and grandparents used to go to the elder-tree which was close at hand, and which served them so cheaply and often much better than the expensive grapes. Some years ago, I was among the Austrian Alps, and saw there to my great joy how the elder -tree was still honoured. "Of that," said on old peasant to me, "we do not let a single berry go to waste." How simple, how sensible! Even the birds before they commence their autumnal travels seek out everywhere the elder-trees in order to purify their blood and strengthen their nature for their long journey. What a pity that man, on account of art and affectation no longer feels or takes notice of all these natural instincts,"the sound mind !"

If the berries are boiled down with sugar, or better still with honey, they will prove especially good in winter time for people who have but little exercise and are condemned to a sedentary mode of life. A spoonful of the above preserve stirred in a glass of water, makes the most splendid cooling and refreshing drink, operates on the secretion of the urine, and has a good effect on the kidneys.

Many country people dry the berries. But whether these dried berries are boiled as porridge, or stewed eat, or eaten dry, in all forms they are an excellent remedy against violent diarrhoea. Because the exceedingly good services rendered by the elder-tree, are no longer remembered; this faithful and formerly so highly esteemed house-hold friend is in many ways rejected. May the old friend be brought once more to honour!

Dwarf Elder. (Sambucus ebulus L.)

On the borders of woods, especially in parts which have been thinned, the dwarf elder may be seen standing above three feet high, bearing in July the great white umbellar blossoms, and in autumn the splendid, heavy, and bright umbellar grapes. Tea prepared from such roots, expels the water, and purifies the kidneys, it is therefore of extraordinary effect in cases of dropsy. I know several cases in which the rather advanced disease has been entirely cured by such tea. Also against other complaints in the abdomen, springing from bad juices, it operates well: it removes the juices through the urine. Dwarf-elder tea prepared from the powder has the same effect. For one cup of tea, which should be taken in two doses at different parts of the day, a pinch of this powder will be sufficient. Late in autumn the roots are gathered and thoroughly dried in the air, and then the dried roots themselves, or the powder made by crushing them, are kept in the house dispensary.

Brother Aloysius wrote of Elder and Dwarf Elder:

Elder flowers are undoubtedly the most well known diaphoretic in use and cam be successfully employed at the onset of all kinds of chills. The inner rind of one year old shoots, mixed with half a quantity of licorice, is an excellent remedy for dropsy. The leaves drunk as tea, are a depurative. The infusion should contain $1/4^{th}$ to $1/3^{rd}$ cup per two cups boiling water.

The well known elder syrup can be made from berries picked in autumn. The infusion of elder flowers contains 4 to 5 tablespoons per two cups boiling water. Elder flowers boiled in milk with a slice of white bread soaked in it, applied between linen cloths on burning eyes soon draws out all burning; sore eyes are also soon healed by this remedy. A good laxative is 4 to 5 teaspoons of elder berries. Elder leaves, boiled in milk, are beneficial for scurf; they are depurative and laxative. The dosage is 1 to 2 cups daily.

Dwarf Elder:

The root is used medicinally and should be gathered in July. The decoction contains 1 to 2 tablespoons per 2 cups water and is very beneficial for the treatment of dropsy. A larger dose acts as a purgative. Gout and podagra are soon cured by the application of elder root, boiled for quite a long time in wine dregs. Flowers and leaves, boiled to a paste, are highly recommended for sciatica, rheumatism and paralysis. This, alone, will cure these complaints. It can also be fruitfully used in the treatment of neuralgia.

Resources of the Southern Fields and Forests states:

The juice of the root has been highly recommended in dropsy as a hydragogue cathartic, sometimes acting as an emetic, in the dose of a tablespoonful, repeated every day with less frequency if it act with violence. Dr. Stratton, of New Jersey, uses a syrup in place of Sarsaparilla, made with the juice of the berries. New Jersey Med. Rep., vii, 466. U. S. Disp. The flowers are excitant and sudorific, and are used in the form of an ointment as a discutient. The inner bark is a hydragogue cathartic and emetic, acting well in drops', and as an alterative in various chronic diseases. The purgation which results from its employment is sometimes, however, too severe. The berries are diaphoretic and aperient and are used as a remedy in rheumatic gout and syphilitic affections. The juice of these diluted with water furnishes a cooling and valuable laxative drink. This plant is employed to some extent in domestic practice for the purposes severally referred to above. A decoction made by pouring boiling water over the leaves, flowers or berries of the elder is recommended as a wash for wounds to prevent injury from flies. An ointment used for the same purpose is prepared by stirring the elder or mixing the juice into lard while boiling, and straining through a coarse sieve. Beeswax may be added. Surg. S. E. Chambers reports in the Confed. States Med. Journal, Jan., 1865. that he has used the following ointment with complete success in at least one hundred cases of camp itch. In ordinary cases it will cure in one week. The patient is first made to wash well with soap and water, to dry the parts affected, and then to rub the ointment on the parts affected with the hand until it is absorbed. One pound of the inner bark of the elder, in two and a half pints of water is boiled down to one quarter of a pint. Then one pound of lard and four ounces of sweet gum are added, evaporate the water and at the same time skim whatever filth may rise to the top of the vessel, after which set it aside to cool. When thoroughly cool add two ounces of basilicon ointment, three of olive oil and half an ounce of flour of sulphur. See, also, Phylotacca decandra, Poke. According to Mr. Cozzens, the ripe berries afford a deli- cate test for acids and alkalies. The elder berry stewed with copperas, vinegar and alum, makes, as I have seen, an excellent ink and a dye.

King's American Dispensatory, 1898 tells us:

Action, Medical Uses, and Dosage.—Sambucus is stimulant to all of the emunctories, increasing secretion. In warm infusion, elder flowers are diaphoretic and gently stimulant; in cold infusion, they are diuretic, alterative, and cooling, and may be used in all diseases requiring such action, as in hepatic derangements of children, erysipelas, erysipelatous diseases, etc. In infusion, with maidenhair and beech-drops, they will be found very valuable in all erysipelatous diseases. The expressed juice of the berries, evaporated to the consistence of a syrup, is a valuable aperient and alterative; 1 ounce of it will purge. An infusion of the young leaf-buds is likewise purgative, and sometimes acts with violence. The flowers and expressed juice of the berries have been beneficially employed in scrofula, cutaneous diseases, syphilis, rheumatism, etc. The inner green bark is cathartic; an infusion of it in wine or cider, or the expressed juice, will purge moderately, in doses of from ½ to 1 fluid ounce; large doses produce emesis; in small ones, it proves an efficient deobstruent, promoting all the fluid secretions, and is much used in dropsy, especially that following scarlatina, and other febrile and exanthematous diseases, as well as in many chronic diseases. Specific Sambucus is largely used as an alterative where there is a tendency to unhealthy deposits in, or depravation of the tissues. The chief indication for sambucus is a fullness or oedematous condition of the parts, giving them a watery and flabby appearance. In these conditions it is a valuable agent in dropsy. Webster asserts that small doses of specific sambucus are valuable in the catarrhal nasal obstructions of infants. The juice of the root in 1 ounce doses, daily, acts as a hydragogue cathartic and diuretic, and will be found valuable in dropsical affections requiring purgation.

Externally, sambucus is a valuable agent, especially for eruptions which appear upon the full, flabby, oedematous tissues as described above, and particularly when attended with abundant discharge of serum. Beaten up with lard or cream, it forms an excellent discutient ointment, which is of much value in burns, scalds, and some cutaneous diseases, such as eczema, milk-scall, old ulcers, with soft, oedematous edges and free secretion of serum, and in mucous patches, with free discharges. The dose of specific sambucus ranges from 1 to 60 drops; decoction (inner bark, 2 ounces, to water, 1 quart, boiled down to 1 pint), from 2 to 4 fluid ounces.

Specific Indications and Uses.—In skin affections, when the tissues are full, flabby, and oedematous; epidermis separates and discharge of serum is abundant, forming crusts; indolent ulcers, with soft, oedematous borders; mucous patches, with free secretions; post-scarlatinal dropsy; low deposits in, or depravation of tissues.

Plants for A Future states:

Medicinal use of Elder: The plant has medicinal qualities. No further details are given but these are the medicinal properties of the closely related S. ebulus:- The leaves are antiphlogistic, cholagogue, diaphoretic, diuretic, expectorant and laxative. The fruit is also sometimes used, but it is less active than the leaves. The herb is commonly used in the treatment of liver and kidney complaints. When bruised and laid on boils and scalds, they have a healing effect. They can be made into a poultice for treating swellings and contusions. The leaves are harvested in the summer and can be dried for later use. The root is diaphoretic, mildly diuretic and a drastic purgative. Dried, then powdered and made into a tea, it is considered to be one of the best remedies for dropsy. It should only be used with expert supervision because it can cause nausea and vertigo. A homeopathic remedy is made from the fresh berries or the bark. It is used in the treatment of dropsy.

The Rodale Herb Book states:

A delightful tea is made from the dried blossoms, and it is helpful for colds and to promote sleep. Elder has been used for many medical purposes, in skin lotions, facials and packs, and as an antiseptic for skin disease.

Elder was widely used by the American Indians, who applied the bark as an antidotal poultice to painful swellings and inflammations. There was some us of a bark tea to ease parturition and a tea made of the dried flowers as a febrifuge. The elder berries were listed in the official pharmacopoeias for a few years during the nineteenth century and the flowers for nearly a century long period spanning the nineteenth and twentieth centuries. The flowers were listed as mildly stimulant, carminative and diaphoretic.

The Physicians' Desk Reference for Herbal Medicine tells us:

Flowers and berries of Sambucus nigra and Sambucus canadensis are used to shorten the duration and severity of flu and cold, to treat eczema and other skin disorders, and to reduce pain and inflammation. Indications and usage approved by Commission E: cough/bronchitis, fevers and cold.. The drug is used for colds and coughs it is a sweat producing remedy for the treatment of feverish colds. Unproven uses: in folk medicine, elderflowers are used internally as a sudorific tea and for colds and other fevers conditions. Elder is also used as an infusion, a gargle, mouthwash and for respiratory disorders, such as coughs, head colds, laryngitis, flu, and shortness of breath. Elder is used occasionally by nursing mothers to increase lactation. Externally, herbal pillows are used for swelling and inflammation. Precautions and adverse reactions: only fully ripe purple berries are used, as red berries can be mildly toxic. Leaves, shoots, bark, roots and raw red berries contain a cyanogenic glycoside, sambunigrin, that can cause dizziness, headache, convulsions, gastrointestinal distress, nausea, vomiting, diarrhea and tachycardia. Bark lectins may stimulate hyperplasia of the small intestine. Data suggest Sambucus may be a source potential harm to diabetic patients in caution should be advised.

Sassafras, Sassafras albidum

Sassafras was once widely used in Herbal Medicine, and its export to Europe was among the first major industries in the North American colonies. Amy Stewart writing in The Drunken Botanist, mentions, "In 173, sassafras was described in an early history of the colonies as being used to 'promote perspiration, to attenuate thick and viscous humours, to remove obstructions, to cure the gout and the palsy,' Godfrey's Cordial, a popular 19th century cure-all, included molasses, sassafras oil and laudanum, an opium tincture."

Unfortunately, it has fallen out of use. The reasoning for this is due to government over-reach and (in my opinion) seriously flawed reasoning.

Frankly, I trust hundreds of years of trial and error by real people far more than I do scientists whose findings are based on giving outrageous amounts of highly concentrated substances to mice, that would have no practical equivalent in real world, human use. I use Sassafras. The old folks in the Appalachian Mountains, many of whom live to be around 100 years old and maintain health and vigor far longer than their "modern" counterparts, consider Sassafras a "Spring tonic". It is believed to cleanse the blood after a long winter of being stuck inside, breathing wood and coal smoke and eating preserved foods. They believe it strengthens immunity. I believe in their wisdom.

Mrs. Grieves listed the medicinal properties of Sassafras as:

Aromatic, stimulant, diaphoretic, alterative. It is rarely given alone, but is often combined with guaiacum or sarsaparilla in chronic rheumatism, syphilis, and skin diseases.

The oil is said to relieve the pain caused by menstrual obstructions, and pain following parturition, in doses of 5 to 10 drops on sugar, the same dose having been found useful in gleet and gonorrhoea.

Safrol is found to be slowly absorbed from the alimentary canal, escaping through the lungs unaltered, and through the kidneys oxidized into piperonalic acid.

A teaspoonful of the oil produced vomiting, dilated pupils, stupor and collapse in a young man.

It is used as a local application for wens and for rheumatic pains, and it has been praised as a dental disinfectant.

Its use has caused abortion in several cases.

Dr. Shelby of Huntsville stated that it would both prevent and remove the injurious effects of tobacco.

A lotion of rose-water or distilled water, with Sassafras Pith, filtered after standing for four hours, is recommended for the eyes.

Brother Aloysius wrote of Sassafras:

Sassafras is a tree that grows in North America. The bark and wood are used medicinally and have stimulating, diuretic, diaphoretic properties. Sassafras is recommended for catarrh, rheumatism and gout, scrofulous skin conditions, scurvy and dropsy. The decoction contains 1 tablespoon per 2 cups water. Dosage: 1 cup daily.

Resources of the Southern Fields and Forests states:

Sassafras (Laiirus).—Whilst engaged in active duties as Surgeon to the Holcombe Legion, whenever a soldier suffered from measles, pneumonia, bronchitis, or cold, his companion or nurse was directed to procure the roots and leaves of Sassafras, and a tea made with this supplied that of Flax Seed or Gum Arabic, The leaf of the Sassafras contains a great amount of mucilage.

After the conquest made by the Spaniards in Florida sassafras was used in the treatment of syphilis, the warm infusion being applicable in cutaneous disease, by acting on the emunctories. The root is employed in the Carolinas in combination with guaiac, sarsaparilla, and China briar, (Smilax.') in the formation of diet drinks. It is diaphoretic and diuretic, useful in rheumatism, and Alibert speaks highly of it in gout. The pith of the young branches, according to Eberle, contains a great deal of mucilage; which is " an exceedingly good application in acute ophthalmia, and no less useful in catarrhal and dysenteric affections;" it is not affected by alcohol; Griffith (Med. Bot. 552) also speaks favorably of it as an application to inflamed eyes, being effectual in the removal of the irritation so constant in this complaint. It is advantageously given as a demulcent drink in disorders of the re piratory organs, bowels and bladder; being more efficacious than that prepared from the leaves of Bene, (Sesamum Indicum.').

King's American Dispensatory, 1898 tells us:

Action, Medical Uses, and Dosage.—Sassafras is a warm, aromatic stimulant, alterative, diaphoretic, and diuretic. It is generally used in combination with other alteratives, particularly podophyllum, whose flavor it improves, in syphilitic affections, chronic rheumatism, scrofula, and many cutaneous eruptions. Stubborn cases require also the aid of vapor, spirit or sulphur baths. The mucilage of the pith (2 drachms to 1 pint of water) is used as a local application in acute ophthalmia, and is a demulcent drink in disorders of the chest, bowels, kidneys, and bladder. The oil, in doses of from 5 to 10 drops on sugar, is used to afford relief in the distressing pain attending menstrual obstructions, and that following parturition; also used in diseases of the kidneys and bladder. I have also derived some benefit from its internal use in gonorrhoea and obstinate gleet; 5 to 10 drops on sugar, 3 times a day (J. King), Externally, as a rubefacient, in painful swellings, sprains, bruises, rheumatism, etc., and is said to check the progress of gangrene. An infusion of the bark (℥j to hot water Oj) administered internally and applied externally is reputed an excellent treatment for rhus poisoning.

Rodale's Illustrated Encyclopedia of Herbs states:

The root bark contains antiseptic constituents, making it an effective remedy for skin wounds and sores. It has been recommended for relief from the itching of poison ivy and poison oak. The gummy core of the branches was once used to soothe tired eyes.

Plants for A Future states:

Medicinal use of Sassafras: Sassafras has a long history of herbal use. It was widely employed by many native North American Indian tribes who used it to treat a wide range of complaints, valuing it especially for its tonic effect upon the body. It is still commonly used in herbalism and as a domestic remedy. The root bark and root pith are alterative, anodyne, antiseptic, aromatic, carminative, diaphoretic, diuretic, stimulant and vasodilator. A tea made from the root bark is particularly renowned as a spring tonic and blood purifier as well as a household cure for a wide range of ailments such as gastrointestinal complaints, colds, kidney ailments, rheumatism and skin eruptions. The mucilaginous pith from the twigs has been used as a poultice or wash for eye ailments and is also taken internally as a tea for chest, liver and kidney complaints. An essential oil from the root bark is used as an antiseptic in dentistry and also as an anodyne. The oil contains safrole, which is said to have carcinogenic activity and has been banned from use in American foods - though it is less likely to cause cancer than alcohol. In large doses the oil is poisonous, causing dilated pupils, vomiting, stupor, collapse and kidney and liver damage. The oil has been applied externally to control lice and treat insect bites, though it can cause skin irritation

Peterson Field Guides Eastern and Central Medicinal Plants tells us:

Root bark tea a famous spring blood tonic an "blood purifier"; Also a folk remedy for stomach aches, gout, arthritis, high blood pressure, rheumatism, kidney ailments, colds, fevers, skin eruptions. The mucilaginous twig pith has been used as a wash or poultice for eye elements; also taken internally, in tea, for chest, bowel, kidney, and liver ailments. Leaves mucilaginous, once used to treat stomach aches, widely used as a base for soup stocks. Warning: safrole (found in oil of sassafras) reportedly is carcinogenic. Banned by FDA. Yet the safrole in a 12 ounce can of old-fashioned root beer is not as carcinogenic as the alcohol (ethanol) in a can of beer.

Botany In a Day states:

Sassafras is usually a small tree found on the edges of forests throughout the east the bark of the root was the first commercial product sent to Europe by the colonist. Its leaves are a key ingredient in gumbo. The leaves as well as the flowers and drupes make a nice tea. The root is recommended as a tea in traditional medicine to help people through transitions between seasons but also during life changes such as a new job or moving homes. Sassafras contains a volatile compound called safrole, which was shown to be carcinogenic in studies with rats and mice in the 1960s, leading to a banned by the FDA on the use of sassafras as a flavoring or food additive. Later research by James Duke debunked the earlier studies, but the ban is still in effect.

Sorbus americana, American Mountain-Ash or American Rowan

Twenty-three varieties of Sorbus have been found useful in Herbal Medicine: Sorbus alnifolia - Korean Mountain Ash, Sorbus americana - American Mountain Ash, Sorbus aria – Whitebeam, Sorbus aucuparia - Mountain Ash, Sorbus austriaca, Sorbus commixta, Sorbus decora - Showy Mountain Ash, Sorbus devoniensis - French Hales, Sorbus domestica - Service Tree, Sorbus gracilis, Sorbus hybrida - Swedish Service Tree, Sorbus intermedia - Swedish Whitebeam, Sorbus japonica, Sorbus lanata, Sorbus latifolia - French Hales, Sorbus mougeotii, Sorbus pohuashanensis, Sorbus sambucifolia, Sorbus scopulina - Western Mountain Ash Synonym: Sorbus sambucifolia, Sorbus sitchensis - Sitka Mountain Ash, Sorbus thibetica, Sorbus torminalis - Wild Service Tree, Sorbus vestita

The only variety native to my region is the American Mountain Ash or American Rowan. Although it is rarely seen around my home, this large member of the Rose Family grows in many parts of the Appalachian Mountains, and was once an important food source.... Now, mostly forgotten.

Dioscorides referred to Sorbus as "Uva":

Uva which are a yellowish colour and not yet ripe, first cut apart and dried in the sun, are astringent for the bowels, ground up and eaten as a meal. It is eaten instead of polenta, and a decoction of them (taken as a drink) does the same.

For Gerard, it was the Service Tree:

A. Service berries are cold and binding, and much more when they be hard, than when they are mild and soft: in some places they are quickly soft, either hanged in a place which is not altogether cold, or laid in hay or chaff: those services are eaten when the belly is too soluble, for they stay the same; and if they yield any nourishment at all, the same is very little, gross, and cold; and therefore it is not expedient to eat of these or other like fruits, nor to use them otherwise than in medicines.

B. These do stay all manner of fluxes of the belly, and likewise the bloody flux; as also vomiting: they stanch bleeding if they be cut and dried in the sun before they be ripe, and so reserved for use:

these we may use divers ways according to the manner of the grief and grieved part.

Culpepper also wrote of the Service Tree:

This grows to be a pretty large tree, whose branches are cloathed with winged leaves, somewhat like those of the ash-tree, consisting of seven or nine serrated pinnæ, each leaf terminating in an odd one. It has several clusters of five-leaved white flowers which are followed by fruit of the shape and bigness of a small pear, growing several together on foot-stalks and inch long; they are of a greenish colour, with a mixture of red, as they have been more or less exposed to the sun; of a rough, austere, choaky taste; but when ripe or mellow, sweet and pleasant.

It is under Saturn, and reckoned to be very restringent and useful for all kinds of fluxes; but when ripe, not altogether so binding. This fruit is seldom or never to be met with in our markets; and therefore, for a succedaneum, we use the following:

MANURED SERVICE TREE - The common service-tree will, in good ground, grow considerably tall, having a whitish bark, and leaves that differ from those of the former, in not being winged, but somewhat like the maple, though larger and longer, being cut into seven sharp-pointed and serrated segments, the two next the stalk being cut in deepest, of a pale green above, and whitish underneath. The flowers grow in clusters like the former, of a yellowish white colour; and the fruit is set in the same manner on long footstalks, more than as big again as the common haws; they are likewise umbilicated at the top, of a harsh restringent taste when green, but when mellowed, sweet and pleasant, having a stony substance in the middle, including two seeds.

Place: It grows frequently in woods and thickets, and flowers with the former, the fruit being ripe as late.

Government and virtues. It is under the dominion of Saturn. The fruit, as I said, is used for the former, being of the same nature, or rather more restringent and binding, being good for all kinds of fluxes, either of blood or homours; when ripe, it is pleasant and grateful to the stomach, promoting digestion, and preventing the too hasty passage of the food out of the bowels; and is commended in fevers attended with a diarrhœa. If they be dried before they be mellow, and kept all teh year, they may be used in decoctions for the same purpose, either to drink, or to bathe the parts requiring it; and are profitably used in that manner to stay the bleeding of wounds, and of the mouth or nose, to be applied to the forehead, and nape of the neck.

Brother Aloysius wrote of Mountain Ash:

Rowan berries are astringent. The sap was formerly recommended for vomiting and heavy bleeding.

King's American Dispensatory, 1898 tells us:

Action, Medical Uses, and Dosage.—The ripe fruit of sorbus, when infused with water, furnishes an acidulous and astringent gargle for acute diseases of the pharyngeal vault and tonsils, with excessive secretion. The bark and the unripe fruit are employed in infusion, or decoction in scurvy and diarrhoea, and topically to relaxations of the anal or vaginal walls and throat, all with profuse secretion. The very astringent qualities of sorbus render it a good agent for poultices when one of such a character is desired.

Related Species.—Pyrus Americana, De Candolle (Sorbus Americana, Marshall), and the Pyrus sambucifolia, Chamisso et Schlechtendal (Sorbus sambucifolia, Roemer), are two indigenous species resembling the European tree but bearing smaller fruits. Both are known as American mountain ash.

Crataegus.—The bark, fruit, and leaves of this genus of plants are sometimes employed as astringents and tonics. (See also Crataegus Oxyacantha.)

Pyrus coronaria, Linné, Crab apple, Pyrus arbutifolia, Linné filius, Chokeberry. Both of these species have the properties of sorbus.

Peterson Field Guides Eastern and Central Medicinal Plants tells us:

American Indians used tea from ripe fruit for scurvy, worms, tea made from inner bark or buds for colds, debility, boils, diarrhea, tonsillitis; also as a blood purifier, appetite stimulant; Astringent, tonic.

Staphylea trifolia, Bladder Nut

Five varieties of Staphylea have been found useful in Herbal Medicine: Staphylea bumalda, Staphylea colchica - Bladdernut, Staphylea emodi, Staphylea pinnata - Bladder Nut, Staphylea trifolia - American Bladder Nut

Only one Staphylea is native to my region, Staphylea trifolia (American Bladdernut). Like many uniquely American trees that are unique to a region, I cannot find much information on its medicinal use. Plants for A Future states only, "An infusion of the powdered bark has been used as a wash for sore faces."   Although, the seed is edible and said to be quite good."

Resources of the Southern Fields and Forests tells us:

STAPHYLEACEJD. {Bladder-nut Family.)

THEEE LEAVED BLADDER-NUT, (Staphylea trifolia, L.)

Damp woods. North Carolina, Tennessee and northward (Chap.) The nut of our tree resembles closely that of the S. pinnata, which is used in Catholic countries for making rosaries. Rosaries are also made of the seeds of the Pride of India tree, {Melia.) The nuts of the S. trifoliata resemble a large, inflated bladder. Cyrilla racemlflora, Walter. Grows in swamps and inundated lands; collected in St. John's, where it is found in abundance; vicinity of Charleston ; Newbern. Fl. July. Ell. Bot. Med. Notes, i, 295. The outer bark of the oldest shrubs, near the root, is extremely light and friable, and absorbs moisture. It has been used with advantage as a substitute for agaric and other styptics. I learn that it is much confided in for this purpose by those living in Darlington District, South Carolina. When rubbed on the hand, it produces a sensation similar to that produced by the application of an astringent fluid. It has also been applied to ulcers when the indication is to cicatrize them. This plant merits further attention. TITI, {Cliftonia ligxistrina, Banks. Mylocarium, Wild.) Pine barren ponds and swamps, Florida and lower districts of South Carolina and Georgia. The stems, when dried, are found to suit admirably for pipe- stems—a heated wire being passed through the pith. Much used by our soldiers in camps ; and now (1868) becoming to some extent an article of trade.

Stewartia

We have two varieties of Stewartia native to our region, Stewartia ovata (Mountain-Camellia) and Stewartia ovata (Mountain-Camellia). These are members of the Tea family, the Camelias and likely have medicinal use, although I have yet to find any documentation.

Styrax, Snowbell

Three varieties of Styrax have been found useful in Herbal Medicine: Styrax japonica - Japanese Storax, Styrax officinalis - Storax Tree, Styrax serrulatus

Two varieties of Styrax are native to my region, but they are not listed above: Styrax americanus (American Snowbell), Styrax grandifolius (Bigleaf Snowbell). They likely share similar properties, but will need further study. Plants for A Future lists Styrax as simply, "A resin obtained from the stems of the plant is antiseptic and expectorant."

Dioscorides wrote of Styrax:

Styrax is the oozing of a certain tree like a quince tree. The best is yellow, fat, full of resin, having white under the clots, which remains a long time in its sweet sauce, and which when it is softened releases a certain honeyish kind of moisture. The gabalites, pissiadicus and the cilicius are like this. That which is black, brittle and like bran (or encrusted) is worthless. An oozing like the gum is also found (transparent like myrrh but there is only a little that grows of this. They counterfeit it with powder from the same tree (made by the boring of worms) by mixing honey with it and the thick matter of iris and certain other things. Some also aromatise wax or tallow in the sharpest sun, work it together with styrax, and press it out into cold water through a colander with broad holes (making as it were little worms of it), and they sell it, calling it vermiculatum [now a name for gum of acacia thorns]. Those who are unskilful approve of it as authentic, not noticing the weak intensity of the smell, for that which is without deceit is very sharp. It is warming, softening and digestive. It cures coughs and dripping mucus, runny noses, hoarseness and loss of the voice. It is good for closures and hardness in the vulva, and taken as a drink and applied it dries out the menstrual flow. It gently softens the bowels if a little of it is swallowed down with resin terminthos. It is also effective mixed with dispersing ointments or plasters and acopon [fatigue removers]. It is burned, roasted, scorched and made into a soot like thus and this soot is good for the same things as thus. But the ointment styracinum [also refered to as oil of crocus] which is made from it in Syria warms and powerfully softens; but it causes pain, heaviness of the head and sleep.

Gerard Listed Storax as:

A. It helpeth the cough, the falling down of rheums and humours into the chest, and hoarseness of the voice: it also helpeth the noise and sounding of the ears, prevaileth against strumas, or the King's evil, nodes on the nerves, and hard swellings proceeding of a cold cause: it prevaileth also against all cold poisons, as Hemlocks and such like.

B. Of this gum there are made sundry excellent perfumes, pomanders, sweet waters, sweet bags, and sweet washing balls, and divers other sweet chains & bracelets, whereof to write were impertinent to this history.

Culpepper wrote of the Storax Tree:

This is a Solar plant, and only the gum is used. It is hot in the second degree, and dry in the first. It heals, molifies, and digests, and is good for coughs, catarrhs, distillations of rheum and hoarseness. Pills thereof, with a little turpentine, gently loosen the belly. It resists cold poisons. Dropped into the ears, it helps the singing and noise in them. Applied to parts afflicted with cold aches, *it gives much comfort and ease, and is good to be put in baths for lameness and weakness. It is also good to put with white frankincense to perfume those that have catarrhs, rheums, and defluxions from the head to the nose, or other parts, by casting it on quick coals, and holding the head over the smoke. It dissolves hard tumours in any part, and is good for the king's evil.*

Mrs. Grieves wrote of Storax as:

A stimulating expectorant and feeble antiseptic, at present very seldom used except as a constituent of the compound tincture of benzoin. Externally, mixed with 2 or 3 parts of olive oil, it has been found a useful local remedy in scabies. It has the same action as balsams of Tolu and Peru and benzoin. It has been recommended as a remedy in diphtheria, in pulmonic catarrhs, and as a substitute for South American copaiba in gonorrhoea and leucorrhoea. Combined with tallow or lard, it is valuable for many forms of skin disease, such as ringworm, especially in children. The taste and smell of opium is well concealed by the addition of Storax in pills, its fragrance being used frequently also in ointments.

King's American Dispensatory, 1898 tells us:

Action, Medical Uses, and Dosage.—Storax is a stimulant, acting more especially upon mucous tissues, as do nearly all balsams. It has been found beneficial as an expectorant in cough, chronic catarrh, asthma, bronchitis, and other pulmonary affections; also in gonorrhoea, leucorrhoea, and gleet, in which it is as efficient, and more pleasant than copaiba. In fact the uses of storax are very similar to those of the latter balsam. Combined with tallow or lard, it forms a valuable application in many forms of cutaneous disease, especially those common to children, as ringworm, tinea, ringworm of the scalp, scabies, etc. It forms a good application for ulcerations, the result of freezing the fingers or toes. It is much used, on account of its fragrance, for compounding ointments and pills, and is an excellent addition to opium in the form of pill, when it is necessary to conceal the taste and smell of this narcotic; 3 or 4 grains of storax may be combined with 1 grain of opium for this purpose. The dose of storax is from 10 to 20 grains, gradually increased.

Symplocos, Sweet Leaf

Four varieties of Symplocos have been found useful in Herbal Medicine: Symplocos microcalyx, Symplocos paniculata - Asiatic Sweetleaf, Symplocos sumuntiia, Symplocos tinctoria - Sweet Leaf

Native to my region is Symplocos tinctoria (Sweetleaf). Of Sweetleaf, Plants for A Future merely states, "The bitter, aromatic roots have been used as a tonic. A decoction of the scraped roots has been used in the treatment of fevers."

Tamarix, Tamarisk

Fourteen varieties of Tamarisk have been found useful in Herbal Medicine: Myricaria elegans, Myricaria germanica, Myricaria squamosa, Reaumuria hypericoides, Tamarix Africana, Tamarix anglica - English Tree, Tamarix aphylla - Athel Tamarisk, Tamarix canariensis, Tamarix gallica - Manna Plant, Tamarix hispida - Kashgar Tree, Tamarix chinensis - Chinese Tamarisk, Tamarix juniperina, Tamarix parviflora - Small-Flowered Tamarisk, Tamarix ramosissima

The number of Tamarisk trees naturalized in my region surprised me: Tamarix canariensis (Canary Island Tamarisk), Tamarix chinensis (Chinese Tamarisk), Tamarix gallica (French Tamarisk), Tamarix parviflora (Smallflower Tamarisk), Tamarix ramosissima (Saltcedar)

Tamarisk was widely used in the ancient world, and continued to be popular well into the middle ages, as it includes the "Myrica Gale" that was a popular and highly intoxicating ingredient in beer before Saint Hildegard popularized hops as the primary bittering agent.

Dioscorides wrote of Tamarisk:

Myrica or myrris is a well-known tree, growing in marshy grounds and standing waters, with a fruit as a flower, of a mossy consistency. Some of it is planted in gardens in Egypt — in other things like the wild, but it bears fruit like a gall [excrescence on oak trees], unequally astringent to the taste, and used instead of galls in medicines for the mouth, eyes and spitting of blood. It is given in drink to women troubled with colic, those who have a flowing-forth from the vulva or sickness of the head, and for those bitten by phalangii [harvest spiders]. Applied as a poultice it stops oedema. The bark does the same things, as well as the fruit. A decoction of the leaves (taken as a drink with wine) melts the spleen, and gargled in the mouth it helps toothache. For hip baths it is good for women troubled with a discharge of fluids from the vulva, and a heated rub of it is good for those with lice and nits. Ash from the wood (applied) stops flows from the uterus. There are some who make cups from the wood which they use for those troubled with spleen (as though the drink given them from such cups should do them good).

Gerard wrote of French Tamarisk and German Tamarisk:

A. Tamarisk hath a cleansing and cutting faculty with a manifest drying; it is also somewhat astringent or binding, and by reason of these qualities it is very good for an hard spleen, being boiled with vinegar or wine, either the root or leaves, or tender branches, as Galen writeth.

B. Moreover Dioscorides teacheth, that the decotion of the leaves made with wine, doth waste the spleen, and that the same is good against the toothache, if the mouth be washed therewith: that it bringeth down the menses, if the patient sit therein; that it killeth lice and nits, if the parts be bathed therewith.

C. The ashes of burnt Tamarisk hath a drying faculty, and greatly scouring withal, and a little binding.

D. The flowers and downy seed of the greater Tamarisk doth greatly bind, infomuch as it cometh very near to the gall named galla omphacitis, but that the roughness of taste is more evident in the gall; the which flowers are of an unequal temperature, for there is joined to the nature thereof a great thinness of parts, and cleansing faculty, which the gall hath not, as Galen writeth.

These flowers we fitly use (saith Dioscorides) instead of gall, in medicines for the eyes and mouth.

F. It is good to stanch blood, and to stay the lask and women's whites, it helpeth the yellow jaundice, and also cureth those that are bit of the venomous spider called Phalangium; the bark serveth for the same purposes.

G. The leaves and wood of Tamarisk have great power and virtue against the hardness and stopping of the spleen, especially the leaves being boiled in water, and the decoction drunk, or else infused in a small vessel of ale or beer, and continually drunk: and if it tbe drunk forth of a cup or dish made of the wood or timber of Tamarisk, is of greater efficacy.

Culpepper wrote:

Government and virtues. A gallant Saturnine herb it is. The root, leaves, young branches, or bark boiled in wine, and drank, stays the bleeding of the hæmorrhodical veins, the spitting of blood, the too abounding of women's courses, the jaundice, the cholic, and the biting of all venomous serpents, except the asp; and outwardly applied, is very powerful against the hardness of the spleen, and the tooth-ache, pains in the ears, red and watering eyes. The decoction, with some honey put thereto, is good to stay gangrenes and fretting ulcers, and to wash those that are subject to nits and lice. Alpinus and Veslingius affirm, That the Egyptians do with good success use the wood of it to cure the French disease, as others do with lignum vitæ or guiacum; and give it also to those who have the leprosy, scabs, ulcers, or the like. Its ashes doth quickly heal blisters raised by burnings or scaldings. It helps the dropsy, arising from the hardness of the spleen, and therefore to drink out of cups made of the wood is good for splenetic persons. It is also helpful for melancholy, and the black jaundice that arise thereof. The ancients believed that swine which fed out of a trough made of this wood, would have no milk. The bark is sometimes used for the rickets in children.

An Irish Herbal states:

The wood, bark and leaves are very good for all disorders of the spleen. Drinking a decoction opens obstructions and is good for coughs and catarrh.

Taxodium

Only one variety of Taxodium is native to my region, Taxodium ascendens (Pond-cypress), but another introduced variety is fairly common, Taxodium distichum (Bald-cypress).

Of Taxodium, Herbs for A Future mentions only the Swamp Cyress (Taxodium distichum), "The resin in the cones is used as an analgesic for wounds."

Tilia, Basswood or Lime

Thirteen varieties of Tilia have been found useful in Herbal Medicine: Tilia americana - American Basswood, Tilia amurensis, Tilia caroliniana - Carolina Basswood, Tilia cordata - Small Leaved Lime, Tilia heterophylla - White Basswood, Tilia chinensis, Tilia japonica - Japanese Lime, Tilia mongolica - Mongolian Lime, Tilia oliveri Synonym: Tilia pendula, Tilia platyphyllos - Large Leaved Lime, Tilia tomentosa - Silver Lime, Tilia tuan,Tilia x europaea - Common Lime

Three Tilias are native to my region: Tilia americana var. americana (American Basswood), Tilia americana var. caroliniana (Carolina Basswood), Tilia americana var. heterophylla (White Basswood)

It should be pointed out that the Tilias called "Lime Tree" are not the citrus trees that bear lime fruit. These trees are predominately called Lime in Europe. They are an important part of the European herbal tradition, so I will include their use along with our native Basswoods. These are trees in the Linden family and are often simply called Linden.

Saint Hildegard von Bingen wrote of Linden:

A person who ails in his heart should take the interior branches of linden root and reduce it to a powder. He should eat this powder often with bread, and his heart will be better. ...In summer, place fresh leaves of linden over your eyes when you go to sleep, and cover your whole face with them. This will clarify your eyes and make them clean. If you are vigichtiget, you should take the earth which lies around the root of the linden, and put it on the fire. Pour water over it when it is hot, and so bathe in a sauna. Do this for nine days, and you will be cured.

Mrs. Grieves writes of Lime Tree:

Medicinal Action and Uses---Lime-flowers are only used in infusion or made into a distilled water as household remedies in indigestion or hysteria, nervous vomiting or palpitation. Prolonged baths prepared with the infused flowers are also good in hysteria.

In the Pyrenees they are used to soothe the temporary excitement caused by the waters, and M. Rostan has used them with success against spasms. The flowers of several species of Lime are used.

Some doctors prefer the light charcoal of lime wood to that of the poplar in gastric or dyspeptic disturbances, and its powder for burns or sore places.

If the flowers used for making the tisane are too old they may produce symptoms of narcotic intoxication.

Fr. Kneipp wrote of Lime Tree:

(Tilia grandifolia and parvifolia Ehrh)

It is almost solely the elderly people of the old school who still gather the once so well liked limetree blossoms. They are quite right and need only remain conservative with regard to their old custom. Lime-blossom-tea together with elder- blossom-tea are the best known teas for producing perspiration. Concerning perspiring, as it is usually carried on, I have my own particular opinion, which is not at all in its favour. On the other hand, I willingly use the blossoms for the vapours which produce, and supply the place of perspiration.

Lime-blossom-tea has excellent effects on such complaints as old coughs, obstructions of the lungs and wind-pipes, troubles of the abdomen which have their origin in obstructions of phlegm in the kidneys. Instead of the limetree- blossoms, I use the St. John's-wort with or without admixture of common yarrow; see St. Johns-wort.

Brother Aloysius wrote of Lime tree:

The blossom of the lime tree is used medicinally for dizziness, migraines, indigestion, chills, nervous complaints; this teas is highly recommended for old people in particular. The infusion contains

1/8 to ¼ cup per 2 cups boiling water. Hot lime blossom baths are highly recommended for convulsions in children. Charcoal powder from lime wood is best for internal use. A cup of lime blossom tea in the evening with ½ to 1 spoonful of honey is very depurative, strengthens the heart, is good for the nerves and promotes sleep. In addition, lime tea is recommended for nervous complaints in general; also for hysteria, hypochondria, migraines, epilepsy, indigestion, colic, coughs, chills, shivering, and to avoid strokes.

Resources of the Southern Fields and Forests tells us:

The flowers of our American Tilia, sent to me from Pendleton District, S. C, I find quite as useful as the imported " Tilleul," a material for quieting, anti-spasmodic teas, which I have repeatedly seen prescribed in France. It is particularly grateful and soothing to lying-in women: quieting nervous excitement, and pleasant to the taste. I would particularly recommend a larger use of these flowers in the Southern States. It can be used wherever a tea is required.

King's American Dispensatory, 1898 tells us:

Action, Medical Uses, and Dosage.—The European species (Tilia europaea) is a common domestic remedy in Europe for the relief of many nervous and catarrhal disorders. The leaves, flowers, and buds are employed, and their properties may be regarded as stimulant, lenitive, tonic, and nervine. The infusion is generally preferred, and may be given to allay irritation and restlessness, and to promote rest and sleep. The hot infusion is employed to check diarrhoea from cold, and in the various forms of colds and catarrhal conditions, while, either hot or cold, it may be used in restlessness, nervous headaches, painful and difficult digestion, and mild hysteria. The effects upon the nervous system are sometimes obtained by an enema, or bath, prepared from the flowers. The infusion is prepared from 30 or 40 grains of the flowers and 1 pint of water. It forms an agreeable vehicle for other medicines. A strong tincture may be prepared of the flowers (℥viij) and strong alcohol (Oj). Dose, 1 to 20 minims. The other species undoubtedly possess similar properties.

Euell Gibbons tells us:

The use of dried flowers of linden or basswood for making a tea-like hot drink is widespread. The French enjoy a number of herbal tisanes, and that made from linden blossoms is one of their favorites..... Medicinally, it is reported to be calmative and restorative, being given as a home remedy for nervousness, hysteria, insomnia and cramps.

Plants for A Future states of Basswood:

Medicinal use of American Basswood: A tea made from the inner bark is applied to burns - it soothes and softens the skin. It is taken internally in the treatment of lung complaints, dysentery, heart burn and weak stomach. The bark is diuretic. An infusion has been taken to promote urination. A decoction of the bark, mixed with cornmeal, has been used as a poultice to draw out boils. A tea made from the fresh or dried flowers is antispasmodic, diaphoretic and sedative. It is used in the treatment of hypertension, hardening of the arteries, digestive complaints associated with anxiety, feverish colds, respiratory catarrh, migraine etc. Lime flowers are said to develop narcotic properties as they age and so they should only be harvested when freshly opened. An infusion of the leaves has been used as an eyewash. A poultice of the leaves has been used in the treatment of burns and scalds, broken bones and swollen areas. A tea or tincture made from the leaves, flowers and buds has traditionally been used for nervous headaches, restlessness and painful digestion. Use with caution, see notes above on toxicity. A decoction of the roots and the bark has been taken in the treatment of internal haemorrhaging. A decoction of the roots has been used as a vermifuge to rid the body of worms.

Medicinal use of Carolina Basswood: A tea made from the flowers is antispasmodic, diaphoretic and sedative.

Medicinal use of White Basswood: A tea made from the flowers is antispasmodic, diaphoretic and sedative. A decoction of the inner bark has been used in the treatment of dysentery. A decoction of the bark, mixed with cornmeal, has been used as a poultice in the treatment of boils. A decoction of the inner bark and twigs has been used during pregnancy to treat heartburn, weak stomach and weak bowels.

The Rodale Herb Book states:

Linden flowers and leaves are an old household remedy for nervousness, colds, headache and indigestion. A hot infusion is used to check diarrhea. It was also used in a hot bath to promote sleep. Linden flower wine is used as a tonic to stimulate appetite and aid digestion.

Peterson Field Guides Eastern and Central Medicinal Plants tells us:

American basswood: American Indians used inner bark tea for lung ailments, heartburn, weak stomach; Bark poultice draws out boils. Leaves, flower and bud tea, or tincture traditionally used for nervous headaches, restlessness, painful digestion. Warning: frequent consumption of flower tea may cause heart damage.

Botany In a Day states:

Tilia, Basswood, Linden tree: Linden trees are native to the eastern forest... medicinally, AT of the inner bark is soothing for burns. A tea of the dried flowers is expectorant, sedative, and diaphoretic an effect.

Tsuga, Hemlock

Five varieties of Tsuga have been found useful in Herbal Medicine: Tsuga canadensis - Canadian Hemlock, Tsuga caroliniana - Carolina Hemlock, Tsuga heterophylla - Western Hemlock, Tsuga chinensis - Chinese Hemlock, Tsuga mertensiana - Mountain Hemlock

Two varieties of Hemlock are native to my region: Tsuga canadensis (Eastern Hemlock) and Tsuga caroliniana (Carolina Hemlock)

It should be noted that these are Hemlock trees, not the "poison hemlock", which is an umbelliferous, herbaceous plant.

The Thomsonian System of Medicine states:

HEMLOCK. Canadensis. INNER BARK. (Dr. Thomson.)

This is the common hemlock tree, and grows in all parts of New England. The best medicine is to peel the bark from the young tree, and shave the dross from the outside, and preserve only the inner bark; dry it carefully, and pound or grind the rind to a powder. A tea made by putting boiling water to this bark is a good medicine for canker, and many other complaints. The first of my using hemlock bark as medicine was in 1814. Being in want of something for canker, I tried some of it by chewing, and found it to answer, and made use of it to good advantage. Since then, have made constant use of it, and have always found it a very good medicine, both for canker and other complaints of the bowels and stomach. A tea made of this bark is very good, and may be used freely ; it is good to give the emetic and No. 2 in, and may be used for drink in all cases of sickness, especially when going through a course of medicine and steaming. This, with bayberry bark and the lily root, forms No. 3, or what has been commonly called coffee, though many other things may be added, or either of them be used to advantage alone. The boughs, made into a tea, are very good for gravel and other obstructions of the urinary passages, and for rheumatism. The dose of the Fluid Ext. or Tincture is from 15 to 60 minims. One of the finest preparations made is Pinus Canadensis, made by the Rio Chemical Company of New York City. It is uniform in strength and gives entire satisfaction

Plants for A Future lists:

Medicinal use of Carolina Hemlock: The bark is astringent, diaphoretic and diuretic. A tea made from the inner bark or twigs is helpful in the treatment of kidney or bladder problems, and also makes a good enema for treating diarrhoea. It can also be used as a gargle or mouthwash for mouth and throat problems or externally to wash sores and ulcers. A poultice of the bark has been used to treat itchy armpits. The powdered bark can be put into shoes for tender or sweaty feet or for foot odour. An infusion of the stem tips has been used to treat kidney problems. A decoction of the roots has been used as a birthing aid to help expel the afterbirth. The roots have been chewed in order to treat diarrhoea.

Edible parts of Carolina Hemlock: Inner bark - raw or dried, ground into a powder and then used as a thickening in soups etc or mixed with cereals when making bread. The leaves and twigs yield "spruce oil", which is used commercially to flavour chewing gum, soft drinks, ice cream etc. A herbal tea is made from the young shoot tips. These tips are also an ingredient of "spruce beer".

Botany In a Day states:

Tsuga is astringent, diarrhetic, and diaphoretic. A tea of the bark or twigs is used for sore mouth or throat, and kidneys or bladder problems. Externally it is used as a wash for sores. The inner bark was reportedly used by the Native Americans for food in the springtime.

The Physicians' Desk Reference for Herbal Medicine tells us:

The active agents are the tannin, hemlock tannin, and picea tannols. The drug has astringent, anti-inflammatory, diaphoretic and diuretic properties. Unproven uses: pinus bark is used for digestive disorders, diarrhea, and diseases of the mouth and throat. It was formerly used to treat scurvy.

Ulmus, Elm

Fourteen varieties of Elm have been found useful in Herbal Medicine: Ulmus alata - Winged Elm, Ulmus americana - American Elm, Ulmus davidiana - Japanese Elm, Ulmus glabra - Wych Elm, Ulmus japonica – Japanese, Ulmus laciniata, Ulmus macrocarpa, Ulmus parvifolia - Chinese Elm, Ulmus procera - English Elm, Ulmus pumila - Siberian Elm, Ulmus rubra - Slippery Elm, Ulmus thomasii - Rock Elm, Ulmus villosa - Cherry Bark Elm, Ulmus wallichiana

Three Elms are native to my region: Ulmus alata (Winged Elm), Ulmus americana (American Elm), Ulmus rubra (Slippery Elm). Three Elms have been naturalized: Ulmus parviflora (Chinese Elm, Lacebark Elm), Ulmus procera (English Elm), Ulmus pumila (Siberian Elm)

Elm is likely the most commonly known and used tree in Herbal Medicine, due to the popularity of Slippery Elm. This common use has led Slippery Elm to be over-harvested in many areas.

Saint Hildegard von Bingen wrote of Elm:

One who is troubled by gicht should burn a fire with its wood only. Soon, he should warm himself by the fire, and the gicht will cease immediately. But for one who is virgichtiget, so tha this tongue fails to speak, fresh new leaves of this tree should be placed in water, and this should be given to him to drink. The gicht in his tongue will cease, and he will recover his speech. One who has freislich on his body should often drink the same water, tempered with those leaves, and the freislich will disappear. If someone burns this wood alone, heats water with it, and takes a bath with this water, it will take away malignity and bad will, and give him benevolence, and make his mind happy. The tree has a certain prosperity in its nature, so that spirits of the air are unable to move phantasms, wrongs, and illusions through it with their many wrathful confrontations.

While I do not know what freislich is… I certainly wish to avoid wrathful confrontations!

Gerard wrote:

A. The leaves and bark of the Elm be moderately hot, with an evident cleansing faculty; they have in the chewing a certain clammy and gluing quality.

B. The leaves of Elm glue and heal up green wounds, so doth the bark wrapped and swaddled about the wound like a bandage.

C. The leaves being stamped with vinegar do take away scurf.

D. Dioscorides writeth, that one ounce weight of the thicker bark drunk with wine or water purgeth phlegm.

E. The decoction of Elm leaves, as also of the bark or root, healeth broken bones very speedily, if they be fomented or bathed therewith.

F. The liquor that is found in the blisters doth beautify the face, and scoureth away all spots, freckles, pimples, spreading tetters, and such like, being applied thereto.

G. It healeth green wounds, and cureth ruptures newly made, being laid on with Spleenwoort and the truss closely set unto it.

Culpepper wrote, of the Government and Virtues of Elm Tree:

It is a cold and Saturnine plant. The leaves thereof bruised and applied heal green wounds, being bound thereon with its own bark. The leaves or the bark used with vinegar cureth scurf and leprosy very effectually: The decoction of the leaves, bark, or root, being bathed, heals broken bones. The water that is found in the bladders on the leaves, while it is fresh, is very effectual to cleanse the skin, and make it fair; and if cloths be often wet therein, and applied to the ruptures of children, it healeth them, if they be well bound up with a truss. The said water put into a glass, and set into the ground, or else in dung for twenty-five days, the mouth thereof being close stopped, and the bottom set upon a lay of ordinary salt, that the foces may settle and become clear, is a singular and sovereign balm for green wounds, being used with soft tents: The decoction of the bark of the root fomented, mollifieth hard tumours, and the shrinking of the sinews. The roots of the elm, boiled for a long time in water, and the fat arising on the top thereof being clean scummed off, and the place anointed therewith that is grown bald, and the hair fallen away, will quickly restore them again. The said bark ground with brine and pickle, until it come to the form of a poultice, and laid on the place pained with the gout, giveth great ease. The decoction of the bark in water, is excellent to bathe such places as have been burnt with fire.

Mrs. Grieves wrote of both "Common" and Slippery Elm:

(Common Elm) Medicinal Action and Uses---Tonic, demulcent, astringent and diuretic. Wasformerly employed for the preparation of an antiscorbutic decoction recommended in cutaneous diseases of a leprous character, such as ringworm. It was applied both externally and internally. Under the title of Ulmus the dried inner bark was official in the British Pharmacopoeia of 1864 and 1867 directions for the preparation of Decoc. Ulmi being as follows: Elm

Bark 1 part, water 8 parts; boil for 10 minutes, strain, make up to 8 parts.

A homoeopathic tincture is made of the inner bark, and used as an astringent.

Fluid extract, dose 2 to 4 oz. three or four times daily.

A medicinal tea was also formerly made from the flowers.

In Persia, Italy and the south of France, galls, sometimes the size of a fist, are frequently produced on the leaves. They contain a clear water called eau d'orme, which is sweet and viscid, and has been recommended to wash wounds, contusions and sore eyes. Culpepper tells us:

'the water that is found in the bladders on the leaves of the elm-tree is very effectual to cleanse the skin and make it fair.'

Towards autumn, these galls dry, the insects in them die and there is found a residue in the form of a yellow or blackish balsam, called beaume d'ormeau, which has been recommended for diseases of the chest.

(Slippery Elm) *Medicinal Action and Uses*---Demulcent, emollient, expectorant, diuretic, nutritive. The bark of this American Elm, though not in this country as in the United States an official drug, is considered one of the most valuable remedies in herbal practice, the abundant mucilage it contains having wonderfully strengthening and healing qualities.

It not only has a most soothing and healing action on all the parts it comes in contact with, but in addition possesses as much nutrition as is contained in oatmeal, and when made into gruel forms a wholesome and sustaining food for infants and invalids. It forms the basis of many patent foods.

Slippery Elm Food is generally made by mixing a teaspoonful of the powder into a thin and perfectly smooth paste with cold water and then pouring on a pint of boiling water, steadily stirring meanwhile. It can, if desired, be flavoured with cinnamon, nutmeg or lemon rind.

This makes an excellent drink in cases of irritation of the mucous membrane of the stomach and intestines, and taken at night will induce sleep.

Another mode of preparation is to beat up an egg with a teaspoonful of the powdered bark, pouring boiling milk over it and sweetening it.

Taken unsweetened, three times a day, Elm Food gives excellent results in gastritis, gastric catarrh, mucous colitis and enteritis, being tolerated by the stomach when all other foods fail, and is of great value in bronchitis, bleeding from the lungs and consumption (being most healing to the lungs), soothing a cough and building up and preventing wasting.

A Slippery Elm compound excellent for coughs is made as follows: Cut obliquely one or more ounces of bark into pieces about the thickness of a match; add a pinch of Cayenne flavour with a slice of lemon and sweeten, infusing the whole in a pint of boiling water and letting it stand for 25 minutes. Take this frequently in small doses: for a consumptive patient, about a pint a day is recommended. It is considered one of the best remedies that can be given as it combines both demulcent and stimulating properties. Being mucilaginous, it rolls up the mucous material so troublesome to the patient and passes it down through the intestines.

In typhoid fever, the Slippery Elm drink, prepared as for coughs, is recommended, serving a threefold purpose, to cleanse, heal and strengthen, the patient being allowed to drink as much as desired until thirst has abated, and other remedies can be used. If the patient is not thirsty, a dose of 2 large tablespoonfuls every hour for an adult has been prescribed.

The bark is an ingredient in various lung medicines. A valuable remedy for Bronchitis and all diseases of the throat and lungs is compounded as follows: 1 teaspoonful Flax seed, 1 OZ. Slippery Elm bark, 1 OZ. Thoroughwort, 1 stick Liquorice, 1 quart water. Simmer slowly for 20 minutes. Strain and add 1 pint of the best vinegar and 1/2 pint of sugar. When cold, bottle. Dose: 1 tablespoonful two or three times a day.

In Pleurisy, the following is also recommended: Take 2 oz. each of Pleurisy root, Marsh Mallow root, Liquorice root and Slippery Elm bark. Boil in 3 pints of water down to 3 gills. Dose: 1/2 teaspoonful every half-hour, to be taken warm.

As a heart remedy, a pint of Slippery Elm drink has been prescribed alternately with Bugleweed compound.

Slippery Elm bark possesses also great influence upon diseases of the female organs.

It is particularly valuable both medicinally and as an injection in dysentery and other diseases of the bowels, cystitis and irritation of the urinary tract. The injection for inflammation of the bowels is made from an infusion of 1 OZ. of the powder to 1 pint of boiling water, strained and used lukewarm. Other remedies should be given at the same time.

An injection for diarrhoea may also be made as follows: 1 drachm powdered Slippery Elm bark, 3 drachms powdered Bayberry, 1 drachm powdered Scullcap.

Pour on 1/2 pint of boiling water, infuse for half an hour, strain, add a teaspoonful of tincture of myrrh and use lukewarm.

As an enema for constipation, 2 drachms of Slippery Elm bark are mixed well with 1 OZ. of sugar, then 1/2 pint of warm milk and water and an ounce of Olive Oil are gently stirred in.

Injection for worms (Ascarides): 1/2 drachm Aloes powder, 1 drachm common salt, 1/2 drachm Slippery Elm powder (fine). When well mixed, add 1/2 pint warm water and sweeten with molasses, stirring well.

Slippery Elm mucilage is also prescribed to be mixed with Oil of Male Fern (2 oz. of the mucilage to 1 drachm of the oil) as a remedy for the expulsion of tapeworm

The Red Indians have long used this viscous inner bark to prepare a healing salve, and in herbal medicine a Slippery Elm bark powder is considered one of the best possible poultices for wounds, boils, ulcers, burns and all inflamed surfaces, soothing, healing and reducing pain and inflammation.

It is made as follows: Mix the powder with hot water to form the required consistency, spread smoothly upon soft cotton cloth and apply over the parts affected. It is unfailing in cases of suppurations, abscesses, wounds of all kinds, congestion, eruptions, swollen glands, etc. In simple inflammation, it may be applied directly over the part affected; to abscesses and old wounds, it should be placed between cloths. If applied to parts of the body where there is hair, the face of the poultice should be smeared with olive oil before applying.

In old gangrenous wounds, an excellent antiseptic poultice is prepared by mixing with warm water or an infusion of Wormwood, equal parts of Slippery Elm powder and very fine charcoal and applying immediately over the part.

A very valuable poultice in cases where it is desirable to hasten suppuration or arrest the tendency to gangrene is made by mixing the Slippery Elm powder with brewer's yeast and new milk.

Compound Bran poultice is made by mixing with hot vinegar equal quantities of wheaten Bran with Slippery Elm powder. This is an excellent poultice for severe rheumatic and gouty affections, particularly of the joints, synovitis etc.

Herbal poultices, generally made from the bruised, fresh leaves of special herbs, are frequently mixed with Slippery Elm and boiling water sufficient to give the mass consistency.

Marshmallow Ointment, one of the principal ointments used in herbal medicine, has a considerable proportion of Slippery Elm bark in its composition. It is made as follows: 3 oz. Marshmallow leaves, 2 OZ. Slippery Elm bark powder, 3 oz. Beeswax, 16 OZ. Lard. Boil the Marshmallow and Slippery Elm bark in 3 pints of water for 15 minutes. Express, strain and reduce the liquor to half a pint. Melt together the lard and wax by gentle heat, then add the extract while still warm, shake constantly till all are thoroughly incorporated and store in a cool place.

The bark of Slippery Elm is stated to preserve fatty substances from becoming rancid.

It has been asserted that a pinch of the Slippery Elm powder put into a hollow tooth stops the ache and greatly delays decay, if used as soon as there is any sign of decay.

Lozenges or troches containing 3 grains of Elm flavoured with methyl salicylate are used as a demulcent.

An Irish Herbal states:

The leaves and inner bark heal and consolidate wounds, bruises and fractured bones. The liquid that is found in the leaves removes freckles, pimples and spreading eruptions. The bark is abstersive and is frequently used in gargles for sore mouths and throats. The *inner bark, being scraped off and steeped in water for 24 hours, is exceedingly good to be applied to burns and scalds.*

Resources of the Southern Fields and Forests states:

SLIPPERY ELM, (Ulmus fulva.) I have observed it in Fairfield District. It is sometimes found in the lower districts, N. C. Am. Herbal. 139; Frost's Elems. Mat. Med. and Therap. 228; U. S. Disp. 727; Dr. McDowell's Med. Exam. 244; West Jour. Med. and Phys. Sc; Michaux, Fl. Americana, i, 172^; and N. Am. Sylva, iii, 89 ; Griffith, Med. Bot. 563. A decoction of the bark was much used by the Indians in the cure of leprosy. It is an excellent demulcent employed as an emollient application, and internally is especially recommended in suppression of urine, inflammation of the bladder, dysentery and diarrhea. A decoction made of this, combined with the root of the sassafras, and guaiac, is esteemed as a valuable drink to increase cutaneous transpiration, and to improve the tone of the digestive organs. Griffith considers it a good substitute for acacia, and he has witnessed its beneficial effects, externally applied, in obstinate cases of herpetic and syphilitic eruptions; he is inclined to ascribe higher curative powers to it than are generally admitted. It forms a good vehicle for enemata, where a mucilaginous fluid is required. The bark, cut in the form of a bougie, has been used in dilating sinuses and contractions of the urethra. The sub- stance exuding from the bark is called ulmin. It could be largely collected for the use of soldiers—suitable wherever a highly mucilaginous substance is required.

I append the following to the second edition: Dr. C. W. Wright, of Cincinnati, states (Western Lancet) that slippery elm bark has the property of preserving fatty substances from rancidity ; a fact derived originally from the Indians who prepared bear's fat by melting it with the bark in the proportion of a drachm of the latter to a pound of the former, keeping them heated together for a few minutes, and then straining off the fat. Dr. Wright tried the name process with butter and lard and found them to remain perfectly sweet for a long time. (Am. J. Pharm. xxiv, 180,) U. S. Disp. 12th Ed. Dr. McDowel, of Virginia, used the bark for the dilatation of fistulas and strictures, (Med. Exam, i, 244,) and Dr. H. E. Storer, of Boston, subsequently for dilating the os uteri. (Bost. Med. And Surg. J. liii, 300.) See U. S. Disp.

WHITE ELM, (Ulmus Americana, Mx.) Vicinity of Charleston; N. C. Mer. and de L. Diet, de M. Med. vi, 799 ; Coxe, Am. Disp. 611; Phil. Med. Mus. 11. The U. fulva probably referred to. The wood of the white elm, like that of the common European elm, is of a dark brown ; and cut transversely, or obliquely to the longitudinal fibres, it exhibits the same numerous and fine undulations, but it splits more easily and has less compactness. It is, however, used at the North for the naves of coach wheels, because it is difficult to procure the black gum. In Maine it is used for the keels of vessels. Its bark is said to be easily detached during eight months of the year; soaked in water and suppled by pounding, it is used in the Northern States for the bottoms of common chairs. Miehaux,

The Thomsonian System of Medicine states:

SLIPPERY ELM BARK. - Ulmus Fulva.

The inner bark of this tree is an article of much value, and may be used to advantage in many different ways. There are several species of the elm that grow common in this country, and there are two kinds of the slippery elm. In one the bark is rather hard and tough, and the other is very brittle; the latter is the best for medicinal uses. The bark should be peeled, the outside rind shaved off, dried, and ground or pounded to a fine powder. If used internally, put a teaspoonful of this powder into a teacup with as much sugar, mix them well together, then add a little cold water and stir it until perfectly mixed, and then put hot water to it and stir till it forms a jelly thick enough to be eaten with a spoon. A teacupful may be taken at a time, and is an excellent medicine to heal soreness in the throat, stomach and bowels, caused by canker; or more hot water may be put to it and made into a drink and freely taken for the same purpose. I have always made much use of this bark for poultices, and have in all cases found it a most excellent article for that purpose. Mixed with pounded cracker and ginger it makes the best poultices I have ever found for burns, scalds, felons, old sores, etc., it is the best thing that can be used to allay the inflammation, ease the pain and heal them in a short time. With Lobelia, it forms an excellent poultice for abscesses and boils. In constipation, dysentery, diarrhoea and cholera infantum, used both internally and per rectal injection, it soothes and relieves the intestinal irritation. It is a nutritious demulcent, soothing to the mucous membrane wherever needed and quieting to the nervous system. In diphtheria, after the throat has been ridded of the decayed membrane, it is quite raw, also during the scaling process in scarlatina and measles and at times in typhoid fever; slippery elm is then a very important agent.

King's American Dispensatory, 1898 tells us:

Action, Medical Uses, and Dosage.—Elm bark is nutritive, expectorant, diuretic, demulcent, and emollient, and is a very valuable remedial agent. In mucous inflammations of the lungs, bowels, stomach, bladder, or kidneys, used freely in the form of a mucilaginous drink (1 ounce of the powdered bark to 1 pint of water), it is highly beneficial, as well as in diarrhoea, dysentery, coughs, pleurisy, strangury, and sore throat, in all of which it tends powerfully to allay the inflammation. A tablespoonful of the powder boiled in a pint of new milk, affords a nourishing diet for infants weaned from the breast, preventing the bowel complaints to which they are subject, and rendering them fat and healthy. Some physicians consider the constant use of it, during and after the seventh month of gestation, as advantageous in facilitating and causing an easy delivery; ½ pint of the infusion to be drank daily. Elm bark has likewise been successfully employed externally in cutaneous diseases, especially in obstinate cases of herpetic and syphilitic eruptions, and certainly possesses more efficient virtues than are commonly supposed. As an emollient poultice, the bark has been found very serviceable when applied to inflamed parts, suppurating tumors, fresh wounds, burns, scalds, bruises, and ulcers; and in the excruciating pains of the testes, which accompany the metastasis of mumps, whether of recent or long standing, the constant use of an elm poultice, regularly changed every 4 hours, will be found a superior remedy. Notwithstanding its general value as an application to ulcers, it will often be found injurious, especially when used as a cataplasm to ulcers of the limbs, rendering the ulcer more irritable and difficult to heal, and frequently converting a simple sore, which might be cured by astringent or other washes, into an almost intractable ulcer; much care is, therefore, required in the application of this bark externally. As an injection, the infusion will prove useful in diarrhoea, dysentery, tenesmus, and hemorrhoids, also in gonorrhoea and gleet. The powder, sprinkled on the surface of the body, will prevent and heal excoriations and chafings, and allay the itching and heat of erysipelas. As the bark increases in bulk by imbibing moisture, it has been recommended to form bougies and tents of it for the dilatation of strictures, fistulas, etc., but in urethral strictures it has proved troublesome, from the liability of the part behind the stricture breaking off in the attempt to withdraw it, and passing into the bladder. The infusion of the bark is the common form of administration, and may be drank ad libitum (J. King). (See Mucilago Ulmi.)

Euell Gibbons tells us:

Medical books list the properties of slippery elm as demulcent, emollient, expectorant, diuretic, soothing and laxative. ...

The early settlers learned from the Indians how to sue slippery elm, and it became one of the most important home remedies in early America. ...It is very good for coughs, colds, influenza, pleurisy, quinsy, dysentery and painful menstruation.

Plants for A Future Lists:

Medicinal use of American Elm: An infusion made from the bark has been used in the treatment of bleeding from the lungs, ruptures, coughs, colds, influenza, dysentery, eye infections, cramps and diarrhoea. An infusion of the bark has been taken by pregnant women to secure stability of children. A decoction of the bark has been used as a wash on wounds. A decoction of the inner bark has been taken in the treatment of severe coughs, colds, menstrual cramps. An infusion of the inner bark has been drunk, and used as a bath, in the treatment of appendicitis. An infusion of the root bark has been used in the treatment of coughs, colds and excessive menstruation. A decoction has been used as an eye wash in the treatment of sore eyes. The inner bark has been used as an emollient on tumours.

Medicinal use of Slippery Elm: Slippery elm bark is a widely used herbal remedy and is considered to be one of the most valuable of remedies in herbal practice. In particular, it is a gentle and effective remedy for irritated states of the mucous membranes of the chest, urinary tubules, stomach and intestines. The inner bark contains large quantities of a sticky slime that can be dried to a powder or made into a liquid. The inner bark is harvested in the spring from the main trunk and from larger branches, it is then dried and powdered for use as required. Ten year old bark is said to be best. Fine grades of the powder are best for internal use, coarse grades are better suited to poultices. The plant is also part of a North American formula called essiac which is a popular treatment for cancer. Its effectiveness has never been reliably proven or disproven since controlled studies have not been carried out. The other herbs included in the formula are Arctium lappa, Rumex acetosella and Rheum palmatum. The inner bark is demulcent, diuretic, emollient, expectorant, nutritive. It has a soothing and healing effect on all parts of the body that it comes into contact with and is used in the treatment of sore throats, indigestion, digestive irritation, stomach ulcers etc. It used to be frequently used as a food that was a nutritive tonic for the old, young and convalescents. It was also applied externally to fresh wounds, burns and scalds. The bark has been used as an antioxidant to prevent fats going rancid.

Peterson Field Guides Eastern and Central Medicinal Plants us:

Slippery Elm: Three tablespoons of inner bark in a cup of hot water makes a thick, mucilaginous tea, traditionally used for sore throats, upset stomach, indigestion, digestive irritation, stomach ulcers, coughs, pleurisy, said to help in diarrhea and dysentery. Inner bark considered edible. Once used as a nutritive broth for children, the elderly, and convalescing patients who had difficulty consuming or digesting food. Externally the thick tea, made from powdered inner bark, was applied to fresh wounds, ulcers, burns, scalds. Science confirms tea is soothing to mucous membranes and softens hardened tissue. Bark once used as an antioxidant to prevent rancidity of fat.

Botany In a Day states:

Slippery Elm: the leaves are edible raw or cooked. The bark may be dried and ground into flour; it is used in times of scarcity. The green fruits are also edible. The slippery Elm, Ulmus fulva, is widely popular as a medicinal plant. The inner bark is highly mucilaginous and somewhat astringent. Other species may be more stringent and less mucilaginous. The Elm is used especially as a soothing remedy, externally as an emollient for burns or internally as a demulcent for sore throats or other internal *inflammations, including diarrhea. It is the kind of remedy that can be used for just about anything. A friend once gave me some in tea to reduce a fever on an expedition. I recall that it was very effective.*

The Physicians' Desk Reference for Herbal medicine tells us of Elm bark:

The drug has diuretic and astringent properties. Unproven uses: internally, the drug is used for digestive disorders and severe cases of diarrhea. Externally it is used to treat open wounds. No health hazards or side effects are known in conjunction with the proper administration of designated therapeutic doses

Vaccinium

Usually considered a bush or shrub, Vaccinum includes such well known and beloved plants as blue berry. But, native to my region is also the Vaccinium arboreum (Sparkleberry, Farkleberry). This bush grows large enough to be considered as a small tree. While other members of this family have wide medicinal use, that is a subject for a future book (God willing). Of the delightfully named Farkleberry, Plants for A Future states:

Medicinal use of Farkleberry: The berries, root-bark and leaves are very astringent and have been used internally in the treatment of diarrhoea, dysentery etc. The infusion is valuable in treating sore throats, chronic ophthalmia, leucorrhoea etc.

King's American Dispensatory, 1898 tells us:

Action, Medical Uses, and Dosage.—Diuretic and astringent. The fruit is very useful, eaten alone, with milk or sugar, in scurvy, dysentery, and derangements of the urinary organs. The berries and roots, bruised and steeped in gin, form an excellent diuretic, which has proved of much benefit in dropsy and gravel. A decoction of the leaves or bark of the root is astringent, and may be used in diarrhoea, or as a local application to ulcers, leucorrhoea, and ulcerations of the mouth and throat.

Viburnum

Forty-one varieties of Viburnum have been found useful in Herbal Medicine: Viburnum betulifolium, Viburnum cassinoides - Withe Rod, Viburnum cordifolium, Viburnum corylifolium, Viburnum cotinifolium, Viburnum cylindricum, Viburnum dentatum - Arrow Wood, Viburnum dilatatum - Linden Viburnum, Viburnum edule – Mooseberry, Viburnum erosum, Viburnum erubescens, Viburnum erubescens gracilipes, Viburnum farreri, Viburnum foetens, Viburnum fordiae, Viburnum furcatum, Viburnum grandiflorum, Viburnum japonicum, Viburnum lantana - Wayfaring Tree, Viburnum lantanoides – Hobbleberry, Viburnum lentago – Sheepberry, Viburnum mongolicum, Viburnum mullaha, Viburnum nudum - Smooth Withe Rod, Viburnum odoratissimum, Viburnum opulus - Guelder Rose, Viburnum phlebotrichum, Viburnum plicatum - Japanese Snowball, Viburnum prunifolium – Stagberry, Viburnum rufidulum - Southern Black Haw, Viburnum sempervirens, Viburnum setigerum - Tea-Leaf Viburnum, Viburnum sieboldii, Viburnum suspensum, Viburnum tinus – Laurustinus, Viburnum trilobum - American Cranberry, Viburnum veitchii, Viburnum wrightii, Viburnum wrightii hessei, Viburnum x bodnantense, Viburnum x juddii

Four Viburnums are native to my region: Viburnum cassinoides (Withe-rod), Viburnum nudum (Possumhaw Viburnum), Viburnum prunifolium (Blackhaw), Viburnum rufidulum (Rusty Blackhaw)

Viburnums are among the most useful plants in Herbal Medicine. They are also among the most varied in their appearance and growth habits. These may be bushes or trees, "cranberries", "haws" or simply ornamental shrubs with flowers much like hydrangea.

Mrs. Grieves writes of the Guelder Rose, the most popular of the Viburnums, often called Cramp Bark:

The bark, known as Cramp Bark, is employed in herbal medicine. It used formerly to be included in the United States Pharmacopoeia, but is now omitted though it has been introduced into the National Formulary in the form of a Fluid Extract, Compound Tincture and Compound Elixir, for use as a nerve sedative and anti-spasmodic in asthma and hysteria.

In herbal practice in this country, its administration in decoction and infusion, as well as the fluid extract and compound tincture is recommended. It has been employed with benefit in all nervous complaints and debility and used with success in cramps and spasms of all kinds, in convulsions, fits and lockjaw, and also in palpitation, heart disease and rheumatism.

The decoction (1/2 oz. to a pint of water) is given in tablespoon doses.

The bark is collected chiefly in northern Europe and appears in commerce in thin strips, sometimes in quills, 1/20 to 1/12 inch thick, greyish-brown externally, with scattered brownish warts, faintly cracked longitudinally. It has a strong, characteristic odour and its taste is mildly astringent and decidedly bitter.

Resources of the Southern Fields and Forests sates:

BLACK HAW, (Viburnum prrumfolium, L) Fruit edible. Dr. Phares, of Newtonia, Miss., calls attention in the Atlanta Med. and Surg. Journ. (1847) to the medical properties of this plant. He regards it as a nervine, anti-spasmodic, astringent, diuretic and tonic, and claims that in the nervous disorders of pregnancy and uterine diseases, it is a valuable remedial agent. He says: "It is particularly valuable in preventing abortion and miscarriage, whether habitual or otherwise ; whether threatened from accidental cause or criminal drugging." The editor of the same journal adds his testimony in favor of the same remedy, and details several cases when threatened miscarriage was promptly arrested by its use. It is given in the form of in- fusion or decoction of the bark, in doses of from one to two ounces, repeated every two or three hours, until the pains cease; then lessen the dose and lengthen the interval according to circumstances. Where there is a tendency to abortion, it may be used as a preventive three or four times daily, for a great length of time. (Richmond Med. J.Jan., 1868, p. 77.) See Hamamelis Virginica, for which the same virtues are claimed. The Black Haw may probably contain viburnic acid, which was thought to be yielded by the Elder, which is closely related to it.

King's American Dispensatory, 1898 tells us:

Viburnum Opulus (U. S. P.)—Viburnum Opulus

Action, Medical Uses, and Dosage.—High cranberry bark is a powerful antispasmodic, and, in consequence of this property, it is more generally known among American practitioners by the name of Cramp bark. It is very effective in relaxing cramps and spasms of all kinds, as asthma, hysteria, cramps of the limbs or other parts in females, especially during pregnancy, and it is said to be highly beneficial to those who are subject to convulsions during pregnancy, or at the time of parturition, preventing the attacks entirely, if used daily for the last 2 months of gestation. Like *Viburnum prunifolium*, it is a remedy for the prevention of abortion, and to prepare the way for the process of parturition. It allays uterine irritation with a tendency to terminate in hysteria, while in the neuralgic and spasmodic forms of dysmenorrhoea, it is a favorite remedy with many physicians. It has been used in spasmodic contraction of the bladder, and in spasmodic stricture. The doses employed are from a fraction of a drop to 20 drops of specific viburnum. The action of this agent closely resembles that of the black haw, and there is reason to believe that they are often used interchangedly for similar purposes (see Viburnum Prunifolium). The following forms an excellent preparation for the relief of spasmodic attacks, viz.: Take of cramp bark, 2 ounces; scullcap, skunk-cabbage, of each, 1 ounce; cloves, ½ ounce; capsicum, 2 drachms. Have all in powder, coarsely bruised, and add to them 2 quarts of good sherry or native wine. Dose, 1 or 2 fluid ounces, 2 or 3 times a day. Dose, of the decoction or vinous tincture of cramp bark, 2 fluid ounces, 2 or 3 times a day; specific viburnum, 1/10 to 30 drops. "It may be proper to remark here that I have found a poultice of low cranberries very efficient in indolent and malignant ulcers; and, applied round the throat in the inflammation and swelling attending scarlatina maligna, and other diseases, it gives prompt and marked relief. Probably the high cranberries will effect the same results" (J. King). (See Vaccinium Macrocarpum and Cataplasma Oxycocci.)

Specific Indications and Uses.—Cramps; uterine pain, with spasmodic action; pain in thighs and back; bearing down, expulsive pains; neuralgic or spasmodic dysmenorrhoea. As an antiabortive.

Viburnum Prunifolium (U. S. P.)—Black Haw

Action, Medical Uses, and Dosage.—Of the physiological action of this agent little is known. To the taste it is bitter, and slightly aromatic. Large doses sometimes produce nausea and vomiting, and by some observers is said to produce contraction of the uterine *muscular tissue. That it has a decided affinity for the female reproductive organs is well established. By Dr. D. L. Phares, of Mississippi, who brought the remedy forward, it was described as having nervine, antispasmodic, tonic, astringent, and diuretic properties. To these Prof. King adds alterative. Decoctions of the drug were formerly used as a gargle in aphthae, as a wash in indolent ulcers, and in various ophthalmic disorders. By its astringency it has proved of value in diarrhoea and dysentery. It has been recommended in jaundice, but we have a better agent in chionanthus. Palpitation of the heart is said to have been relieved by it. Such cases are sympathetic disturbances, generally near the menstrual period. Its principal use at the present day is in disorders of the female organs of reproduction. As a uterine tonic it is unquestionably of great utility. It restores normal innervation, improves the circulation, and corrects impaired nutrition of these organs. In the hyperaesthetic, or irritable condition of the uterus incident to highly nervous women, or as the result of overwork, it will be found an admirable agent. It is called for in weakened conditions of the body, with feeble performance of the uterine functions. In dysmenorrhoea, with deficient menses, uterine colic, and in those cases where there are severe lumbar and bearing-down pains, it will prove an efficient drug. Helonias is also an excellent agent in the latter condition. It is specifically indicated in cramp-like menstrual pains—pains decidedly expulsive and intermittent in character and in the various painful contractions of the pelvic muscles, so common to disorders of women. Uterine congestion and chronic uterine inflammation are often greatly relieved by specific black haw. It acts promptly in spasmodic dysmenorrhoea, especially with excessive flow. Menorrhagia due to malaria is promptly met with Viburnum prunifolium. It is a good remedy for uterine hemorrhage, attending the menopause. In amenorrhoea in pale, bloodless subjects, the menses are restored by it. Cramps of limbs attending pregnancy yield to both black haw and cramp bark. It is considered almost specific for cramp in the legs, not dependent on pregnancy, especially when occurring at night. The condition for which black haw is most valued is that of threatened abortion. It is the most prompt drug in the materia medica to check abortion, provided the membranes have not ruptured. In all cases of habitual abortion it should be given in small doses for a considerable length of time. The abundant testimony as to its value in this condition alone gives it a high place among drugs. By its quieting effects upon the irritable womb, women who* have previously been unable to go to full term have been aided by this drug to pass through the pregnancy without mishaps which would otherwise have proven disastrous to both child and mother. Small doses of the specific black haw should be administered throughout the dangerous period, and may be continued with good results until parturition. Dr. Phares, who introduced it as all antiabortive, states that it will prevent abortion, whether habitual or otherwise-whether threatened from accidental cause or criminal drugging. He considered it to completely neutralize the effect of the cotton bark when this is used for the purpose of causing abortion. It was for a long time customary for planters to compel their female slaves "to drink an infusion of black haw daily whilst pregnant to prevent abortion, from taking the cottonroot" (Scudder, Spec. Med., 266). It has been used to control postpartum hemorrhage, but is less effective than ergot and cinnamon. It assists in reducing the size of the womb in subinvolution of that organ. Viburnum is of some value in nervous disorders, and has been advised in chorea, hysteria, hystero-epilepsy, petit mal, and paralysis agitans. It is of service only when these troubles are associated with menstrual wrongs. Viburnum Opulus resembles this agent very closely in its effects, and may be used in the above-named conditions, for which the black haw is useful.

Black haw is said to be of value in sterility. Some cases of spermatorrhoea are benefited by it. False pains of pregnancy are readily controlled, and for after-pains it is nearly as valuable as macrotys, or actaea. Black haw promptly allays ovarian irritation. The late Prof. Howe considered it one of the very best uterine tonics, and incorporated it with wild cherry and aromatics in his Black Haw Cordial. This he recommended to allay the pangs of dysmenorrhoea; to arrest leucorrhoea, and to alleviate pelvic discomfort; and as a remedy of value in chlorosis and the debility of the second climacteric. Prof. Howe compounded the cordial to meet the wants of the alcoholic tippler. It allays the gnawing sensations in the stomach, and relieves the faucial discomfort met with in the inebriate. Specific black haw, in drop doses, is a valuable drug in obstinate singultus. The black haw is steadily growing in favor with all schools of medicine. The usual prescription is: Rx Specific black haw, ʒss to ʒi, aqua ℥iv. Mix. Sig. Teaspoonful every 1 to 4 hours, according to case under treatment. The infusion may be given in ½-fluid-ounce doses, several times a day; or the tincture in doses of 1 fluid drachm, 4 or 5 times a day. The powder may be given in ½ or

1-drachm doses; specific black haw, 1/10 to 30 drops; Howe's black haw cordial, 1 to 2 fluid drachms.

Specific Indications and Uses.—Uterine irritability, and hyperaesthesia; threatened abortion; uterine colic; dysmenorrhoea, with deficient menses; severe lumbar and bearing-down pains; cramp-like, expulsive menstrual pain; intermittent, painful contractions of the pelvic tissues; after-pains and false pains of pregnancy; obstinate hiccough.

Plants for A Future states:

Medicinal use of Guelder Rose: Guelder rose is a powerful antispasmodic and is much used in the treatment of asthma, cramps and other conditions such as colic or painful menstruation. It is also used as a sedative remedy for nervous conditions. The bark is antispasmodic, astringent and sedative. The bark contains "scopoletin", a coumarin that has a sedative affect on the uterus. A tea is used internally to relieve all types of spasms, including menstrual cramps, spasms after childbirth and threatened miscarriage. It is also used in the treatment of nervous complaints and debility. The bark is harvested in the autumn before the leaves change colour, or in the spring before the leaf buds open. It is dried for later use. The leaves and fruits are antiscorbutic, emetic and laxative. A homeopathic remedy is made from the fresh bark. It is used in the treatment of menstrual pain and spasms after childbirth.

Medicinal use of Withe Rod: The bark and root bark is antispasmodic, diaphoretic, febrifuge and tonic. An infusion has been used to treat recurrent spasms, fevers, smallpox and ague. The infusion has also been used as a wash for a sore tongue.

Medicinal use of Smooth Withe Rod (Possumhaw): A tea made from the bark is antispasmodic, diuretic, tonic and uterine sedative.

Medicinal use of Stagberry (Blackhaw): Stagberry was used by the North American Indians to treat dysentery and to arrest haemorrhage of the uterus. It is now considered to be a specific treatment for the relief of menstrual pain - the bark contains "scopoletin", a coumarin that has a sedative affect on the uterus and salicin, a painkiller that is used in making aspirin. The bark of the root and stems is abortifacient, anodyne, antispasmodic, astringent, nervine and sedative. A tea is used internally in the treatment of painful or heavy menstruation, prolapse of the uterus, morning sickness, to prevent miscarriage and to relieve spasms after childbirth. It is also used to treat convulsive disorders, colic and other cramping pains that affect the bile ducts, hysteria, asthma and palpitations of a nervous origin. The stem bark is harvested in the autumn before the leaves change colour, or in the spring before the leaf buds open. The root bark is only harvested in the autumn. Both barks can be dried for later use.

Medicinal use of Southern Black Haw (Rusty Blackhaw): The bark is antispasmodic and has been used in the treatment of cramps and colic.

The Physicians Desk Reference for Herbal Medicine tells us:

Blackhaw: Effects. The drug has a spasmolytic and to date, undefined effect on the uterus. Unproven uses: black haw is used for complaints of dysmenorrhea. No health hazards or side effects are known in conjunction with the proper administration of designated therapeutic dosage.

Vernicia fordii, Tung Tree

This naturalized tree is the source of Tung Oil. Plants for A Future states:

Medicinal use of Tung Tree: The oil from the seed is used externally to treat parasitic skin diseases, burns, scalds and wounds. The poisonous oil is said to penetrate the skin and into the muscles, when applied to surgical wounds it will cause inflammation to subside within 4 - 5 days and will leave no scar tissue after suppressing the infection. The plant is emetic, antiphlogistic and vermifuge. Extracts from the fruit are antibacterial.

Zanthoxylum clava, Hercules Club

Resources of the Southern Fields and Forests states:

The species belonging to this order are generally aromatic and pungent.

PRICKLY ASH; TOOTH-ACHE BUSH

Barham's Hortus Americanus. The scraped root is applied to ulcers in order to heal them. The plant possesses stimulating powers, and is a "powerful sudorific and diaphoretic;" remarkable, according to Barton, for its extraordinary property of exciting salivation, whether applied immediately to the gums, or taken internally. It is reported to have been used successfully in paralysis of the muscles of the mouth, and in rheumatic affections. Also, in low forms of fever; the tincture of the berries being sometimes employed as a carminative in doses of ten to thirty drops, increasing the quantity when its stimulating effect is desired. Dr. King, of Cincinnati, states that it wasbeneficially employed in cholera in teaspoonful doses. See Dr. Bates' article ; Tildeu's J. Mat. Med., April, 1867. Mer. and de L. Diet, de M. Med. vi, 179; Journal Gen. de Med. xl, 226. Dr. Gillespie asserts that it is a good tonic and febrifuge. According to Cam, the Indians employed the decoction as an injection in gonorrhoea : "Voyage to Canada." It has been given in syphilis as a substitute for guaiacum, and also for mezereon. See Anc. Journal de Med. ii, 314. A peculiar principle, xanthopicrite, is afforded by it. U. S. Disp. Its acrimony is impartedto boiling water, and to alcohol. According to Dr. Staples, besides fibrous substances, it contains volatile oil, a greenish, fixed oil, resin, gum, coloring matter, and a peculiar crystallizable principle, which he calls xanthoxylin. The latter is given in doses of two to six grains. Journal Phil. Coll. Pharm. i, It is stimulating ; producing, when swallowed, a sense of heat in the stomach, arterial excitement, and a tendency to diaphoresis. It enjoys considerable reputation in chronic rheumatism. Dose of powder from ten grains to half a drachm. It has been tried by many with advantage in this disease. Barton's Collec.i, 25, 52 ; Thacher's Disp. sub. A. spinosa ; Big. Am. Med. Bot. iii, 162. A fluid extract is also prepared and given in doses of fifteen to forty-five drops. (Tilden's Jour. Mat. Med.) In rheumatism an infusion is given, made of one ounce of the bark to one quart of boiling water; one pint to be administered in divided doses during the twenty-four hours. Rep. from Surgeon-Gen. Office, 1862. It should not be confounded with Aralia spinosa, sometimes called prickly ash. X. Carolinianum, Lam.

and T. and G. X tricarium, Ell. Sk. This species is supposed to be possessed of similar properties with the above. It is the Prickly Ash of the Southern States. T. and G. Chapman, in his Flora of the Southern States, does not include X. Americanum among our Southern plants, but what is said of the medicinal properties of X. Americanum, applies to this plant. These plants have the reputation in America of being powerfully sudorific and diaphoretic, and excite copious salivation, not only when made to act directly on the mouth, but when taken internally, and have been found highly efficacious in paralysis of the muscles of the mouth. Rural Cyc. This may account for their utility in toothache. I have ascertained (1868) that the decoction of this plant is extensively used by physicians in South Carolina as a remedy in dropsy. In a letter from a medical friend, he reports to me an aggravated case which recovered under its use. A saturated tincture of the berries or root made with whiskey is also given.

King's American Dispensatory, 1898 tells us:

Action, Medical Uses, and Dosage.—Physiologically, prickly ash acts upon the secretions, the nervous and circulator systems. The bark, when chewed, imparts an aromatic, sweetish taste, followed by bitterness and persistent acridity. Its sialagogue properties are remarkable, inducing a copious flow of saliva, together with a great quantity of mucus from the buccal glands. This is brought about both by its local and systemic action. In the stomach it creates a sense of warmth, and the flow of both gastric and intestinal juices is augmented. There is increased biliary and pancreatic activity. Under its action the kidneys become more active, and an increased urinary product results. Cardiac action is increased, the pulse becomes slightly accelerated, and the integumentary glands give out an abundant secretion. Therapeutically, the bark is sialagogue, alterative, diaphoretic, and especially stimulant to the mucous surfaces. It is also emmenagogue and carminative, and the berries are said to possess antiseptic properties. To increase its diaphoretic power, it should be administered with plenty of hot water, at the same time subjecting the patient to a warm foot-bath. Prof. King cautions us that there is a material difference, in their influence on the system, between the tincture of the bark, or that of the berries, which should always be kept in view. The properties of the bark, as given by him, are stimulant, tonic, alterative, and sialagogue; of the berries, stimulant, carminative, and antispasmodic, acting especially on mucous tissues. Prickly ash has been deservedly valued in domestic practice as a remedy for chronic rheumatism, and was once quite popular as a masticatory for the relief of toothache. It undoubtedly has some value in rheumatic complaints, and may be combined with phytolacca when the indications for that drug are present. Its value in chronic rheumatism is very likely due to its eliminative power. It is best adapted to debilitated patients, and to cases of transient and fugitive forms of rheumatism, particularly lumbago, torticollis, myalgia, and muscular rheumatism. It may be used externally and administered internally, and in many cases will assist the action of macrotys. Its use in odontalgia will be confined to those cases where there is dull, grumbling pain due to peridental inflammation, the parts being dry and shining, and the buccal secretions scanty. Owing to its eliminative powers, it has been quite extensively used in constitutional syphilis and scrofula, and as a remedy for the former ranks with guaiac, stillingia, sarsaparilla, and mezereon. It is one of the constituents of "Trifolium Compound," and other alterative mixtures. Prof. King states that "combined with equal parts of pulverized blue flag and mandrake, it will bring on salivation, and is useful on this account in the treatment of scrofulous, syphilitic, and other diseases where there is a want of susceptibility to the influence of other alterative agents; the mixture must be given in small doses, and repeated at short intervals. Externally, it forms an excellent stimulating application to indolent and malignant ulcers." Xanthoxylum is serviceable in many disorders of the mouth and throat, as well as of the entire alimentary tract. It has some reputation as a local stimulant for paralysis of the tongue, though its value here is overrated. In like manner it has been employed in neuralgia, and paralytic conditions of the vocal apparatus and organs of deglutition. That it will relieve an unpleasant dryness of the mouth and fauces is well established. It is a remedy of value in pharyngitis, especially the chronic variety, the mucous surfaces presenting a glazed, shining, dry condition, with thin, adherent scales of dried mucus. In both pharyngitis and post-nasal catarrh a decoction locally, and specific xanthoxylum (bark) internally, will be found to aid a cure in those cases having dryness of mucous membranes as a distinctive feature. Prickly ash is unmistakably an admirable gastro-intestinal tonic. It will find a place in the treatment of atonic dyspepsia and gastric catarrh. Many chronic affections of the mucous tissues are benefited by it, the cases being those of enfeeblement and relaxation, with hypersecretion. Constipation due to deficient intestinal secretion has been overcome by its use alone. It is more especially indicated when accompanied by a flatulent distension of the abdomen. As an agent for flatulence, the preparation from the berries will give the best results. Lack of secretion in any part of the intestinal tract calls for a preparation of prickly ash bark. Both the bark and the berries may be required in some instances. Icterus, the result of biliary catarrh, is specifically influenced by xanthoxylum, as well as that form resulting from malarial impression. In spasm of the bowels, colic, cholera infantum, and cholera morbus, specific xanthoxylum (berries) will be found valuable in atonic cases. It is useful to restore the bowels to their normal state after severe attacks of dysentery, and has been of particular service as a remedy for epidemic dysentery. Prof. John King introduced the saturated tincture of the berries to the profession in Cincinnati, in 1849, as a remedy for Asiatic cholera. In his article on prickly ash berries in the College Journal for 1856 (p. 86), he writes: "I have used this tincture for some years past, and had the pleasure to introduce it to the profession in this city during the year 1849, both in the treatment of tympanitic distension of the bowels during peritoneal inflammation and in Asiatic cholera. In tympanites it may be administered by mouth and by injection; internally, from ½ to 1 fluid drachm may be given in a little sweetened water, repeating the dose every ½ or 1 hour. At the same time, ½ fluid ounce may be added to the same quantity of water and used as an injection, repeating it every 15 or 30 minutes, according to its influence and the severity of the symptoms, and should there be pain 10 to 20 drops of laudanum may be added to every third or fourth injection. The action is usually prompt and permanent, and, as far as my experience has gone, I prefer it, in a majority of cases, to oil of turpentine and other remedies advised in this condition. In Asiatic cholera during 1849-50 it was much employed by our physicians in Cincinnati, and with great success—it acted like electricity, so sudden and diffusive was its influence over the system. In this disease the tincture was given in teaspoonful doses, and repeated, according to circumstances, every 5, 10 or 20 minutes, at the same time administering an injection, prepared as above, after each discharge from the bowels, and causing it to be retained by the bowels as long as possible." Prof. King likewise valued it in atonic diarrhoea and in typhoid conditions requiring a stimulant, believing it to have an advantage over all other drugs for that purpose. In the tympanitic conditions incident to cholera infantum and other forms of diarrhoea, he combined equal parts of olive oil and tincture of prickly ash berries and had the little patient's abdomen freely rubbed with it, in a downward direction only, for 1 or 2 hours, until the flatulent state was over, claiming thereby to have saved many a little one who would otherwise have gone to an early grave. To prevent a return of the tympanitic distension he used the tincture by mouth and per rectum. Combined with diuretics and tonics, prickly ash has been employed in dropsy and in malarial manifestations, and is in good repute as a remedy for functional dysmenorrhoea. For the latter purpose about 20 drops of specific xanthoxylum (bark) should be administered at a dose, and repeated as often as necessary. Both the bark and berries give good results in neuralgic dysmenorrhoea with marked pain and hypersensitiveness. Xanthoxylum is a valuable nerve stimulant, and may be administered for some length of time without ill effects. It is valuable in all cases of prostration, and has been recommended in "hemiplegia, locomotor ataxia, and all depressed conditions of the vital forces." Pains down the anterior portions of the thighs, as well as after-pains, accompanied with dorsal or sacral pain, are relieved by it. It relieves neuralgic pains in anemic and delicate persons. Owing to its action on blood stasis, overcoming capillary engorgement, it has been found useful in determining the rash to the surface in the eruptive diseases, and is especially serviceable in cases of retrocession of the eruption. It is a remedy that is neglected, but should be borne in mind during the prevalence of summer diseases. The dose of specific xanthoxylum (berries) is from 5 to 30 drops; of specific xanthoxylum (bark), from 2 to 20 drops; of the powder, from 10 to 30 grains, 3 times a day. The oil of xanthoxylum may be used for the same purpose as the berries, in doses of from 2 to 10 drops, in mucilage, or on sugar; and its tincture, made according to the formula below (see Preparation), may be administered in the same doses as the tincture of the berries.

Specific Indications and Uses.—Xanthoxylum is specifically indicated (in the smaller doses) in hypersecretion from debility and relaxation of mucous tissues; atonicity of the nervous system (larger doses); in capillary engorgement in the exanthemata, sluggish circulation, tympanites in bowel complaints, intestinal and gastric torpor (with deficient secretion), dryness of the mucous membrane of mouth and fauces (with glazed, glossy surfaces), flatulent colic, Asiatic cholera, uterine cramps, and neuralgia. For

the painful bowel disorders, the preparations of the berries are to
be preferred.

Plants for A Future states:

*Medicinal use of Hercules Club: This species is quite widely used in
herbal medicine, it has the same properties as Z. americanum, but
is said to be more active. All parts of the plant, but especially the
bark and roots, contain the aromatic bitter oil xanthoxylin. This has
a number of applications in medicine. The fruit has a similar
medicinal action to the bark. The bark and roots are irritant,
odontalgic and antirheumatic. Along with the fruit they are
diaphoretic, stimulant and a useful tonic in debilitated conditions of
the stomach and digestive organs. They produce arterial
excitement and are of use in the treatment of fevers, ague, poor
circulation etc. The fruits are considered more active than the bark,
they are also antispasmodic, carminative, diuretic and
antirheumatic. The pulverized root and bark are used to ease the
pain of toothache. One report says that it is very efficacious, but the
sensation of the acrid bark is fully as unpleasant as the toothache.
Chewing the bark induces copious salivation. Rubbing the fruit
against the skin, especially on the lips or in the mouth, produces a
temporary loss of sensation. A tea or tincture of the bark has been
used in the treatment of rheumatism, dyspepsia, dysentery, heart
and kidney troubles etc. A tea made from the inner bark has been
used to treat itchy skin.*

Wood Ash

Wood Ash and Charcoal are very important to Herbal Medicine.

Brother Aloysius wrote of Wood Ash:

*The remains of burned plants, typically wood, are called ash. It
purifies and desiccates. Ash from oak is an excellent styptic; when
mixed with vinegar it is even more efficacious. Footbaths from
wood ash and salt are highly recommended if the sweating of the
feet has been suppressed or expelled; in addition, footbaths can
bee used for congestion of blood in the head and to draw the blood*

away from the chest. Ash is also recommended for inflammation of the eyes, headache and toothache. Put 2 handfuls of wood ash and 1 handful of salt in a bucket of warm water and keep the feet in it for 10 to 12 minutes. Note: Footbaths should never be taken hot lukewarm is best and the best time is before retiring.

Charcoal

Charcoal is among the most effective and simple natural remedies. Specifically, Activated Charcoal is used as a first aid in many situations. Activated Charcoal is very porous. It is used in cases of poisoning, snake bites, insect stings, food poisoning, bad water, etc. Activated charcoal works by absorbing toxins and gasses, and helping eliminate them from the body. For cases of food poisoning and other internal toxins, it is taken orally. A poultice of charcoal is used for bites and stings.

Mistletoe

This is a warning. American Mistletoe is very different from European Mistletoe. Most European herbals recommend European Mistletoe for many conditions, and it is a very useful herb. American Mistletoe is poisonous! The two must never be confused as even small amounts of American Mistletoe can be deadly. Although the plant does have some historical use in herbal medicine, it is far too dangerous to include any recommendation for its use in this book.

Afterward

I hope, in writing this book, that I have accomplished two goals. The first is that I have shared with you the vast and powerful medicine chest that we walk among daily. Look up, it is over your head! So long as there are woods and forests, parks and landscaping, there will be trees. So long as there are trees, there will be free and readily accessible herbal medicine available for all. As the Bible states, "My people perish for lack of knowledge." The trees are the most easily identifiable wild cultivated plants we are likely to encounter. Perhaps, for this reason they have been taken for granted. How many have been sick, dying or going to doctors when the simple cures for simple ailments grew in their back yards? When you learn to identify a tree, you may discover a pharmacy within it…. when you plant a tree, you may do far better than buying health insurance!

Beyond that mission though, I hope to have transferred to my readers my love of "herbals", books about herbal medicine. I began my herbal apprenticeship at around age 15, in the oral tradition of Appalachian folk medicine. There were no books. I was taught what grandmothers and grandfathers had passed down to their descendants for generations. It was wonderful and magical, practical and thoroughly imbued with simple wisdom. Too soon, it was over. The older folks passed away and took their way of life with them. With that, my herbal mentors were gone. All the bearers of the folk wisdom of the Scottish, Irish, English, Cherokee and Catawbas that I knew, was gone. No longer could I ask questions. No longer would they show me the plants in the woods and tell me how to use them. It happened so quickly! I was left with tears and fond memories.

After my time spent with the Hicks family of Beech Creek, NC, I wandered in my herbal journey. I spent approximately a decade studying Traditional Chinese Medicine. I spent time not thinking about herbs much at all. Often times, a friend or even a stranger would ask my advice about an illness or about a plant, and I would answer at length, with facts and authority that surprised me. Time had passed, but my memory was so very connected to the herbs… Immediately, I was back in the mountains, my mentors and loved ones there with me, the smells, the songs and stories, the accents, the feel of the cool air, warm sun and moist, rich earth… autumn leaves and woodsmoke. Eventually, enough people said, "You should teach", that I began writing about herbs. I hesitated for years, until I picked up a book by Maria Treben. Mrs. Treben was the Austrian herbalist who revived the tradition of German Folk Medicine. As I read her books, the memories came flooding back. She convinced me that, just as she had presented her tradition of herbalism to new generations, I should as well. Beyond that though, I found a "friend" in her writing. Her personality came through in her words. I truly enjoyed reading her books.

Mrs. Treben mentioned Saint Hildegard, Fr. Kneipp and Fr. Künzle, so I read their books. There, I found irascible old priests, full of humor, wisdom and common sense knowledge. I also found a visionary saint and hero, whose works leave me in awe. The writings of these people reminded me of the many Germans, Swiss and eastern European folks who lived in my home town when I was a child, and of many lessons I had forgotten. The German folk medicine was very much a part of my childhood, but it was presented as simple "home remedies"… I took it for granted. In reading Fathers Kneipp and Künzle, I came to understand that German Folk Medicine was intended to be home medicine, or "Kitchen Medicine." This great herbal tradition was humble by intent.

Reading the herbals in the German tradition began me on a path that led me to co-author a book on Fr. Künzle, which was my first work as an herbal author. It also led me to begin reading the great herbals of history. Perhaps, many of us take herb books for granted. We are are fortunate to have been born into a time when herbals are not uncommon. There were several decades in the middle of the century that was 1900, when the federal government tried to blot out our folk medicine traditions. We find a vibrant tradition up to around 1920, then a good deal of silence until certain herbalists rediscovered and revived herbalism in the 1960s -90s. Although that era of silence was brief, the force of law was heavy handed in its attempt to make off limits thousands of years of herbal knowledge. The "age of science" simply had no tolerance for anything unproved in a laboratory… truth be damned. So along with Mrs. Treben, and a few others who sought to preserve tradition and folk knowledge, we also owe a large debt of gratitude to the naturalists like Jethro Kloss and Euell Gibbons and the hippies – Michael Moore, Rosemary Gladstar, Susan Weed, Stephen Harron Buhner, Howie Brounstein, 7 Song, etc, who dug up the old books by Mrs. Grieves, Native Americans and the Eclectics, etc., and re-introduced herbalism to the "modern" world. The Foxfire series also did a great deal to preserve the wisdom of my mentors and their contemporaries and present it to the rest of America in the 1970s, because the old ways lived on in the Appalachians.

When I was a kid though, there were few… if any, herbals to be found. Herb books were expensive luxuries that I really couldn't afford. The few that appeared on the shelves of a local bookstore were little more than pamphlets meant to sell products. The libraries didn't have them… or, if they did, I never found them! In my 30s, I discovered the herbals. I tried to begin with the ancient Greeks and Romans, but that was disappointing – there are far fewer herbs discussed, with their uses, in Hippocrates' works than one may be led to believe…. And, those so often attributed to Pliny and Galen are remarkably hard to source. Dioscorides became my favorite reference from that era. The monastic medicine followed, beginning with the monk, Walafrid Strabo, born in 808 AD, tutor in the house King Louis, son of Emperor Charlemagne and one of the most influential minds in the post Roman era. His Hortulus, a brief work on gardening and medicinal herbs is a true delight written in poetry and full of humor. From there, I began to read the works of the herbalists century by century, country by country. I love these books. In them, I find a wealth of knowledge. I also have come to think of the authors as my friends. I read Culpepper and spend some time with my mischievous, brilliant and rebellious friend who died far too young. I read I read Fr. Kneipp, and listen to him poke fun at the pace of modern life and the foolish hurry of chasing after the almighty dollar! In each author, I find a mentor and companion. Opening a new book, to me, is like unwrapping a gift.

So, it is in this spirit that I present to you a description of the works cited in my little book. My hope is that you may find in them the joy I have come to know. I hope you will make all of this a part of your own folk tradition and pass it on to future generations. If my book can be but a guidepost along the way, I will be pleased. In many ways, I feel that I am as William F. Buckley described, "standing athwart the back of history, yelling STOP!" But in this case, my message is, "Stop. Look up. See what God has provided. Look around and realize the profound beauty of nature. Sit down and read a good, old book."

Sources:

Pedanius Dioscorides, de Materia Medica:

(40–90 AD) was a Greek physician, pharmacologist, botanist, and author of De materia medica —a 5-volume Greek encyclopedia about herbal medicine and related medicinal substances (a pharmacopeia), that was widely read for more than 1,500 years. He was employed as a physician in the Roman army. A native of Anazarbus, Cilicia, Asia Minor, Dioscorides likely studied medicine nearby at the school in Tarsus, which had a pharmacological emphasis, and he dedicated his medical books to Laecanius Arius, a medical practitioner there. Though he says he served in the Roman army, his pharmacopeia refers almost solely to plants found in the Greek-speaking eastern Mediterranean, making it unlikely that he served in campaigns (or traveled) outside that region. The name Pedanius is Roman, suggesting that an aristocrat of that name sponsored him to become a Roman citizen. Between AD 50 and 70 Dioscorides wrote a five-volume book in his native Gree, known in Western Europe more often by its Latin title De Materia Medica ("On Medical Material"), which became the precursor to all modern pharmacopeias. In contrast to many classical authors, Dioscorides' works were not "rediscovered" in the Renaissance, because his book had never left circulation; indeed, with regard to Western materia medica through the early modern period, Dioscorides' text eclipsed the Hippocratic corpus. In the medieval period, De Materia Medica was circulated in Greek, as well as Latin and Arabic translation. - Wikipedia

Saint Hildegard von Bingen, Physica

Saint Hildegard was born a sickly and weak child around 1098 AD. She was entrusted to the care of the Benedictines. Her illness caused her to be often bed-ridden and even blind. She was unable to pursue formal education. But, from an early age she began having mystical visions:

From my early childhood, before my bones, nerves and veins were fully strengthened, I have always seen this vision in my soul, even to the present time when I am more than seventy years old. In this vision my soul, as God would have it, rises up high into the vault of heaven

and into the changing sky and spreads itself out among different peoples, although they are far away from me in distant lands and places. And because I see them this way in my soul, I observe them in accord with the shifting of clouds and other created things. I do not hear them with my outward ears, nor do I perceive them by the thoughts of my own heart or by any combination of my five senses, but in my soul alone, while my outward eyes are open. So I have never fallen prey to ecstasy in the visions, but I see them wide awake, day and night. And I am constantly fettered by sickness, and often in the grip of pain so intense that it threatens to kill me, but God has sustained me until now. The light which I see thus is not spatial, but it is far, far brighter than a cloud which carries the sun. I can measure neither height, nor length, nor breadth in it; and I call it "the reflection of the living Light." And as the sun, the moon, and the stars appear in water, so writings, sermons, virtues, and certain human actions take form for me and gleam.

Around the age of 40, Saint Hildegard began to write or dictate her visions:

But I, though I saw and heard these things, refused to write for a long time through doubt and bad opinion and the diversity of human words, not with stubbornness but in the exercise of humility, until, laid low by the scourge of God, I fell upon a bed of sickness; then, compelled at last by many illnesses, and by the witness of a certain noble maiden of good conduct [the nun Richardis von Stade] and of that man whom I had secretly sought and found, as mentioned above, I set my hand to the writing. While I was doing it, I sensed, as I mentioned before, the deep profundity of scriptural exposition; and, raising myself from illness by the strength I received, I brought this work to a close – though just barely – in ten years. [...] And I spoke and wrote these things not by the invention of my heart or that of any other person, but as by the secret mysteries of God I heard and received them in the heavenly places. And again I heard a voice from Heaven saying to me, 'Cry out, therefore, and write thus!'.

She became the most influential and popular author and speaker of the era. She wrote mystical books on theology and the cosmos, man and nature, sickness and health, science and herbal medicine. She also composed the largest body of religious music of the era, wrote a play and created an entirely new written language! Encouraged by the Pope and the Church leaders of her time, she founded several nunneries, traveled as widely as possible to preach in Catholic churches throughout central Europe and became known as the "Sybil of the Rhine". Those who could afford to make such a journey flocked to her for her advice, wisdom and insight that she always credited as coming from a Divine source. Over the centuries, devotion to Hildegard continued and many miracles, especially for healing, have been attributed to prayers asking for her intercession. She was named a Doctor of The Church and canonized as a saint.

I ask this amazing woman, and another Patron Saint of herbalism, Saint Fiacre (an Irish hermit born around 600 AD) to pray for me daily. As with everything I do in regard to herbs, this book is under the patronage of Saint Fiacre and Saint Hildegard of Bingen. These are Catholic Patron Saints of Herbal Medicine, devout people who dedicated their lives to the study of herbs and their uses in healing mankind. Saints Fiacre and Hildegard, pray for us, as we pray for our family. For, as our Lord said, "'I am the God of Abraham, and the God of Isaac, and the God of Jacob'? He is not God of the dead, but of the living." Now, in Heaven, they see God face to face and dedicate eternity to praising God and praying for us, their family still in this world... for ever so short a time. May we spend our lives in service to others, in study of God's great creation, seeking the Wisdom of Solomon, who knew all plants and all their uses, in hopes of spending eternity in the fulness of Truth and Love in the family of God.... the God who gave his Saints such power to intervene for his people on earth that the dead man whose body touched the bones of the prophet Elisha came to life... may Saint Fiacre and Saint Hildegard intervene so powerfully for us as we seek to understand and use... as Maria Treben said, "God's Pharmacy".

German Folk Medicine:

With the ebbs and flows of history and political upheaval for which Central Europe is so rightly known, much was not written down over the centuries, and the Monastic Medicine became "folk medicine." This deep and rich herbalism became part of the lives of common people. The term, "kitchen medicine" came into use for the teas and poultices one would employ to treat ailments within the family.

Father Sebastian Kneipp:

In the 1800s, a new force came on the scene. The dynamic and brilliant Father Sebastian Kneipp became, arguably, the most famous herbalist in the western world! While a seminary student, the future Fr. Kneipp contracted tuberculosis. His case was dire, and no medical treatment could help. He was informed by doctors, in no uncertain terms, that he would die before he graduated.

Although, Fr. Kneipp was likely well steeped in the German Folk Medicine tradition even as a youth, it was advice he found in an old book that proved to be his cure. The book advised the sick to "toughen the constitution" by swimming regularly in cold water. The young Fr. Kneipp did so, daily swimming in the frigid river… and his condition improved. A fellow seminarian was even sicker than he, so he began bringing his friend along on his daily swims. Soon, both young men were fully recovered, healthy and ready for graduation! This led to Fr. Kneipp's classic book, My Water Cure.

My Water Cure was a book of instruction on the systematic use of (mostly) cold water baths that Fr. Kneipp developed in treating the multifarious illnesses of his parishioners. It was also, a comprehensive herbal. Fr. Kneipp's stated goal was to provide an apothecary, and instructions for use, for the common man. His vision was the ideal of German Folk Medicine: Children, having been thoroughly instructed by their parents, gathering herbs from among the wildflowers, as they walked barefoot in the morning dew. Kitchens, fully stocked with well ordered and properly prepared herbs. Parents, acting as effective physicians for their families, and passing on that wisdom.

My Water Cure Became the first international "best seller". The book was so popular that flawed counterfeits were sold in multiple languages. Even today, Fr. Kneipp's cold water therapies are still popular among people in the region, and his more elaborate treatments are performed in spas that are a regular part of life in that beautiful part of the world.

Father Johannes Künzle:

In 1911, Fr. Johannes Künzle published what would become one of the most important books written on Herbal Medicine in the 20th Century. This bold and outspoken Swiss priest wrote what was little more than a pamphlet on herbs and their use. His brief booklet, of fewer than 40 pages, sought to educate the common people of central Europe about the flowers, weeds and trees that grew in abundance, and how they may be used to treat common illnesses. Like his predecessor, Fr. Kneipp, his vision was of kitchen medicine, folk medicine, and a firm faith that God had provided all an individual of family could need for general health in the "Herbs and Weeds". His little book became a best seller. This led to fame that he generally did not desire, and to clashes with the medical establishment. He challenged that establishment and won court battles, proving that his herbs were sometimes even more effective than their medicine. This made Fr. Künzle an international figure.

Fr. Künzle revitalized the tradition of "German Folk Medicine", and his booklet was likely to be found in any German speaking home. Unfortunately, then came the World Wars. Much of the world was at war with Germany and its allies. Books written in the German language were not to be seen in homes in America, England or France (etc.). Fr. Künzle's little booklet was never translated into English during his lifetime; only one such effort was made decades later, and that disappeared quickly. By the 2,000s, only scarce reference was found of Fr. Künzle, even online. I only became aware of his work through Maria Treben, the great Austrian herbalist who once more brought German Folk Medicine to the collective consciousness of the modern world.

Thanks to the shared efforts of my co-author, Austrian herbalist, Jolanta Wittib, Fr. Künzle's work is now available in English. All credit for the translation and the photos goes to Jolanta. What became evident to us early on was that the simple translation of the work was not sufficient. The brief booklet assumed a regional knowledge of plants. Some plants and many terms would be unfamiliar to English readers. Moreover, much has been learned about herbs and illnesses since Fr. Künzle's time. We decided to write our own commentary on his work, and expand on many points, as professional herbalists. The result was an entirely new work of more than 150 pages! Do not fear though, Fr. Künzle's words are still there, intact. His wisdom and delightful character shine through.

If you enjoyed this book, I hope you will consider purchasing The Herbs and Weeds of Fr. Johannes Künzle, a new book by Judson Carroll and Jolanta Wittib!

Brother Aloysius:

Comfort To The Sick was published in Holland in 1901. It was written by Brother Aloysius, who was a member of the monastery Monseigneur Savelberg in Heerlen. He came to be interested in the study of herbs and The Water Cure, because he healed himself of consumption using the Kneipp Water Cure. This brought him to study with Msgr. Kneipp, and to eventually work with common herbs – plants found in the local woods and fields – to help people maintain health when the energies of the body are out of balance. – from A Healer's Herbal, Recipes for Medicinal Herbs and Weeds by Brother Aloysius (English translation of Comfort To The Sick).

Maria Treben:

Treben was born in 1907 in Žatec, Bohemia, then Austria-Hungary, the middle of three daughters of the owner of a printing shop who died when she was 10. After the Great War, the Sudetenland became part of the newly founded Czechoslovakia. In 1945, at the end of the Second World War, she and her husband Ernst Gottfried Treben were victims of the Expulsion of Germans from Czechoslovakia. For several years they lived in refugee camps until they found refuge in Austria and settled down in Grieskirchen in 1951. She died in 1991. Treben became famous through her two books: Health Through God's Pharmacy and Maria Treben's Cures. The first was translated into 24 languages and sold over 8 million copies.

Treben addressed seminars and presented at natural health conferences in Germany, Austria and across Europe, attracting hundreds of people. She is perceived as a pioneer of the renewed interest for natural remedies and traditional medicine at the end of the 20th century. Treben used traditional German and Eastern European remedies handed down from previous generations. She only used local herbs and always accompanied her remedies with advice on diet. She commonly used Thyme, Greater Celandine, Ramsons, Speedwell, Calamus, Chamomile, Nettle and Lady's Mantle. She treated a broad range of conditions from psoriasis to constipation and diabetes to insomnia. She used her own recipes as well as traditional healing remedies like Swedish bitters that she used as a cure-all. ...To this day she is widely read and referred to for her knowledge of European medicinal herbs. (Wikipedia).

The British Tradition:

John Gerard, Herball

Gerard published hi classic work in 1597. Although it was heavily reliant on Rembert Dodoens's 1554 herbal, Gerard was a great plant collector and herbalist in his own right. His chief contribution of herbalism and botany was as a plant collector. He grew rare and exotic specimens collected from throughout the British empire and beyond. In 1586, he established a "Physic Garden" for The College of Physicians and was its curator. He later established gardens on property adjoining Somerset House for the royal family. Described as, "a worshipful gentleman and one that greatly delighteth in strange plants", his Herball continues to be beloved not only for the information it contains about plants, but its flights of fancy and the delightful beauty with which it was written.

Nicholas Culpepper, The English Physitian (1652), later entitled The Complete Herbal

Culpepper was quite the character. Earlier in this book, I mentioned him a puckish and rebellious.

From the age of 16 he studied at Cambridge, but it is not known at which college, although his father studied at Queens', and his grandfather was a member of Jesus College. He was then apprenticed to an apothecary. After seven years his master absconded with the money paid for the indenture, and soon after, Culpeper's mother died of breast cancer.

In 1640, Culpeper married Alice Field, the 15-year-old heiress of a wealthy grain merchant, which allowed him to set up a pharmacy at the halfway house in Spitalfields, London, outside the authority of the City of London, at a time when medical facilities in London were at breaking point. Arguing that "no man deserved to starve to pay an insulting, insolent physician" and obtaining his herbal supplies from the nearby countryside, Culpeper could provide his services free of charge. This and a willingness to examine patients in person rather than simply examining their urine (in his view, "as much piss as the Thames might hold" did not help in diagnosis), Culpeper was extremely active, sometimes seeing as many as 40 patients in a morning. Using a combination of experience and astrology, he devoted himself to using herbs to treat his patients. -(Wikipedia)

Culpepper scandalized the medical and academic establishments by translating the London Directory from Latin into English, making medical knowledge available to the common man. He further infuriated the educated classes by introducing British folklore, astrology and the Doctrine of Signatures into his works on herbal medicine…. likely, at least in part, to tweak those who saw themselves as his betters. His efforts were met with great condemnation and even accusations of witchcraft by the Society of Apothecaries and attempts to ban him from publishing by the College of Physicians. He served as a battlefield surgeon in the Battle of Newbury and was wounded in the chest. He later died from those injuries at the age of 37.

Culpepper's legacy would strongly influence later herbalists both in England and the colonies. He left us these words which would be a fitting creed for many who have felt pressure to join the establishment or conform their ideals to a culture with which they find themselves irreconcilably out of step:

"This not being pleasing, and less profitable to me, I consulted with my two brothers, Dr. Reason and Dr. Experience, and took a voyage to visit my mother Nature, by whose advice, together with the help of Dr. Diligence, I at last obtained my desire; and, being warned by Mr. Honesty, a stranger in our days, to publish it to the world, I have done it."

John K'eogh, The Botanalogia Universalis Hibernica or A General Irish Herbal

This is the best example of the tradition of Irish Herbalism that I have found. Written in 1735, this it is a straight-forward materia medica of the native plants and their uses. K'eogh wrote, There is not an herb, shrub or tree in nature but that is serviceable to man either for food or medicine, or for both. Unfortunately, this is but a glimpse into what may have once been the among the most rich and profound traditions of herbalism the world has ever known. We know from the ancient historians that Ireland was the seat of a great amount of herbal wisdom, but it is often only included in tales of Druid rituals. It is very likely from this tradition that Saint Fiacre drew his knowledge. It would be fascinating to learn how pagan herbal wisdom translated into Catholic practice. But Ireland has been the most invaded, persecuted and enslaved nation the world may have ever known. Most of its indigenous culture was purposefully and violently stamped out by the "civilized and enlightened" English long before the printing press was invented. My heritage includes both Irish and English ancestry (as well as French)... I can say, without any hesitancy that the English were on the wrong side of history and morality in their violent and inhumane subjugation of the Celtic peoples, Catholics within their own borders and others throughout the colonies. I respect English history and am proud of my ancestors who were of the House of Wessex, but I do not worship the English as many American do.

Maude Grieves, A Modern Herbal.

Mrs. Grieves, as I always call her out of profound respect, gave a great service to the world when she published her two volume work in 1931. In the immense turmoil of World War 1, she devoted herself to the study and teaching of herbal medicine. She fully realized that the knowledge of herbs had faded from collective memory, and knew that her nation and the innocent peoples of the world who found themselves in extreme danger needed the collective wisdom of European and British herbalism, presented in an easy to understand and utilize, accessible format.

In A Modern Herbal, Mrs. Grieves gives us the history of each plant, information about its cultivation and the herbal uses for more than 800 herbs! She quotes freely from Pliny, Galen, Dioscorides, Parkinson, Gerard and Culpepper, in a style that was a major inspiration for this book. Moreover, she references the Medical texts of the day to give us formulas and instructions for use of the herbs.

In many ways, Mrs. Grieves was the pivotal figure in preserving tradition and promoting modern herbalism.

The Americans:

Obviously, herbalism was a tradition in North America long before the Portuguese, Spanish, French and English ever set foot on our soil. It is well documented that the early European settlers learned life-saving remedies from the Native Americans. Too often, such favors were not returned. However, early American herbalism must be seen in the light of a blending of British herbalism with native wisdom.

In this book, drew from two Native American Herbals. Obvious by omission is the Cherokee tradition that made up so much of what I was taught via Appalachian folk medicine. I am still researching recorded sources and will likely update this book with that tradition in the future. Half my life was spent in southeastern NC, among my many relatives and friends in the Lumbee Tribe. We are very fortunate to find much of the Lumbee tradition of herbalism in one volume:

Arvis Locklear Boughman, Herbal Remedies of the Lumbee Indians

"There's nothing happens to a person that can't be cured if you get what it takes to do it. We come out of the earth, and there's something in the earth to cure everything ... I don't fix a tonic until I'm sure what's wrong with a person. I don't make guesses. I have to be sure, because medicine can do bad as well as good, and I don't want to hurt anybody.... Maybe it takes some herbs. Maybe it takes some touching. But most of all, it takes faith"--Vernon Cooper, Lumbee healer. The Lumbee Indian tribe has lived in the coastal plain of North Carolina for centuries, and most Lumbee continue to live in rural areas of Robeson County with access to a number of healing plants and herbs used in the form of teas, poultices, and salves to treat common ailments. The first section of this book describes and documents the numerous plant and herbal remedies that the Lumbee have used for centuries and continue to use today. There are remedies for ailments relating to cancer (external and internal), the circulatory and digestive systems, the heart, hypertension and hypotension, infections and parasitic diseases, asthma, pregnancy, sprains, swellings, and muscle, skeletal and joint disorders, to name just a few. The second portion of this work records the words, recollections and wellness philosophies of living Lumbee elders, healers, and community leaders.

Tis Mal Crow, Native Plants, Native Healing: Traditional Muskagee Way

Tis Mal Crow studied the medicinal use of plants and traditional native root doctoring techniques from childhood. He shared his knowledge and insights on how to gather herbs respectfully and use them to make tinctures, teas, liniments, oils, lotions and salves for medicinal use. Twenty-two Eastern Woodland plants are profiled and identified by their doctrine of signature, which ailments respond to their treatment, and what type of application works best. The importance of responsible harvesting is stressed, as a number of wild medicinal plants face extinction due to overharvesting.

The most Prominent American school of Herbalism in early America was the Thomsonian and Eclectic tradition. The term, Eclectic, was coined by a Transylvanian botanist who studied Native American plants and herbalism. But, it was John Thomson who really founded this school of herbalism. Thomson was born in the New Hampshire wilderness in 1769. A life-long curiosity about plants led him to study with a "root doctor' in his teens. After a rather tragic early life beset by illnesses and injury that took most of his loved ones – experience all too common in early America – he renewed his study with two local herbalists. Eventually, he opened his own practice and founded the "Thomsonian System."

Much of what is at this day called medicine, is deadly poison, and were people to know what is offered them of this kind they would absolutely refuse ever to receive it as a medicine. This I have long seen and known to be true; and have laboured hard for many years to convince them of the evils that attend such a mode of procedure with the sick; and have turned my attention to those medicines that grow in our own country, which the God of nature has prepared for the benefit of mankind. Long has a general medicine been sought for, and I am confident I have found such as are universally applicable in all cases of disease, and which may be used with safety and success, in the hands of the people.

After thirty years study and repeated successful trials of the medicinal vegetables of our country, in all the diseases incident to our climate; I can, with well grounded assurance, recommend my system of practice and medicines to the public, as salutary and efficacious.

Thomsonian medicine was based on traditional herbalism, with special emphasis placed on ridding the body of toxins and protection/recovery from the cold weather for which New Hampshire is known. His books were very popular, and like Culpepper had done generations before in England, he promoted an anti-establishment egalitarianism. In many ways, Thomson was to America what Fr. Kneipp was to the German speaking world. The books written by Thomson and his followers were many. For this book, I decided to quote The Thomsonian System of Medicine by R. Swineburn Clymer, Phd, MD, as it gives us an authoritative view into the Thomsonian system at its heyday, written by a medical physician, before the modern medical establishment was able to quash it through rule of law and, often, baseless slander. While I do not fully ascribe to the Thomsonian model, it is likely that Thomson and the Eclectics healed at least as many people than the mainstream medical establishment of their day, and killed far fewer.

The Southern folk medicine tradition is as varied and vast as the people who settled my homeland. It encompasses British and Celtic traditions, Native American traditions, African and Caribbean herbalism. Some has been documented, but much has been lost. The Foxfire books helped preserve the Appalachian tradition. Unique among the Southern works though is Resources of the Southern Fields and Forests. During the Civil War, when the Union blockaded Southern Ports and roads, the intent was to cut of the South from all commerce, including imported medicine and food. The Confederacy fired a French botanist to research our native plants with the goal of replacing all imports. By then, a tradition of French botanists researching plants in the American South had been established for more than a century. Francis Peyre Porcher had immense resources and knowledge upon which to draw as he wrote this massive work in the general vicinity of Charleston, SC. The learned Frenchman did not disappoint! He wrote over 800 pages in extreme detail, with extensive sources and person experience on how our native plants could be used for medicine, food, fiber, fuel, etc… and how we could grow opium, with instructions to process it, in the South sufficient to drive the rest of the world's production out of business – a resource sorely needed as men were having limbs blown off with no other means of anesthetic. Resources of The Southern Fields And Forests stands as one of the most significant books ever published and should be on everyone's shelf… not just herbalists! One never knows what disasters and upheavals may come our way. This book goes far beyond what any "prepper" could ever envision.

By no means though was herbalism confined only to "alternative medicine" populists in New England or to the rural South. The "modern medicine" of America in the 1800s found its "drugs' in the plants of herbal medicine. King's American Dispensatory of 1898 proves that the "mainstream" doctors and pharmacies of the time created their "medicaments" from the very same plants we use today. This invaluable work gives modern herbalists the knowledge that doctors had just over 100 years a go and detailed instruction for how we can use herbs to make those very same medicines. It is my pleasure to present excerpts from this book here. I would encourage all modern herbalists to obtain a copy of this book and others like it, to show any doubters and skeptics who scoff at herbal medicine in their ignorance.

Modern works.

I have been hesitant to quote modern works, as the authors are (mostly) living and I do not wish to take away from their livelihood. Our Lord said, "The worker is due his pay." I would not wish for someone to read enough in my book to discourage them from buying the source from which I quote. Therefor, I only chose a few of my "go to" books, the ones I reference frequently, and have refrained from taking too much from them. I encourage my readers to buy these books. I believe them to be indispensable, and they include far more information than just what they state on trees.

Euell Gibbons, Stalking The Healthful Herbs

Gibbons has long been a hero of mine. I love his books. They are well written and enjoyable to read. He and Bradford Angier likely did more to lead generations into the woods for adventure, food and medicine than anyone other than the great George L. Herter. Herter didn't write about herbs though – Gibbons and Angier did. Gibbons wrote more on the medicinal use of trees. Anyone who spends any time in nature should have Euell Gibbons' books on his shelf. He should also have Bradford ANgiers' books…. And George

Herter's books if he has a good sense of humor, doesn't take life too seriously and has a big appetite for wild foods!

Peterson Field Guides Eastern and Central Medicinal Plants

The Peterson Field Guides are excellent. This one, on herbs, is indispensable. I take it with me everywhere and cannot recommend it highly enough!

Thomas J. Elpel, Botany In A Day

No, you will not learn botany in a day from this book. You will, if you are smart, read it and then spend months using it as a field guide. Elpel teaches us how to identify plants through the characteristics of their "plant families". He makes identifying herbs easy and tells us their medicinal used. I consider this book essential.

Plants for A Future is a book and "plant data base' website that seeks to inform us of every useful attribute for every plant. It is a vast and remarkable work. Whenever I need to look up an herb, it is my go-to. The herbs can be found at: naturalmedicinalherbs.net

Many of the trees mention in my book have found use in alcoholic beverages. I cite two books on herbal wines, beers and related drinks: The Drunken Botanist by Amy Stewart, and the remarkable Sacred and Healing Herbal Beers by Stephen Harrod Buhner which is absolutely one of the best and most surprising herbals in my library.

Rodale has long been the leader in organic gardening in America. As such, it is no surprise that they would write good books on growing and using medicinal herbs. While I quote occasionally form Rodale's Illustrated Encyclopedia of Herbs, it is far less useful that The Rodale Herb Book. The Rodale Herb Book is one of the very best herbals written in the 1970s.

Finally, the Physicians' Desk Reference for Herbal Medicine. While this is one of my least favorite herb books, it is certainly useful, and my copy is well worn. It is nearly 900 pages of dry, dull information. It is comprised of information sourced from peer reviewed studies. It gives the official uses of each herb, any potential hazards and contraindications. I think every herbalist should have a copy of this book... if for no other reason, than that its massive bulk could be used to silence a doubter of herbal medicine through physical means, even if the extensive medical information it contains failed so to do.

I think that about wraps it up, folks. Thank you for joining me in this journey and for buying my book!

About the Author

Judson Carroll

I am a certified Master Herbalist and Permaculturist from the Blue Ridge Mountains of North Carolina, USA. I began learning about herbs and their uses from the old Appalachian folks, especially the Hicks family of Beech Creek, when I was around 15.

I host the Southern Appalachian Herbal Podcast: Southern Appalachian Herbs https://www.spreaker.com/show/southern-appalachian-herbs

I teach free, online herbal medicine classes: Herbal Medicine 101 https://rumble.com/c/c-618325

I also write a weekly article on herbs and their properties: https://southernappalachianherbs.blogspot.com/

My passion is being outside, enjoying the woods, the water and the garden. My mission is to revive the tradition of "folk medicine" in America, so families can care for their own ailments at home, using the herbs God gave us for that purpose.

You can join me on The Grow Network forums – I am a moderator and contributor there. https://thegrownetwork.com/

My email address is southernappalachianherbs@gmail.com

www.ingramcontent.com/pod-product-compliance
Lightning Source LLC
Chambersburg PA
CBHW050643270326
41927CB00012B/2849